C0-AWB-477

Cross-National Study of Health Systems: Concepts, Methods, and Data Sources

HEALTH AFFAIRS INFORMATION GUIDE SERIES

Series Editor: Winifred Sewell, Health Science Information Consultant, currently associated with the University of Maryland and the National Health Planning Information Center

Also in this series:

BIOETHICS—*Edited by Doris Goldstein**

CROSS-NATIONAL STUDY OF HEALTH SYSTEMS BY COUNTRY AND WORLD REGIONS—*Edited by Ray H. Elling**

EDUCATION IN THE HEALTH PROFESSIONS—*Edited by Elizabeth A. Martinsen**

HEALTH CARE ADMINISTRATION—*Edited by Dwight A. Morris and Lynne Darby Morris*

HEALTH CARE COSTS AND FINANCING—*Edited by Rita Keintz**

HEALTH CARE POLITICS, POLICY, AND LEGISLATION—*Edited by Joel M. Lee**

HEALTH MAINTENANCE THROUGH FOOD AND NUTRITION—*Edited by Helen Ullrich**

HEALTH PLANNING—*Edited by Lewis Lefko**

HEALTH SCIENCES AUDIOVISUALS—*Edited by Laura P. Barrett**

HEALTH STATISTICS—*Edited by Frieda O. Weise*

HUMAN ECOLOGY—*Edited by Frederick Sargent II**

INTERFACE OF MEDICINE AND THE LAW—*Edited by Sal Fiscina, James Zimmerly, Paul Connors, and Janet B. Seifert**

MEDICAL INFORMATION TRANSFER—*Edited by Winifred Sewell and Marie Dickerman**

THE PROFESSIONAL AND SCIENTIFIC LITERATURE ON PATIENT EDUCATION—*Edited by Lawrence W. Green and Connie C. Kansler**

QUALITY MAINTENANCE AND EVALUATION OF HEALTH CARE—*Edited by Jay Glasser and Irene Eastling**

SURVEY OF EMERGENCY MEDICAL SERVICES SYSTEM RESOURCES—*Edited by Carlos Fernandez-Caballero and Marianne Fernandez-Caballero**

THERAPEUTIC MATERIALS IN THE HEALTH SYSTEM—*Edited by Winifred Sewell and Marie Dickerman**

*in preparation

The above series is part of the
GALE INFORMATION GUIDE LIBRARY

The Library consists of a number of separate series of guides covering major areas in the social sciences, humanities, and current affairs.

General Editor: Paul Wasserman, Professor and former Dean, School of Library and Information Services, University of Maryland

Managing Editor: Denise Allard Adzigian, Gale Research Company

Cross-National Study of Health Systems: Concepts, Methods, and Data Sources

A GUIDE TO INFORMATION SOURCES

Volume 2 in the Health Affairs Information Guide Series

Ray H. Elling

Professor and Director
Program in Cross-National Study of Health Systems
Department of Community Medicine
University of Connecticut Health Center
Farmington

Gale Research Company
Book Tower, Detroit, Michigan 48226

VANDERBILT UNIVERSITY
MEDICAL CENTER LIBRARY

APR 28 1982

NASHVILLE, TENNESSEE
37232

Library of Congress Cataloging in Publication Data

Elling, Ray H   1929-
    Cross-national study of health systems: concepts, methods, and
data sources.

    (Health affairs information guide series ; v. 2)
(Gale information guide library)
    Includes index.
    1. Medical care—Bibliography. 2. Medical
care—Cross-cultural studies—Bibliography.
    3. Medical care—Comparative method—Bibliography.
    4. Medicine, State—Comparative method—
Bibliography. 5. Medical care—Information
services—Directories. I. Title. II. Series.
Z6673.4.E43   [RA394]   016.3621   79-24028
ISBN 0-8103-1449-5

Copyright © 1980 by
Ray H. Elling

No part of this book may be reproduced in any form without permission in
writing from the publisher, except by a reviewer who wishes to quote brief
passages or entries in connection with a review written for inclusion in a
magazine or newspaper. Manufactured in the United States of America.

VITA

Ray H. Elling holds an M.A. from the University of Chicago, 1955, in sociology, and a Ph.D., Yale University, 1958, in medical sociology. He is professor of sociology and director of the Ph.D. program in social sciences and health care and of the program in cross-national study of health systems (CNSHS), Department of Community Medicine, University of Connecticut Health Center, Farmington, Connecticut. He is coordinator of the steering group of the New England program for CNSHS conducted by individual scholars in several New England Universities. Elling's published works related to this subject include edited volumes COMPARATIVE HEALTH SYSTEMS, supplement to INQUIRY 12 (June 1975); NATIONAL HEALTH CARE; a monograph, CROSS-NATIONAL STUDY OF HEALTH SYSTEMS (expected 1980, Transaction Books); and several articles on framework and approaches to CNSHS. From 1971 to 1973 he served as chief of the Behavioural Science Unit, Division of Research in Epidemiology and Communications Sciences (RECS), World Health Organization, Geneva. From 1968 to 1971 he served as secretary-treasurer, Medical Sociology Section, American Sociological Association. He is a fellow of the American Sociological Association; and of the American Public Health Association; and member of the Medical Sociology Research Committee, International Sociological Association.

CONTENTS

FOREWORD

Interest in health and the resources and activities that make it possible is not new. However, the concepts of health as a national resource and as a human right have emerged in the recent past. Legislation during the last two decades has led from these concepts to a complex system with some unsurprising growing pains.

Many people have come into the field, bringing a multiplicity of backgrounds to supplement the traditional health sciences. In addition, today's laymen must make decisions on health care at all levels--from voting for or against legislators who will shape health laws, through serving on local health planning boards, to becoming participants in informed decisions on their own health care. The new recruits and the laymen have in common the need for all kinds of information on social, business, legal, ethical, and other aspects of medicine.

Much of this information has previously been unavailable and not readily understandable to the new audiences. Attempts to satisfy the need have resulted in burgeoning publications on a variety of subjects, ranging from the broad to the specific. These new publications are in many forms, from carefully edited, important texts to poorly conceived and executed technical reports, with a vast array in between. There are journals, newsletters, association and university guidebooks and models, statistical reports, and audiovisuals--all with varying quality and format.

Several problems have resulted. In the first place, there has not yet emerged a major bibliographic resource, such as the National Library of Medicine and Excerpta Medica provide for the clinical and research aspects of medicine. In addition, some of the novices in the field are not accustomed to using published literature in any form, let alone the complex of primary, secondary, and tertiary publications with which their counterparts in clinical medicine and research have become familiar.

It is the purpose of the Health Affairs Series in the Gale Information Guide Library to provide a guide for all participants in the complex health care system to information on the system itself--on the process of the delivery of health care. We are concerned with the management of the system and with how researchers, educators, and practitioners assure the best health possible to each individual. We are not concerned with the content of the information with which the researcher, educator, or practitioner deals, but rather with his mode of functioning in a real world of people with different racial, ethnic, sexual, financial, and geographic backgrounds. For example, we are not interested in how a surgical procedure is carried out, but we are concerned with its availability to those who need it. If one understands the social sciences broadly, then the Health Affairs Series covers the social aspects of medicine.

Among those social aspects we include ones which are focused on the individual in relation to his environment, his education for full participation in his own health care, and his social, political, legal, and ethical responsibilities. In addition, we include all components involved with providing facilities and resources necessary for health care delivery. Individual volumes cover: health statistics; human ecology--both man-environment interactions and manipulations and their outcomes and intervention strategies; health maintenance through food and nutrition, the professional and scientific literature of patient education; health care politics, policy, and legislation; cross national study of health systems; health planning; health care costs and financing; quality maintenance and evaluation of health care; health care administration; emergency medical service systems; preventive, diagnostic, and therapeutic materials in the health system; education in the health professions; health sciences audiovisuals; medical information transfer; and interface of medicine and the law.

Thus, just as the Gale Information Guide Library encompasses a broad spectrum of all fields of knowledge, the Health Affairs Series endeavors to be comprehensive with respect to the social aspects of medicine.

The user may ask: "Why another bibliography when there are already so many?" We agree, but the Health Affairs guides are much more than bibliographies. All contain a careful selection of materials for the intended audience, an evaluation of these materials in annotations and introductory paragraphs, and directions for finding further information. There are lists of many sources of information, such as information centers, schools, publishers, and audiovisuals. The journals which one should read regularly to keep up with the field are mentioned and annotated. In short, the reader will find specific resources for the present, and, for the future, methods of finding new sources as they are developed.

Because all of the social sciences dealing with health affairs are interrelated, it is both impossible and undesirable to prescribe strict limits for each individual volume, excluding from one anything included in another. Instead, each volume of the series is complete for the individual who is interested in only one specific subject. At the same time, other volumes serve as excellent supplements when the user wishes to go into related topics in greater depth.

A person interested in any of the social aspects of medicine should be able to find a volume that focuses on that interest, though the depth of coverage will vary with the topic. In some instances the amount of literature available determined the division of the series into specific volumes, and coverage of materials is highly selective; in other cases, the choice of volume topic was somewhat arbitrary, determined by the independence or cohesiveness of a subject, and a smaller quantity of literature may have allowed for greater depth of coverage of a topic. The series editor takes responsibility for the general organization and coverage of the series, but has left to the judgment of the volume editors decisions on individual items to be included or excluded. The series should thus be helpful to the user not only for what he is able to find in the individual volumes, but for how it has been sifted to exclude those materials that would send him down blind alleys.

We hope that our audience for the series will consist of newcomers to the fields involved, as well as researchers and practitioners who have worked with health affairs in the past but need to renew their familiarity with resources in some aspect of their major current interests. We hope especially that the guides will be useful in the education of students who have chosen one or more of the fields covered for their future careers. And finally, we have tried to make the volumes simple and direct enough that they will provide the informed layperson with access to the information resources needed to make decisions about future procedures and policies in assurance of the best match between national resources and the health care of the nation.

The two volumes by Dr. Elling bring some new dimensions to this beginning series. They are the only ones with major emphasis on health affairs outside the United States. They demonstrate that the editors are well aware that a great deal of important work that may influence United States practices has been done in other countries, even though most other individual volumes in the series are restricted to American materials. Dr. Elling discusses foreign aspects of many of the subjects to be covered in other individual volumes.

Another way in which Dr. Elling introduces volumes to come is that his two volumes, taken together, provide a clear example of two perspectives--materials and methods--that will be explicit or implicit in most of the following Health Affairs Series volumes. Sometimes the primary approach will be from the format of the materials in a field (journals or journal articles, monographs, bibliographies, and so forth) and sometimes methods or processes will predominate.

I am particularly glad to have Dr. Elling as an author in the series since he has had long experience in his field and in the thinking that has gone into it. This experience gives his ideas authority, and allows him to evaluate the

Foreword

sources he includes critically. His annotations should stimulate original thinking by users of the volumes, even when they do not agree with him. Certainly, Dr. Elling's comments will provide a background for all in the explor-
ation of cross-national aspects of health care studies.

Winifred Sewell, Series Editor
Cabin John, Maryland

ACKNOWLEDGMENTS

This work is an enlarged, more fully selected and annotated outgrowth of an initial classified bibliography compiled with Nancy Prouser under a grant from the University of Connecticut Research Foundation. The author has benefited in its preparation from exchanges with the steering group of the New England program for CNSHS and with graduate students and colleagues in the Department of Community Medicine, University of Connecticut, as well as with colleagues at WHO and scholars in other countries. Certain resource materials have been especially helpful and deserve special mention. This is particularly true of the two Akhtar bibliographies (see chapter 9) issued by IDRC--LOW-COST RURAL HEALTH CARE AND HEALTH MANPOWER TRAINING and HEALTH CARE IN THE PEOPLE'S REPUBLIC OF CHINA. Of greatest assistance has been the help my wife, Margit E. Elling, has given in typing and copy editing. The diligent and able assistance of my secretary, Nataly Maysonet, is also much appreciated.

LIST OF ABBREVIATIONS

AAA	American Anthropological Association
AAMC	Association of American Medical Colleges
AFRO	African Regional Office, WHO
AID	Agency for International Development (U.S.)
AJPH	AMERICAN JOURNAL OF PUBLIC HEALTH
AJS	AMERICAN JOURNAL OF SOCIOLOGY
AMA	American Medical Association
APHA	American Public Health Association
ASA	American Sociological Association
ASR	AMERICAN SOCIOLOGICAL REVIEW
Assn.	association
AUPHA	Association of University Programs in Health Administration
Bul.	bulletin
BUL. N.Y. ACAD. MED.	BULLETIN OF THE NEW YORK ACADEMY OF MEDICINE
CNSHS	cross-national study (or studies) of health systems
DHEW	Department of Health, Education and Welfare (U.S.)
Ed.	education
EEC	European Economic Community
EMRO	Eastern Mediterranean Regional Office of WHO
EURO	European Regional Office of WHO
FRG	Federal Republic of Germany (West Germany)
GDR	German Democratic Republic (East Germany)
GNP	gross national product

Abbreviations

GPO	Government Printing Office (U.S.)
HEW	Department of Health, Education and Welfare (U.S.)
HMSO	His or Her Majesty's Stationery Office
IDRC	International Development Research Centre (Canada)
IEA	International Epidemiological Association
ILO	International Labour Organization
Int'l.	international
INT'L. J.H. SERV.	INTERNATIONAL JOURNAL OF HEALTH SERVICES
IPPF	International Planned Parenthood Federation
ISA	International Sociological Association
J.	journal
JAMA	JOURNAL OF THE AMERICAN MEDICAL ASSOCIATION
J. MED. ED.	JOURNAL OF MEDICAL EDUCATION
LDCs	less developed countries
MDCs	more developed countries
Med.	medical or medicine
MILBANK MEM. FUND Q.	MILBANK MEMORIAL FUND QUARTERLY
MNCs	multinational or transnational corporations
NCHSR	National Center for Health Services Research
NEJM	NEW ENGLAND JOURNAL OF MEDICINE
NHI	National Health Insurance
NHS	National Health Service
NIH	National Institutes of Health, USPHS, DHEW
PAHO	Pan American Health Organization (AMRO–American Regional Office of WHO)
PRC	People's Republic of China
Pub. H.	public health
Q.	quarterly
Ref.	reference
Rev.	review
SEARO	South East Asia Regional Office, WHO
SOC. SCI. MED.	SOCIAL SCIENCE AND MEDICINE
UDCs	underdeveloped countries
UK	Britain or United Kingdom of Great Britain, Scotland and Northern Ireland

Abbreviations

UN	United Nations
UNESCO	United Nations Education and Scientific Organization
UNICEF	United Nations International Children's Emergency Fund
UNRISD	United Nations Research Institute for Social Development
USPHS	United States Public Health Services
USSR	Union of Soviet Socialist Republics
WHO	World Health Organization
WPRO	Western Pacific Regional Office, WHO

Chapter 1
INTRODUCTION

This is intended as a bibliography for researchers, teachers, and students of cross-national studies of health systems (CNSHS). I have found such a resource particularly helpful in assisting students and research colleagues to pursue either general comparisons of health systems, such as in some of the more exemplary works found in chapter 4, or specific problems. But there are general works included which are not highly theoretical, methodological, or technical. Thus this book may prove useful to health policymakers and interested citizens. In an attempt to increase the book's general usefulness, brief introductions are offered for each chapter and section to highlight key characteristics of systems or issues surrounding particular problems. There is no intent on my part to limit use to the small group of researchers and scholars in this field. The problems of human health and health services are too serious to be left to the experts alone.

Cross-national study of health systems (CNSHS) as a field of research and scholarship shares most concerns with cross-cultural studies of health orientations and behaviors. However, CNSHS is focused more on the planning, organization, and financing of health services than is the case in most cross-cultural or anthropological studies of health systems. Cross-cultural studies have devoted most attention to relations between traditional and modern systems of care and to the orientations of recipients of care, whether of traditional or modern care. These concerns are in no way irrelevant. Adequate health care coverage of all the people of a nation cannot be achieved where resources are very scarce (as they are for more than three-fourths of the world's people) without taking traditional health and medical resources into account. Also, traditional orientations and health behaviors will be part of the understanding, confidence, and acceptance of whatever mix of traditional and modern care is offered. But the macrolevel--planning, organization, and financing of services--usually plays a key role in determining health orientations and behaviors.

The focus of CNSHS on structural arrangements of health and medical care systems as well as the focus on national entities brings one to direct consideration of political economic systems and their influences on variations in health services organization as well as on orientations of providers and users of care. This focus on the political and economic systems of nations (as distinct from, but not ex-

1

clusive of or opposed to the study of cultural variations) is appropriate because
it is the governing structures of nations which make major decisions to allocate
scarce resources for health in one way or another.

There is a growing acceptance, even active demand for "modern" medicine, by
people at all levels--from the bush to the city--who have experienced or heard
of its dramatic positive effects. This rising demand occurs even as health care
costs rise rapidly, with serious political and economic consequences for national
governments and political leaders. The desire to provide coverage for all people
within a country at costs that can be locally borne is leading to a vigorous search
for new modes of organizing and delivering care. Eventually, this search is
likely to encourage and draw upon further study of the 140 or so "natural labo-
ratories" found in the actual health systems of the countries of the world.

Attempts to meet these demands confront a number of sociotechnical problems
having to do with making appropriate information and materials available and
acceptable. Questions of physical access, financing, citizen and health pro-
vider sophistication, and human dignity are involved. An adequate framework
for dealing with these and other central problems has yet to be developed as the
reader will see in chapter 5.

Above all, the mobilization of people to confront and solve problems is at issue.
The concept of "national will" has been sued as shorthand to express this need.
But this may be too mystical a term, reminiscent of earlier, philosophic discussions of "free will." The term may carry with it the mistaken belief that
such mobilization can occur in any system, it being only a matter of finding the
touchstone to get it started. But if a society is enervated by exploitation and
inequity, its health system can hardly be mobilized to serve the people, as is
now the case, by all appearances, in the PRC. In a situation such as China's,
there is a tremendous release of creative human energy, carrying with it the
hope and invention necessary to solve problems even when resources are minimal.
In the face of a rash of serious apocalyptic predictions,[1] it is important to have
at least this one positive case with which to ward off visions of doom and keep
alive one's search for alternatives.

With strains toward the development of some form of national health insurance
in the United States,[2] with the need, as Ann Somers points out, for rationalization of services in all developed countries,[3] and with the desperate lack of resources in underdeveloped lands to meet the basic health needs of the people,[4]
the world could well use some more continuous, systematic approach to the cross-
national study of health systems. Such work would collect available information
on countries' health systems in relation to their socioeconomic, political, cultural, and epidemiologic contexts, and would generate new information, carry
out analyses, and formulate better frameworks for understanding health systems
in relation to their contexts.[5] From such work, inferences could be drawn to
assist health services development efforts in different countries to be more critical
and creative.

2

This volume represents a small step in the direction of developing such work. This bibliography is drawn from a wide range of sources--collections of descriptions of health systems in different countries, research monographs, journal articles, official reports, unpublished dissertations, and so forth. Rather than limiting the work strictly to studies which actually compare or contrast two or more health systems, descriptions and or analyses of single systems are included as a way of providing an assemblage of data to encourage CNSHS.

This book is sharply limited by being almost exclusively composed of works in English, though it is true that the vast majority of work in CNSHS is in this language. It is limited also in the period covered. Most publications included in this volume fall between 1965 and 1977; no thorough search has been made to uncover earlier studies or works primarily of historical interest (though many of the best-known works of this genre are included in chapter 3.1). In this rapidly growing field of study, new works are being published constantly; a book like this could be kept up to date only if it were in looseleaf form.

The limitation to modern studies seems justified as the field is relatively new, and health systems and their national contexts change rapidly enough to warrant a focus on the current situation, though it should be clear that anyone making a contrasting or comparative study of two or more systems is well advised to look closely into the historical development of those systems. In the absence of historical analysis, current institutional arrangements cannot be clearly understood. Even in countries where a major political economic revolution has taken place, elements of the present system will be taken from the past. For example, in the Soviet Union, the feldsher (a relatively autonomously acting medical practitioner with training somewhat intermediate to that of a nurse and physician) was first developed under the czars to provide care in rural areas.

Because each health and medical care system is vitally embedded in its surrounding national context, a certain number of items are included in chapters 2 and 3 to provide material on the socioeconomic, political, cultural, and epidemiologic environments of the health and medical care systems in particular countries. This contextual coverage is more exemplary than thorough. Each subject, such as the world capitalist political economy, population, food, and epidemiology, would warrant a volume to approach any acceptable degree of thoroughness.

I want to further emphasize here the crucial importance of the political, economic and associated aspects of national context. One of the major lessons which can be drawn, even now, from CNSHS is the necessity of dealing with problems in an interrrelated rather than a problem-specific or fractionated way. The problems of health, nutrition, population growth, economy, and social security are inextricably bound together. Systems that confront one of these while ignoring the others are doomed to fail in anything beyond the short-run spurt of initial enthusiasm for this program or that campaign.

A small number of items are not annotated, for a variety of reasons, mainly because the title is adequately descriptive. A few items have not been consulted.

NOTES

1. Geoffrey Barraclough, "The Great World Crisis I," NEW YORK REV. OF BOOKS 21 (January 23, 1975): 20-29; Philip Handler, "On the State of Man," speech presented at the Annual Convocation of Markle Scholars, The Homestead, Virginia, September 29, 1974; Robert L. Heilbronner, INQUIRY INTO HUMAN PROSPECTS (New York: Norton, 1974).

2. "Albert Says National Health Insurance Will Pass in 1975," NEW YORK TIMES, November 23, 1974, p. 34. For an examination of issues involved, see R.H. Elling, ed., NATIONAL HEALTH CARE, ISSUES AND PROBLEMS IN SOCIALIZED MEDICINE (New York: Atherton, 1973).

3. Anne R. Somers, "The Rationalization of Health Services: A Universal Priority," INQUIRY 8 (March 1971): 48-60. See also Robert Maxwell, HEALTH CARE: THE GROWING DILEMMA, NEEDS VERSUS RESOURCES IN WESTERN EUROPE, THE US AND THE USSR (New York: McKinsey, 1974).

4. The priority of achieving adequate coverage for all peoples--rural as well as urban, migrant as well as stationary populations--is indicated by the WHO/UNICEF "Joint Study of Alternative Approaches to Meeting Basic Health Needs of Populations in Developing Countries," JC 20/UNICEF-WHO/75.2 (Geneva, 1975). Issued as a book with this title under the editorship of V. Djukanovic and E.P. Mach (see chapter 3.3).

5. The desirability of improving our understandings along these lines is called for in "Organizational Study on Methods of Promoting the Development of Basic Health Services," Annex II to OFFICIAL RECORDS OF THE WORLD HEALTH ORGANIZATION, no. 206 (Geneva: WHO, 1973), especially paragraph 4.3.1, p. 110.

6. The segmental approach carried out under the ideology of a "campaign" as inherited from colonialist military influences is sharply criticized by D. Banerji, "Social and Cultural Foundations of the Health Systems of India," in Ray H. Elling, ed., COMPARATIVE HEALTH SYSTEMS, supplemental volume of INQUIRY 12 (June 1975): 70-85.

Chapter 2

WORLD POLITICAL ECONOMY, POPULATION,

RESOURCES, DEVELOPMENT, AND HEALTH

The topics of this chapter each deserve considerably more attention than they can receive here. Many publications exist on the world capitalist political economy and its effect on both developed and underdeveloped countries (UDCs). The works reflect sharply divergent positions. Perhaps the best scholarly overview of these is given in Brookfield's book. In brief, and without the ability to do justice to the different positions, the key issue is whether the developed capitalist economies are aiding the UDCs to "develop" by investing capital and making loans, or do these acts entail controlling, exploitative relations which suppress development and generate disparities, including extreme differences in health and health services between client elites and the masses of peasants and workers. The first view is variously termed the modernization or diffusion approach, resting upon consensual or other forms of integrative theory in which development is seen as due to peoples assuming new values and technologies which allow them to use capital (seen as neutral regardless of source) to good advantage. Because this has been the prevailing view in the West and works such as those by Walter W. Rostow, suggesting a "take-off" stage, are generally familiar, selection here has been in the other direction.

This second view rests on dependency, neo-Marxian, or other forms of conflict theory in which inequalities between classes and class struggle is primary. State power is the force allowing control of capital and the means of production to the advantage of a ruling elite. Thus capital transfers internationally are not seen as neutral but as advantageous or disadvantageous to the masses depending on whether state power has been assumed by the masses in a particular country. This conception is perhaps most generally and best presented in the works of Wallerstein and Frank. Recent, very significant empirical tests of this view are given in the articles by Chase-Dunn and Rubinson. From the perspective of this latter position, development involves revolution; some items are therefore included on revolution (e.g., Fanon or Paige).

If the political economic structure orders relations in the world and within countries, the pressures of population and resources cannot be ignored. Views on this range from the possibly apocalyptic (e.g., Heilbronner or Mesarovic and Pestel) to the more hopeful view expressed by the Chinese at Bucharest (see Hofsten).

5

The study of demography is a whole field in itself and cannot be covered here. Similarly, some general items on nutrition are given to reflect the concern for food as a world political economic resource as well as a central concern in relation to population growth and human survival.

Perhaps the key point for our concerns here is the embedded nature of health and health care systems in their surrounding political, economic, cultural, and epidemiologic contexts and the relation of health to development.

Almeida, Silvio, et al. "Analysis of Traditional Strategies to Combat World Hunger and Their Results." INT'L. J.H. SERV. 5 (1975): 121-41. 14 refs.

> During the years 1969-71, fifty-seven UDCs, out of a total of ninety-seven countries studied, had supplies below basic requirements for their populations. This calculation presupposes an equal distribution of the total quantity of food, which in practice is far from being the case. The traditional strategies proposed for development of the agricultural production of the UDCs are examined in this article. The limitations of these strategies are discussed and proposals are made for achieving the agricultural development in the underdeveloped world that will be necessary to eliminate hunger in the near future. This article is based on part 2 of WORLD HUNGER: CAUSES AND REMEDIES, which was prepared by the staff of the Transnational Institute for presentation at the UN World Food Conference in Rome in November 1974.

_____. "Assessment of the World Food Situation--Present and Future." INT'L. J. H. SERV. 5 (1975): 95-120.

> Discusses several issues regarding the problem of hunger: the creation of international grain reserves; problems concerning world trade of foodstuffs; the current difficulties with certain key agricultural production factors, such as fertilizers; the necessity for organizing a worldwide information system on the situation; and prospects of various harvests and threats of famine in UDCs. This article is based on part 1 of WORLD HUNGER: CAUSES AND REMEDIES, which was prepared by the staff of the Transnational Institute for presentation at the UN World Food Conference in Rome in November 1974. Transnational Institute report states, "For hunger is caused by plunder and not by scarcity; the fruits of the earth and of generations of toil are unjustly divided up; the earth is the birthright of all human beings; and what comes from the earth can and must provide nourishment for all the earth's children rather than private gain for the few."

Amin, Samir. ACCUMULATION ON A WORLD SCALE. New York: Monthly Rev. Press, 1974.

> Links military and political power and the "decapitalization" of UDCs through the MNCs seen by other authors (see Frank; Beckford; and Pinto and Knakal, this chapter).

Arrighi, Giovanni. "International Corporations, Labour Aristocracies, and Economic Development in Tropical Africa." In IMPERIALISM AND UNDERDEVELOPMENT, edited by Robert Rhodes, pp. 220-67. New York: Monthly Rev. Press, 1970.

Baldwin, R., and Weisbrod, B. "Disease and Labor Productivity." ECONOMIC DEVELOPMENT AND CULTURAL CHANGE 22 (1974): 414-34.

Inconclusive treatment of a number of discrete indicators for developing countries attempting to relate health to development potential. The problem of circularity cannot be ruled out; that is, there is little rewarding, life-sustaining opportunity for labor, so there is poor health, so there is poor labor productivity.

Barnet, R.J., and Muller, R.E. GLOBAL REACH: THE POWER OF THE MULTINATIONAL CORPORATIONS. New York: Simon and Schuster, 1974.

Comprehensive overview and penetrating analysis of MNCs and their relations to national governments, local industry, and agriculture. Includes case examples of illegal avoidance of national tax laws and pressures on client governments in UDCs. Clearly some MNCs control more resources and are more powerful than most sets of UDCs taken together. Gives no specific attention to health, but there are implications for health in terms of the MNCs' impact on environments, living standards, and labor conditions.

Barraclough, Geoffrey. "The Great World Crisis I." N.Y. REV. OF BOOKS 21 (January 23, 1975): 20-29.

Examines a growing awareness of world crisis in relation to resources and political machinery precipitated by the oil embargo of 1974.

_____. "Wealth and Power: The Politics of Food and Oil." N.Y. REV. OF BOOKS 22 (August 7, 1975): 23-30.

Identifies the brutal trade-offs behind the smokescreen of diplomatic and presumably humanitarian concerns. The increasingly difficult position of the UDCs is described and explained. For example, as oil prices increase, so do fertilizer prices, but the UDCs products generally do not bring higher prices. Thus, unable to produce enough food by present land distribution and cultivation methods, they become more and more dependent on the United States not only for technology but also for food.

Beckford, George. PERSISTENT POVERTY: UNDERDEVELOPMENT IN PLANTATION REGIONS OF THE WORLD. New York: Oxford Univ. Press, 1971.

Although this book gives no special attention to health, it is relevant because there is such a close link generally between poor health and poverty. Nearly three-quarters of the world's population lives in agricultural areas. The role of MNCs in agriculture

VANDERBILT MEDICAL CENTER LIBRARY

in UDCs is examined. The MNCs are interested in keeping labor cheap, taxes low, and markets imperfect (subject to their manipulation through political controls). These interests are inimical to balanced development of the peripheral countries in which the MNCs control the best land and produce their cash crops (crops not usually designed to feed the masses of people of the country itself). Beckford calls this distortion of resource use a state of "dynamic underdevelopment." Distortion is seen to occur in these ways: overspecialization in raw material production (low differentiation); outward-oriented infrastructure (low integration--see Frank, this chapter); and the creation of resource use patterns which retard economic development. In short, countries exposed to the exploitation of MNCs cannot appropriate their own surplus capital to invest in balanced development. MNCs further their own growth but not that of countries in which they locate.

Behm, Hugo, et al. "Demographic Trends, Health, and Medical Care in Latin America." INT'L. J.H. SERV. 2 (1972): 13-22.

The relationship of changing demographic characteristics to health status and medical care in Latin America is examined in this article. The rapid demographic growth, high birth and death rates (although with a downward trend), excessive expansion of the large cities, and dispersion of the rural population are correlated with the unsatisfactory levels of health and living of the masses of the population and the limitations of the health systems. The authors contend that the situation described is basically due to inefficient social, economic, and political structures and an unhealthy dependence on external forces. Only radical structural changes will enable millions of Latin Americans to have access to medical care, health, and life itself.

Black, Cyril E., et al. THE MODERNIZATION OF JAPAN AND RUSSIA. New York: Free Press, 1975.

One of the many works viewing development from the perspective of modernization theory. Modernization is defined simply as societal achievement of or adaptation to "the scientific and technological revolution." The view is that the whole world is on a single course of "development" generally following what the West has achieved, even though different institutional arrangements may be devised. Japan and Russia are studied as "followers" rather than "firstcomers" to national industrialization and are seen as having institutions characteristic of the former type. The work completely ignores and indeed, is opposed in basic theoretical assumptions to the world capitalist system view. (For examples of this view see Frank; Wallerstein; and others, this chapter.) As a consequence, political forms are given little attention and, quite surprisingly, the revolution of 1917 in the USSR and the rise of fascism and World War II in Japan are hardly recognized in this work.

Blasier, Cole. THE HOVERING GIANT: U.S. RESPONSES TO REVOLU-
TIONARY CHANGE IN LATIN AMERICA. Pitt Latin American Series. Pittsburgh: Univ. of Pittsburgh Press, 1976.

> Comprehensive, comparative study of US responses to revolutions in
> Latin American countries. The analysis is based on previously un-
> used sources in German and Russian as well as Spanish and English.
> The revolutionary process in these countries has tended to pass
> through three stages: rebellion, reformism, and revolutionary change.
> Blasier describes the extensive and complex relations between Latin
> American and US leaders in these stages in Mexico (1910-40),
> Bolivia (1943-64), Guatemala (1944-54), and Cuba (1957-61). He
> explains why US leaders sponsored paramilitary units to overthrow
> revolutionary governments in Guatemala and Cuba and compromised
> their differences with revolutionary governments in Mexico and
> Bolivia. In an epilogue, the author skillfully compares US responses
> to these four revolutions with US responses since 1961 in the Do-
> minican Republic, Peru, and Chile. The policy implications of
> his conclusions are discussed in a final section, "Lessons of History."

Brookfield, Harold C. INTERDEPENDENT DEVELOPMENT. Pittsburgh: Univ.
of Pittsburgh Press, 1975.

> The best scholarly survey and analysis of theories of development
> including such popular, but probably wrong, notions as Rostow's
> "stages of growth." The author tentatively offers his own view
> that "development" for some, in the sense of greater GNP or
> similar measures, has always entailed expropriation and underde-
> velopment for others.

Brown, E. Richard. "Public Health in Imperialism: Early Rockefeller Programs
at Home and Abroad." AJPH 66 (September 1976): 897-903.

> An exchange of letters relating to the thesis of this article that
> US public health intervention has often gone along with imperialism.
> See also AJPH 67 (February 1977): 190-92.

Caldwell, John C., et al., eds. POPULATION GROWTH AND SOCIOECO-
NOMIC CHANGE IN WEST AFRICA. New York: Columbia Univ. Press, 1975.

> A large work (763 p. and 25 x 18 cm) with forty-four writers and
> thirty-seven chapters put together by the five editors. While the
> descriptions and discussions are very valuable for the area and for
> particular countries, dependable data are scarce. Particularly good
> for purposes of CNSHS in that public health measures and conditions
> are considered along with numerous other factors. Remarkable pos-
> sibilities and insights abound on fertility of polygynous women,
> effect of lactation on reproduction, catastrophic mortality at young
> ages, lower fertility among nomads, instances of higher urban than
> rural fertility, and so forth.

Candau, Marcolino G. "Keynote Address: Knowledge, the Bridge to Achievement." ISRAEL J. MED. SCIENCE (Jerusalem) 4 (May-June 1968): 343-49.

Presented at the Fourth Rehovoth Conference on Health Problems in
Developing States, Rehovoth, Israel, August 15-23, 1967. Statement by the director general of WHO recognizing the complex and
varied nature of health problems in UDCs and the need for innovative approaches. An ecological, interdisciplinary view is rec-
ommended.

Carr-Saunders, A.M. THE POPULATION PROBLEM: A STUDY IN HUMAN
EVOLUTION. Oxford: Clarendon, 1922.

Important historically.

Chase-Dunn, Christopher. "The Effects of International Economic Dependence
on Development and Inequality: A Cross-National Study." ASR 40 (December
1975): 720-38.

Especially valuable empirical test supporting dependency theory
rather than neoclassical and modernization theories. The latter see
capital flows from core (dominant) countries in the world capitalist
political economic system as leading to growth and greater equality
in income within peripheral countries. This study finds by panel
regression analysis of data for LDCs (those with less than $406 GNP
per capita in 1955) reflecting the period 1950-70 (income inequality
data reflect only one period around 1965) that those with the greatest
investment and debt dependence showed the slowest growth and
greatest income inequalities. Gives very useful brief review of
alternative theories of development and/or exploitation. Consideration of methods and data sources for cross-national studies is also
valuable. No consideration of health.

Cibotti, R. "Introduction to the Analysis of Development and Planning." INT'L.
J. H. SERV. 1 (August 1971): 201-24.

Underdevelopment may be characterized in numerous ways, according to the vantage point from which it is analyzed. Social, political, cultural, and demographic elements may all be taken into
account. An economic point of view emphasizes the phenomenon
of low availability of goods and services for the satisfaction of the
needs and aspirations of the population. Underdevelopment is analyzed here from the point of view of an economic planner. Integration of health services planning into the total development plan
is also discussed.

Cline, William. "Distribution and Development: A Survey of Literature." J.
OF DEVELOPMENT ECONOMICS 1 (1975): 1-42.

Commoner, Barry. THE CLOSING CIRCLE: NATURE, MAN AND TECH-
NOLOGY. New York: Alfred A. Knopf, 1971.

> Inquires into the environmental crisis by describing patterns of eco-
> logical destruction due to technological stress and the social, po-
> litical, and economic forces at work. Survival will be managed
> by restoring to nature what man takes from it. Employs the con-
> cept of biological capital and examines the many ways the indus-
> trialized world is using this capital up by polluting it, while the
> "poorer" part of the world is producing human population at rates
> which are not sustainable in the long run.

Coppock, J.B.M. "The Green Revolution Seen through British Eyes." ROYAL
SOCIETY OF HEALTH J. 94 (December 1974): 269-70, 277.

deAlneida, M. Ozorio, et al. ENVIRONMENT AND DEVELOPMENT. THE
FOUNEX REPORT ON INTERNATIONAL CONCILIATION. No. 586. New
York: Carnegie Endowment for Int'l. Peace, January 1972.

Dubos, Rene. MAN ADAPTING. New Haven, Conn.: Yale Univ. Press, 1965.

> Extends the understanding of his famous MIRAGE OF HEALTH by
> examining man as increasingly the creator of his own environment
> and health problems.

Eberstadt, N. "Myths of the Food Crisis." N.Y. REV. OF BOOKS 23 (February 19, 1976): 32-37.

> Without discounting the gravity of the world population-food supply
> problem, provides critical examination of the interest groups in-
> volved and the inflated, or sometimes understated figures they offer.

Ehrlich, Paul R. THE POPULATION BOMB. Rev. ed. New York: Ballantine
Books, 1972.

> From possibly 10 million people living in 40,000 B.C., the world's
> human population grew to more than 400 million by 1650 A.D.
> Then in less than 400 years it grew tenfold to 4 billion by 1975.
> The lack of completely agreed understanding of this remarkable
> curve is discussed as well as implications for the future of mankind.

The Environmental Fund. WORLD POPULATION ESTIMATES, 1977. Washington, D.C., 1977.

> An annual country-by-country table giving population, growth rate,
> percentage of population under age 15, percentage urban, and so forth,
> and certain other useful data such as energy use. Also gives a
> graph useful in computing the time necessary for a population to
> double according to its growth rate. Not all categories are re-
> peated each year; thus earlier issues may be useful.

Fanon, Frantz. DYING COLONIALISM. New York: Grove Press, 1965.

> A historical analysis of the Algerian revolution, focusing on social
> and political factors. Analyzes the role of western medicine as a
> mistrusted feature of colonialism, and the position of the European
> minority in the fight for independence.

_____. THE WRETCHED OF THE EARTH. New York: Grove Press, 1968.
First published as LÉS DAMNÉS DE LA TERRE by Francois Maspero, Paris, 1961.

> A classic. This as well as most of Fanon's other writings derive
> from his experience as a black psychiatrist in Algeria during the
> struggle for liberation from colonialist France. The contents deal
> with the awakening of a people and their moves toward self-respect
> and self-determination. Points out the need for class and cultural
> consciousness and solidarity of organization to wage a successful
> struggle, rather than individual spontaneity and outbursts of vio-
> lence. From this work one can abstract an analytic, perhaps over-
> lapping and intermixed set of phases of decolonization: "thingifi-
> cation" and "exploitation"; initial resistance and partial accommo-
> dation; the search for cultural roots and group pride; boundary
> crossing and repression; underground development of culture and
> organization; open armed struggle; liberation and extension of con-
> sciousness internationally to other repressed peoples and classes.

Frank, Andre Gundar. "The Development of Underdevelopment." In DEPEN-
DENCE AND UNDERDEVELOPMENT, edited by J.D. Cockcroft et al., pp.
3-17. New York: Doubleday, 1972.

> Discusses distortions which arise through external control (see entry
> below) and notes that many of the poorest areas of Latin America
> today were once highly active centers of raw material production
> in the world economy. But when demand for these materials de-
> clined, the external capital and organization which exploited them
> were withdrawn.

_____. LATIN AMERICA: UNDERDEVELOPMENT OR REVOLUTION. New
York: Monthly Rev. Press, 1969.

> Documents how the economies of Latin America have become out-
> wardly oriented toward the exploiting external capitalist sources of
> investment and control, mostly in the United States. The infra-
> structures--railroads, roads, telegraph lines, and so forth--all are
> oriented toward the ports of exit and function to carry raw materials
> out of the country and return processed goods. Export-oriented
> merchants combine with the landed gentry to prevent the emergence
> of a domestic manufacturing bourgeoisie by politically defeating
> tariffs which would protect infant domestic industry against compe-
> tition from industry core nations. Frank sees this process through-
> out the history of Latin America. For example, civil wars occur-
> ing around 1830 in the newly independent republics involved the

issue of internal versus external orientation. In every case, the forces of external orientation and "free" trade won. Frank terms the penetration of the periphery by core capital in such a way as to create obstacles to development, "the development of underdevelopment." No special discussion of health.

Fucaraccio, A. "Birth Control and the Argument of Saving and Investment." INT'L. J. H. SERV. 3 (1973): 133-44.

From the author's summary: "This paper critically analyzes the thesis that birth control is a valid means of increasing saving and investment to stimulate growth in underdeveloped countries. . . . It is shown that, first, there is not a scarcity of capital in Latin America, but rather a great underutilization of capital; that is, capital appears scarce because it is being considerably underused. Second, part of this underuse occurs because control of capital is limited to the high-income sector of the population, as a result of a highly skewed distribution of income in those countries. . . . The strategy of birth control, aimed especially at those who are unable to save, will obviously increase neither investment nor saving. The so-called savings on education and public health are bound to be minimal because in the present distribution of resources these sectors consume very little of the national product. In this analysis it is thus concluded that the assumptions underlying the argument of population control do not hold for Latin America and do not have a scientific basis."

George, Susan. HOW THE OTHER HALF DIES, THE REAL REASONS FOR WORLD HUNGER. New York: Universe Books, 1977.

A thorough analysis of the world capitalist political economy, the UN, UDCs and other factors such as expensive oil-based fertilizers and single-crop, wage-based economies in the creation of hunger in UDCs.

Gouldner, Alvin W., and Peterson, R.A. NOTES ON TECHNOLOGY AND THE MORAL ORDER. Indianapolis: Bobbs-Merrill, 1962.

Raises and examines the question of "progress."

Goulet, Denis. THE CRUEL CHOICE: A NEW CONCEPT IN THE THEORY OF DEVELOPMENT. New York: Atheneum, 1975.

An important book effectively challenging the direction of the world economy toward unlimited growth.

Griffith, D.H.S., et al. "Contribution of Health to Development." INT'L. J. H. SERV. 1 (August 1971): 253-70.

Health planners in developing countries face the following problems among others: defining the role of health in economic growth, obtaining recognition of the effects of ill health upon economic development, and quantifying health benefits. Three examples of these problems stated in simple health and economic terms are developed in this paper: (1) production function, health expenditures, and investment in Ceylon from 1947-48 to 1958; (2) effects of ill health on the growing of rice in Southeast Asia in 1957; and (3) the health benefits and cost-benefit ratio achieved by malaria prophylaxis in a small mining concern in Thailand in 1969-70. It is suggested that further studies in the fields exemplified will aid health planners in finding ways and means for better justification of programs.

Handler, Phillip. "On the State of Man." Speech presented at the Annual Convocation of Markle Scholars, The Homestead, September 1974. Reproduced. Available from the Markle Foundation.

Highlights the problems of population growth, and the role of science and technology in dealing with the rising demands for agriculture, energy, and water. Calls for immediate worldwide political commitment and action. Considers, but does not accept the notion of "triaging" (writing off) whole sections of the human population such as in South Asia.

Hardin, Garrett. "Lifeboat Ethics: The Case against Helping the Poor." PSYCHOLOGY TODAY 8 (September 1974): 38 ff.

Argues the case for "triage" applied to whole nations and parts of the world. In short, writes off whole sections of humanity. Sees aid to Bangladesh, India, Pakistan, and other parts of South Asia as likely only to create a bigger problem which will draw needed resources from solving population and resource problems in the rest of the world. Conceives of the MDCs as a lifeboat which is full of people surrounded by a sea of people in the LDCs and UDCs seeking to climb aboard. This brutal and inhumane view is sharply attacked on both technical and moral grounds in a number of letters to the editor in the December 1974 issue of this journal. Among points of disagreement: the whole world is one lifeboat with a single ecology; portable atomic weaponry will soon be available in some UDCs and they would not accept "triage"; Hardin is presumptuous as UDCs will decide for themselves.

Harvey, David. "Ideology and Population Theory." INT'L. J.H. SERV. 4 (Summer 1974): 515-37. 41 refs.

Examines the ideological and ethical foundations of population theory in the light of the supposed ethical neutrality of scientific enquiry. Contrasts the works of Malthus, Ricardo, and Marx and shows that their theories of population resulted in each case from the adoption of a particular kind of method--empiricism in Malthus,

normative analytic "model building" in Ricardo, and dialectical
materialism in Marx. It is shown that a Malthusian or neo-Malthusian
view of the population problem is inevitable if enquiry is founded
in empiricism or in normative analytics. Concludes that the choice
of scientific method does not produce unbiased results and that
the dominance of a certain conception of scientific method leads
to the "scientific" support of a viewpoint used to justify repression
of the underprivileged in society.

Hayter, Teresa. AID AS IMPERIALISM. Harmondsworth, Engl.: Penguin, 1971.

Heilbronner, Robert. "The Human Prospect." N.Y. REV. OF BOOKS 20
(January 24, 1974): 21-34.

Inquires into world population and resources and the pessimistic
mood of humanity. Comments on the demographic outlook, un-
interrupted industrial growth, technological imperatives, and unpredictable political behavior. Suggests that postindustrial society
may move toward ritual and tradition, qualities of preindustrial
societies. Suggests the possibility of 40 billion people on earth
in the next 100 years. But concludes that ultimately there is hope
in man to alter the directions in which he is headed.

Heinild, Svend. "Health and the Population: Structure and Substance."
SCANDINAVIAN J. OF SOCIAL MED. 1 (1973): 13-16.

Hirsch, Fred. SOCIAL LIMITS TO GROWTH. A Twentieth Century Fund Study.
Cambridge, Mass.: Harvard Univ. Press, 1976.

The first part of this book deals with disappointment that has accompanied growth as a general social objective. A distinction is
made between use of products not affected by one's position in
society (e.g., enjoyment of a TV program is independent of others'
enjoying that program) and use of products whose enjoyment is affected by position in society (e.g., the pleasure of an especially
well prepared and served meal in a fine restaurant is at least partly
dependent on the consumer's awareness that it is available only to
the rich). As "lower" class incomes are improved, personal, especially menial service, will be less and less offered. The competition over income to maintain such "pleasures" based on the inequalities has serious consequences. In the second half of the
book, the deterioration of the moral foundation of expansive capitalism is examined. An excellent review of this work is given by
Robert L. Heilbronner, author of AN INQUIRY INTO THE HUMAN
PROSPECT, among other works, under the title, "The False Promise
of Growth" in N.Y. REV. OF BOOKS 24 (March 3, 1977): 10-
12.

Hofsten, Erland. "Population Growth--A Menace to What?" INT'L. J. H. SERV. 5 (1975): 417-24. 11 refs.

Originally, many of the initiators of the 1974 World Population Conference had hoped that the conference would bring a final breakthrough for the view that family planning measures should be given top priority in all LDCs. In fact, however, the Plan of Action passed by the conference contained very little relating to population and family planning. Instead, the document is dominated by wordy phrases about the necessity of attaining social and economic development in those countries. The reasons for the underdevelopment of Third World countries cannot be removed through such UN resolutions, according to Hofsten.

Hughes, Charles C., and Hunter, Jane M. "Disease and 'Development' in Africa." SOC. SCI. MED. 3 (March 1970): 443-93.

Unanticipated consequences of development require health programs to be ecologically informed. Gives examples of diseases fostered by development programs, particularly the Aswan Dam and the problem of schistosomiasis, and the role of urbanization and migration patterns.

Illich, Ivan. "Outwitting the 'Developed' Nations." In NATIONAL HEALTH CARE: ISSUES AND PROBLEMS IN SOCIALIZED MEDICINE, edited by Ray H. Elling, pp. 263-76. New York: Atherton, 1973.

Criticizes the inappropriate adopting of ideologies and technologies of developed countries to the problems of underdeveloped nations. Concentrates on the issues of the population explosion and the atrophy of social imagination. Defines underdevelopment as an imposition upon the population through their needs remaining unsatisfied. Research should concentrate on alternatives to prepackaged solutions and avoidance of mimicking.

Inkeles, Alex, and Smith, David H. BECOMING MODERN: INDIVIDUAL CHANGES IN SIX DEVELOPING COUNTRIES. Cambridge, Mass.: Harvard Univ. Press, 1974.

One of many works seeking to understand development as dependent upon social psychological change. Reports on empirical studies of value changes (greater appreciation of science, technology, education, etc.) and their correlates (urbanization, secularization, etc.) in different countries. The introductory chapter appeared in the INT'L. J. OF COMPARATIVE SOCIOLOGY 14 (1973): 157-62.

INT'L. J.H. SERV. 1 (August 1971): entire issue.

Special issue devoted to "Health and Socioeconomic Development." Includes an editorial on this subject by the editor of this journal,

Vicente Navarro, and a brief statement introducing the issues involved in this theme by the health economist A. Peter Ruderman. Other relevant items from this issue are cited elsewhere in this chapter.

Jelliffe, D.B. "Commerciogenic Malnutrition." FOOD TECHNOLOGY 25 (1971): 55-56.

Uncovers the practices of MNCs selling bottle feeding and commercial foods in poor countries and to poor populations who have not the necessary refrigeration, other sanitary means, or cash to support such. Consequences include higher infection, poorer nutrition, and higher mortality. Moreover, because the mother goes off breast feeding too early, there may be population increases in areas where needs are already exceeding available resources.

Kaplan, Barbara Hocking, ed. SOCIAL CHANGE IN THE CAPITALIST WORLD ECONOMY. Political Economy of the World-System Annuals, edited by Immanuel Wallerstein, Vol. 1. Beverly Hills, Calif.: Sage Publications, 1978.

The series editor, Immanuel Wallerstein, is among the contributors to this first volume.

Karefa-Smart, John. "Health and Manpower: Inter-relationship between Health and Socioeconomic Development." ISRAEL J. OF MED. SCIENCE (Jerusalem) 4 (May-June 1968): 586-98. From the Fourth Rehovoth Conference on Health Problems in Developing States, Rehovoth, Israel, August 15-23, 1967.

Health and economic development are interrelated. Health protection of workers is important in assisting production. Malaria, chronic diseases, malnutrition, and tuberculosis are some of the conditions affecting development. Developing countries need to consider whether they can afford to sustain the heavy economic losses resulting from lack of health services. Auxiliary health manpower is essential, especially in rural areas. Social reform and economic development as well as health care must focus on the development of human potential.

Kuehner, A. "The Impact of Public Health Programs on Economic Development: Report of a Study of Malaria in Thailand." INT'L. J.H. SERV. 1 (August 1971): 285-92.

Based on an attempt to describe the economic effects of a health program and to measure these effects. Multiple and complex factors make it difficult to determine the economic value of health investments. This problem of measurement may be solved by considering that any improvement of health means an increase and any deterioration of health indicates a decrease in the working capacities of the labor force. The paper suggests that death and disease cause losses of working time and gross domestic product (GDP).

Lappe, Francis Moore, and Collins, Joseph. FOOD FIRST. New York: Institute of Food and Development Policy, 1978.

An authoritative work covering the central issues related to food, nutrition, and the world system.

Ledogar, Robert J. HUNGRY FOR PROFITS. U.S. FOOD AND DRUG MULTINATIONALS IN LATIN AMERICA. Introduction by Ralph Nader. New York: Int'l. Documentation/North America, 1975.

A critical and penetrating analysis of the role of US drug and food firms in LDCs of Latin America. Among major problems are the creation of dominant single-crop economies for export with peasants moving into low wage employment and unable to purchase enough imported food to feed their whole families; and "dumping" of unsafe or outmoded drugs.

Lenin, V[ladimir]. I[llich]. [Nikolai]. IMPERIALISM: THE HIGHEST STAGE OF CAPITALISM. Peking: Foreign Language Press, 1965.

While Marx saw the expropriative relations between core (dominant) capitalist nations and peripheral nations (colonies) as a passing phase after which the cheap prices of capitalist goods would turn colonies themselves toward a capitalist form of production, Lenin added the notion of imperialism as a relatively enduring aspect of capitalism. He saw monopoly capitalism as needing to export capital and to appropriate raw materials and markets in the peripheral countries. He predicted interimperialist wars resulting from the division and redivision of the periphery by the advanced capitalist powers. Lenin expected that the original centers of capitalism in Europe would become decadent and that the source of industrial strength would move to the periphery. Transfers of productive capacity to LDCs by MNCs, but maintenance of political control in the "home" country and extraction of greater profits than investments (see Barnet and Muller; also Turner; Moran; and Sunkel) suggest some need for revision in this latter notion.

Levi-Strauss, Claude, and Aron, Raymond. "Dynamique culturelle et valeurs" [Cultural dynamics and values]. In APPROACHES DE LA SCIENCE DU DÉVELOPMENT SOCIO-ÉCONOMIQUE, edited by Peter Lengyel, pp. 257-92. Paris: UNESCO, 1971. In French.

An important statement by the two most outstanding French social scientists of the time--an anthropologist (Levi-Strauss) and a sociologist (Aron). Attempts to apply abstract theory of cultural forms and values to practical issues of development. Diffusionist (idealistic) in orientation rather than dependency oriented (political economy).

McNamara, Robert. ONE HUNDRED COUNTRIES, TWO BILLION PEOPLE: THE DIMENSIONS OF DEVELOPMENT. New York: Praeger, 1973.

> An important statement by the president of the World Bank. Gives no particular attention to health, but there is an awareness of the nexus of population, nutrition, infectious disease, health services, family planning, and productivity. This awareness is carried further in the World Bank policy statement on health (see World Bank, below, this chapter).

Malenbaum, W. "Health and Economic Expansion in Poor Lands." See Chapter 3.3.

Marshall, Carter L. "Health, Nutrition, and the Roots of World Population Growth." INT'L. J.H. SERV. 4 (1974): 677-90. 48 refs.

> Well-documented refutation of the thesis that world population growth can be traced to medical programs such as malaria eradication, immunization, improved sanitation, and use of antibiotics. These have not been widely and uniformly applied; yet population growth has been general. The author suggests better food production, distribution, and improved nutrition as more fundamental factors.

Marx, Karl. CAPITAL. Vol. 1. Translated by Samuel Moore and Edward Aveling. Chicago: Charles H. Kerr and Co., 1906. Reprint. New York: Int'l. Publishers, 1967. First published in 3 vols. in German in 1867 as DAS KAPITAL.

> In this first of three volumes on the nature of capitalist political economy Marx identified a law of uneven development and pauperization. While this law may have turned out to be only partially correct for core (dominant) nations of world capitalism, because of union organization, social welfare arrangements, and class struggle generally, it appears correct on a world scale with dependent nations becoming poorer relative to "advanced" (exploiting) nations (see Chase-Dunn, this chapter). In any case, Marx predicts the development of a single world history (Weltgeschichte) as world capitalism transforms separate economies into "the international capitalistic regime":
>
> > "Hand in hand with this centralisation, or this expropriation of many capitalists by few, there develops, on an ever-extending scale, the cooperative form of the labour-process, the conscious technical application of science, the methodical cultivation of the soil, the transformation of the instruments of labour into instruments of labour only usable in common, the economizing of all means of production by their use as the means of production of combined, socialized labour, the entangle-

ment of all peoples in the net of the world-market, and with this, the international character of the capitalistic regime" (vol. 1, p. 763).

Mass, Bonnie. "An Historical Sketch of the American Population Control Movement." INT'L. J.H. SERV. 4 (1974): 651-76.

Effectively links this movement to the ideology, interests, and concerns of the ruling class in the United States. The author reassesses Malthus and neo-Malthusianism, which are based upon the assumption that economic and social irrationalities are invincible and eternal. The author agrees with this assumption only in regards to capitalist society. As she indicates, neither capitalist society nor plans of action that seek to prolong its existence can offer solutions for today's pressing problems of famine and impoverishment in vast portions of the world.

Mathews, William H., ed. OUTER LIMITS AND HUMAN NEEDS, RESOURCE AND ENVIRONMENTAL ISSUES OF DEVELOPMENT STRATEGIES. Uppsala, Sweden: Dag Hammarskjoeld Foundation, 1976.

Contents: "The Concept of Outer Limits"; "Environment and Styles of Development"; "The Interaction of Ecological and Social Systems: Local Outer Limits in Development"; "A Methodological Approach for Estimating Outer Limits: The Example of Energy Production." A second volume edited by Marc Nerfin, entitled ANOTHER DEVELOPMENT: APPROACHES AND STRATEGIES, appeared in 1977.

Mead, Margaret. CULTURAL PATTERNS AND TECHNICAL CHANGE. New York: Mentor Books, 1955.

A work of historical interest for considering the optimistic period when development was conceived more or less as an agricultural extension problem. Ignores the dependency relations in and exploitative character of the world capitalist political economic system.

Meadows, Paul. "Development: Some Perspective Orientations." INT'L. J. OF COMPARATIVE SOCIOLOGY 14 (1973): 19-34.

Valuable examination of different theoretical assumptions behind governmental and other policies and actions for development.

Mesarovic, Mihajlo, and Pestel, Edward. MANKIND AT THE TURNING POINT: THE SECOND REPORT TO THE CLUB OF ROME. New York: E.P. Dutton; Reader's Digest Press, 1974.

Presents the notion of solving problems in an interrelated or integrated rather than an isolated way. Employs computers to project an optimistic and a pessimistic scenario for mankind on earth. Very clearly written. Useful for an overview of world population, resources, and possibilities.

Meyer, John, et al. "Convergence and Divergence in Development." In ANNUAL REVIEW OF SOCIOLOGY, edited by Alex Inkeles, vol. 1, pp. 223-46. Palo Alto, Calif.: Annual Reviews Press, 1975.

Very useful comparison of theories and evidence for and against dependency (or conflict) theory, modernization (or value concensus) theory, and neoclassical economic theory. The weight seems to fall in the direction of a dependency theory of development.

Moore, Wilbert, and Feldman, David. LABOR COMMITMENT AND SOCIAL CHANGE IN DEVELOPING AREAS. New York: Social Science Research Council, 1960.

One of several modernization theories which attribute development to some combination of psychological and technological change. Ignores world political economic relations as dealt with by Wallerstein (see below, this chapter). Emphasizes the transfer of advanced technology, modern "rational" forms of organization, labor habits which fit in well with industrial production, and modern (generally individualistic and entrepreneurial) "attitudes" toward self, family, and society. This view would support penetration of the peripheral nations by core capital and one would predict more rapid development in nations in which such transfers have been greater. Exactly the opposite has been found (see Chase-Dunn; and Rubinson, this chapter).

Moran, Theodore H. "Transnational Strategies of Protection and Defense by Multinational Corporations." INT'L. ORG. 27 (1973): 273-301.

The large scale upon which MNCs operate gives them an advantage over small peripheral countries in which the client ruling elites can be played off against one another. This Balkanization of the periphery makes solidarity difficult. Competition for foreign investment, rather than common regulation of it, has been the main picture.

Myrdal, Gunnar. THE CHALLENGE OF WORLD POVERTY: A WORLD ANTI-POVERTY PROGRAM IN OUTLINE. New York: Vintage Books, 1970. Notes, index, appendix.

Explores the myth of nationally aggregated figures (national averages) as measuring development. Instead, points to the importance of "real progress at the local level." This book was one of the first warnings that the only thing some countries may be "developing" is great disparity and mass poverty. Identifies inequality as a block to productivity; outlines needed radical reforms in UDCs; assigns responsibilities to MDCs. The appendix describes Latin America as "a powder keg." No particular focus on health.

Navarro, Vicente. "The Underdevelopment of Health or the Health of Under-development: An Analysis of the Distribution of Human Health Resources in Latin America." INT'L. J.H. SERV. 4 (1974): 5-27.

A broad and valuable consideration of the interweaving of socio-economic and political conditions with health and health services. The same external world capitalist forces which exploit and ap-propriate from these countries economically are seen to cause un-even distribution of different health conditions and types of health care by social class, urban-rural regions, public versus private sectors, and so forth. Excellent literature review.

North American Congress on Latin America. "U.S. Grain Arsenal." LATIN AMERICA AND EMPIRE REPORT 9 (October 1975): entire issue.

Explores the use of the US grain monopoly as a political and dip-lomatic weapon; how US government policies have contributed to the food crisis; how the secretive corporations that dominate the world's grain trade operate. The NACLA is an independent re-search organization which probes the forces shaping and profiting from US policies. This is the first publication of their Agribusiness Project. Senator James Abourezk of South Dakota said of this report: "I would certainly encourage anyone interested in U.S. foreign policy to read the Report as one of the best sources of information anywhere."

Paige, Jeffrey M. AGRARIAN REVOLUTION: SOCIAL MOVEMENTS AND EXPORT AGRICULTURE IN THE UNDERDEVELOPED WORLD. See Chapter 5.

Park, Robert M. "Not Better Lives, Just Fewer People: The Ideology of Popu-lation Control." INT'L. J. H. SERV. 4 (1974): 691-700. 19 refs.

Overpopulation is interpreted as a consequence, not a cause, of problems (e.g., disparities and poverty) which themselves must be attacked in spite of entrenched elites who seek to secure the cur-rent order.

Parsons, Talcott. THE SYSTEM OF MODERN SOCIETIES. Englewood Cliffs, N.J.: Prentice-Hall, 1971.

Presents one of several essentially idealistic theories of development, attributing development to the diffusion and acceptance of modern values--economic development, education, political independence, and some form of "democracy"--by ruling elites in UDCs. Main-tains that "the 'imperialist' phase of Western society's relationship with the rest of the world was transitional." Apologetic on be-half of the ruling classes in core nations of the world capitalist political economy and directly contradictory to Marx, Lenin, Wallerstein, and others (this chapter).

Pinto, Anibal, and Knakal, Jan. "The Centre-periphery System 20 Years Later." SOCIAL AND ECONOMIC STUDIES 22 (1973): 34-89.

Shows, among the many valuable facts presented, that between 1960 and 1968 profits sent to the United States from Latin America exceeded new investment by $6.7 billion.

Ravel, Roger. "The Balance between Aid for Social Economic Development and Aid for Population Control." INT'L. J. H. SERV. 3 (1973): 667-74.

From the author's summary: "For the people most directly concerned, a reduction in the rate of population growth is not an end in itself but only one of the factors needed to improve their conditions of life. These factors include, besides a lower ratio of children to adults, the following: rational urbanization, rising incomes, introduction of modern agricultural practices, more education, improved health services, higher levels of employment and education for women, better communications, greater opportunities for socio-economic mobility, and reduction in infant and child mortality. Undue concentration on population control will be counterproductive in the long run, even in purely pragmatic terms, and it can have little moral justification."

One of a collection of articles on population, family planning, and health services and development in a special issue of this journal.

Riding, A. "In El Salvadore, 'The peasants live like serfs 400 years ago.'" NEW YORK TIMES, August 27, 1975, p. 15.

Reveals living and working conditions in rural El Salvadore, where there has been no genuine land reform. Peasant farmers' movement seeks to improve conditions of workers by breaking the feudal system of land ownership.

Rodney, Walter. HOW EUROPE UNDERDEVELOPED AFRICA. Dar es Salaam: Tanzania Publishing House, 1972.

A ringing indictment of the exploitation and leftovers of colonialism. For example, "Colonialism created conditions which led not only to famine, but to a chronic undernourishment, malnutrition, and deterioration of the physique of the African people. If such a statement sounds intellectually extravagant, it is only because bourgeois propaganda has conditioned even Africans to believe that malnutrition and starvation were the natural lot of Africans from time immemorial."

Rohrlich-Leavitt, Ruby, ed. WOMEN CROSS-CULTURALLY, CHANGE AND CHALLENGE. The Hague: Mouton; Chicago: Aldine, 1975.

A somewhat disparate collection of papers examining the position and struggle for equality by women in different countries. Lacks any systematic treatment of this important worldwide problem, but it is useful for introducing the problem.

THE ROLE OF SOCIAL SECURITY AND IMPROVED LIVING AND WORKING STANDARDS IN SOCIAL AND ECONOMIC DEVELOPMENT. Report III, Part 1. Eighth Conference of American States Members of ILO, Ottawa, 1966. Geneva: ILO, 1967.

Rubinson, Richard. "The World-Economy and the Distribution of Income within States: A Cross-National Study." ASR 41 (August 1967): 638-59.

An extremely important work employing data from forty-seven countries showing that income inequalities (by household units within quintiles) increase, even in spite of economic growth, when a country's dependence increases or its position in the world capitalist system weakens. The literature review on income inequalities, economic development, and the world capitalist political economy and imperialism is very valuable. Also valuable are the considerations of methods and citation of data sources. No consideration is given to health or health services data, but data cited here could be used to update and enrich a study of contrasting cases in health, particularly by examining income inequalities. Perhaps the key point for general theory is that the effects of capital or wealth depend not simply on amount but on the sociopolitical organization producing and controlling that capital or wealth.

Russel, D.E.H. REBELLION, REVOLUTION AND ARMED FORCES: A COMPARATIVE STUDY OF FIFTEEN COUNTRIES WITH SPECIAL EMPHASIS ON CUBA AND SOUTH AFRICA. New York: Academic Press, 1974.

An important empirical work on factors related to change in political contexts.

Schachter, Oscar. SHARING THE WORLD'S RESOURCES. New York: Columbia Univ. Press, 1977.

A lucid and succinct discussion of the principles of equity and distributive justice and their practical implications for the resolution of international disputes relating to the use and allocation of global resources. Schachter's discussion shows that the ideal of distributive justice is "grounded in the rocky soil of international conflict and the felt necessities of collaboration."

Schumacher, E.F. SMALL IS BEAUTIFUL, ECONOMICS AS IF PEOPLE MATTERED. Introduction by Theodore Roszak. New York: Harper and Row, Harper Torchbooks, 1973.

Presents an economist's fundamental challenge to the inherent expansionism of capitalism in a modern world of limited resources. Sections include "The Modern World," "Resources," "The Third World," and "Organization and Ownership."

Scott, W. "Cross-National Studies of the Impact of Levels of Living on Economic Growth: An Example." INT'L. J. H. SERV. 1 (August 1971): 225-32.

The paper describes a study carried out at the UN Research Institute for Social Development, located in Geneva, to discover a few of the conditions that in six developing countries affected the linkage between certain social levels or "inputs," such as the level of education and health as well as educational and health services, on the one hand, and economic growth, on the other. The conditions that were found to be important, to various degrees, and that should be considered in subsequent analyses (and policy-making) of the relationships of levels of living to economic growth include the structure of production, selected aspects of the social structure, and the nature and distribution of the social characteristics themselves.

Sharpston, Michael. "Health and the Human Environment." FINANCE AND DEVELOPMENT 13 (March 1976): 24-38.

Good overview of the interwoven nature of ill health, poor nutrition, poor sanitation, poverty, high fertility, and the need for "a balanced socio-economic development in the human environment." Discusses the limitations of conventional health services in developing countries. Good conceptual diagram (p. 25).

Sigerist, Henry E. CIVILIZATION AND DISEASE. Ithaca, N.Y.: Cornell Univ. Press, 1944.

One of the early works clearly identifying infections and nutritional diseases as the dominant afflictions of poverty and underdevelopment while chronic diseases, especially heart disease, cancer, and stroke, are those of industrialized societies. The profound implication is that disease is resident in the body social and not only in the cell, organ, or body of the individual person.

Simon, Julian L. THE EFFECTS OF INCOME ON FERTILITY. Chapel Hill: Univ. of North Carolina, 1974.

Almost half of this short book is made up of tables. Organized in chapters dealing with short-run and longer-run relationships in MDCs and LDCs. In both wealthier and poorer countries a rise in income is associated in the short run with a rise in fertility. In the MDCs, in the longer run, increases in aggregate income seem associated with indirect effects which could decrease fertility such as higher education for women and access to abortions. Also in the LDCs in the longer run there is an eventual depressing effect of higher income on fertility but in the interim period fertility rises with higher aggregate income. This corresponds to demographic transition theory. This book gives some important methodological critiques of usual approaches to handling such cross-national data. The work suffers from lack of adequate consideration of income distribution and political economic arrangements within countries. In short, some countries (e.g., the PRC) may control fertility through successful health, women's rights, and contraception programs before full industrialization is reached.

Sivard, Ruth. WORLD MILITARY AND SOCIAL EXPENDITURES, 1974. New York: Institute for World Order, 1975.

Excellent assemblage and presentation of data on expenditures, manpower, and so forth by major economic sectors such as military, education, health, as well as by sectors of the world, mainly 28 developed as compared with 104 developing countries. Shows disparities increasing. Was updated and reissued in 1975, 1976, and 1977.

Sunkel, Oswaldo. "Transnational Capitalism and National Disintegration in Latin America." SOCIAL AND ECONOMIC STUDIES 22 (1973): 132-76.

As summarized by Chase-Dunn (cited above, this chapter):

"Sunkel claims that the connections of ruling groups in the dependent periphery with core-states and transnational corporations create a political structure which keeps wages low and concentrates development in the international sector. The links between the core and elites in the periphery increase income inequality by (1) raising the incomes of elites and (2) keeping the wages of workers low. The power of the elites in dependent peripheral countries is backed by their alliances with the core, so they are able to suppress demands for higher wages and income redistribution. Thus dependence creates a political situation which retards development by linking elites in the periphery to the interests of the core. This prevents the emergence of autonomous forces seeking to mobilize balanced development and maintains extreme inequalities in the periphery" (p. 724).

SYNCRISIS: THE DYNAMICS OF HEALTH: AN ANALYTIC SERIES ON THE INTERACTION OF HEALTH AND SOCIOECONOMIC DEVELOPMENT. See Chapter 3.3.

Taussig, Michael. "Nutrition, Development, and Foreign Aid: A Case Study of US-Directed Health Care in a Colombian Plantation Zone." INT'L. J. H. SERV. 8 (1978): 101-21.

Adds importantly to our understanding of how the U.S. and its agencies, including foundations, may be exacerbating the problem of malnutrition and creating greater dependency in other countries through so-called aid efforts.

Thomlinson, Ralph. POPULATION DYNAMICS: CAUSES AND CONSEQUENCES OF WORLD DEMOGRAPHIC CHANGE. 2d ed. New York: Random House, 1976.

Good textbook for courses on population issues. The first part offers theory, method, and data sources. The theory chapter is useful but not particularly well rounded. Parts 2-4 examine the three demographic variables, mortality, natality, and migration. Parts 5-7 cover population composition, distribution, and national trends in relation to present and prospective living levels. The last part covers policies and programs with emphasis on birth control policies in selected countries, including recent limited data on China.

United Nations (UN). Department of Economic and Social Affairs. DECENTRALIZATION FOR NATIONAL AND LOCAL DEVELOPMENT. New York: UN, 1962.

Considers the advantages of decentralizing major aspects of planning and decision making to subnational regional and local levels.

Viner, Jacob. "America's Aims and the Progress of Underdeveloped Areas." In THE PROGRESS OF UNDERDEVELOPED AREAS, edited by Bert F. Hoselitz, pp. 179-95. Chicago: Univ. of Chicago Press, 1952.

One of a large number of neoclassical economic works which see loans and investments simply as capital transfers which will aid development. Sees as paranoid and reactive the notion that foreign investment and credit are a form of domination and suggests that this view is merely a remnant of an unfortunate but now gone colonial past.

Wallerstein, Immanuel. "Dependence in an Interdependent World: The Limited Possibilities of Transformation within the Capitalist World Economy." AFRICAN STUDIES REV. 17 (1974): 1-26.

_____. THE MODERN WORLD SYSTEM. New York: Academic Press, 1974.

One of the best overviews of the world capitalist political economic system including insights on capitalist development in sixteenth-century Europe. For example, the relatively retarded position of Poland's economy can be understood in terms of the "peripheralization" of this country in relation to "core" capitalist countries in Europe. It is in this work that the author defines the so-called developed countries as the "core" of the world capitalist system, the less dominant, poor, so-called less developed countries as the "periphery". While "backwash" effects (drain of resources and concentration of them) have been most evident in the periphery, in the core, political processes and class struggle generally, including the ruling elite's response of social welfare arrangements (one is reminded of the first compulsory national health insurance which Bismark introduced in 1883 to undercut socialism), have had spread effects (general strengthening of the economy) and ameliorated income disparities.

Weinraub, B. "The Year 2000 in India: Experts Paint Grim Picture." NEW YORK TIMES, June 19, 1974, p. 3.

Panel of economists and sociologists depict a dark future. They urge compulsory population control and other planned changes in society. Fuel is seen as a major problem to be contended with, and all proposals for the future must involve social planning.

Weisbrod, B., et al. DISEASE AND ECONOMIC DEVELOPMENT: THE IMPACT OF PARASITIC DISEASES IN ST. LUCIA. Madison: Univ. of Wisconsin Press, 1967.

Wolf, A.C. "A Strategy for Investment in Health." INT'L. J. H. SERV. 1 (August 1971): 196-200.

The views expressed here were first given at a conference on international health sponsored by the AMA. The author was an officer of the Inter-American Development Bank. Investment in health in developing countries is an indispensable concomitant of economic investment. Together with education, health forms the social infrastructure required for development. Investment in human capital alone is not determinant of improved living conditions in developing countries, but must be complemented by investments in agriculture, industry, and economic infrastructure in order to create jobs for a healthier, growing work force. Investments in health by external agencies are modest when measured by need, and by the investment efforts of the countries themselves. In order to optimize these external investments, an investment strategy is called for, consisting of these elements: (1) Health planning should be a prerequisite for the efficient use of external financial assistance. The health plan of a country should be part of a national development plan. (2) Preference in the allocation of resources should be given to those countries, or regions within countries, whose health situations are least satisfactory. (3) Availability of skilled health manpower needs to be assured for the implementation of health plans. (4) External investment should avoid structures and equipment of a prestige nature. Preference should be given to facilities designed to implement health plans. (5) Opportunities in the industrial infrastructure of health programs--pharmaceutical, biologic, nutritional, and medical equipment industries--should be encouraged. (6) Special concern should be exercised with respect to the health aspects of industrial and physical infrastructure projects. The overall goal of the investment strategy should be improved health for the greatest number.

World Bank. HEALTH SECTOR POLICY PAPER. Washington, D.C.: March 1975.

> Chapters are "Health Conditions in Developing Countries"; "Causes of Poor Health" (including subheadings on demographic factors, malnutrition, unsanitary conditions, unsanitary housing, and causes of improved health); "Approaches to Health Policy"; "Present Policies of Developing Countries" (including subheadings on expenditures on health, resources for medical care, coverage of official health services); "Health Policy for the Future"; "World Bank Lending for Health-related Projects"; and "Policy Alternatives for the Bank." Includes useful annexes giving data on health expenditures and selected health outcomes by country and emigration of doctors to the developed world.

World Health Organization (WHO). INTERRELATIONSHIPS BETWEEN HEALTH PROGRAMMES AND SOCIO-ECONOMIC DEVELOPMENT. Public Health Papers, no. 49. Geneva, 1973.

> Perhaps the most complete apolitical statement on the interwoven nature of economic, population, nutrition, family planning, disease, and health services problems.

Chapter 3
GENERAL WORKS

This chapter includes work in four categories: 3.1, Historical and Early Studies of National Health Systems; 3.2, Developed Countries; 3.3, Underdeveloped Countries; and 3.4, General. Some works which overlap more than one category have been placed according to their predominant emphasis. For example, the important UNICEF/WHO study edited by Djukanovic and Mach has been placed under 3.3 even though it includes principles relevant to developed countries as well as an appendix on a project in Yugoslavia. Section 3.4 includes several works relevant both to developed and to underdeveloped countries such as HEALTH SERVICES PROSPECTS edited by I. Douglas-Wilson and Gordon McLachlan. Works treating experience in several countries are often included under particular problem areas such as "Utilization of Health Services" in Ray H. Elling, CROSS-NATIONAL STUDY OF HEALTH SYSTEMS BY COUNTRY AND WORLD REGIONS INCLUDING SPECIAL PROBLEMS (Detroit: Gale Research Co., 1980). For underdeveloped countries special problems of particular import covered in the work just cited include auxiliary personnel, nutrition, population-family planning, traditional and modern medicine, nomads and special groups, and health and liberation movements. Other special problems are more relevant to developed countries--among them hospitals and health services utilization. Some special problems are about equally related to developed and underdeveloped countries, for example, education of health personnel, health planning, and regionalization of health services.

3.1 HISTORICAL AND EARLY STUDIES OF NATIONAL HEALTH SYSTEMS

Abel-Smith, Brian. PAYING FOR HEALTH SERVICES: A STUDY OF THE COSTS AND SOURCES OF FINANCE IN SIX COUNTRIES. Public Health Papers, no. 17. Geneva: WHO, 1963.

> A ground-breaking study which prepared the way for Abel-Smith's later work on more countries (see chapter 3.4). Collates and analyzes data on costs and payments for medical care from field visits and available reports for Ceylon (now Sri Lanka), Chile, Czechoslovakia, Israel, Sweden, and the United States.

General Works

Allen, C.E. "World Health and World Politics." INT'L. ORGANIZATION 4 (February 1950): 27-43.

> An early statement recognizing the link between political interests and international health programs.

Armstrong, Barbara W. THE HEALTH INSURANCE DOCTOR, HIS ROLE IN GREAT BRITAIN, DENMARK, AND FRANCE. Princeton, N.J.: Princeton Univ. Press, 1939.

Beck, A. A HISTORY OF THE BRITISH MEDICAL ADMINISTRATION OF EAST AFRICA, 1900-1950. Cambridge, Mass.: Harvard Univ. Press, 1970.

Beveridge, W. SOCIAL INSURANCE AND ALLIED SERVICES. New York: Macmillan Co., 1942. Tables, appendixes.

> Surveys national systems of social insurance and allied services in Great Britain, noting interrelation among systems. Indicates assumptions basic to study of social security and social policy. Offers recommendations for improvement of national social insurance scheme, noting previously unmet needs for government consideration. Describes principal changes to existing system, explanations for these, proposed finance mechanisms, and problems particular to social security (benefit rates, alternative remedies, and age of population).

Brand, Jeanne L. DOCTORS AND THE STATE: THE BRITISH MEDICAL PROFESSION AND GOVERNMENT ACTION IN PUBLIC HEALTH, 1870-1912. Baltimore: Johns Hopkins Univ. Press, 1965.

Brockington, Fraser. WORLD HEALTH. London: Whitefriars Press, 1958.

> An excellent overview of health conditions in the world to the date of writing. Draws on WHO perspectives and data sources. Notes the remarkable differences in health patterns between rich and poor nations.

Burdett, H.C. HOSPITALS AND ASYLUMS OF THE WORLD. 3 vols. London: J. and A. Churchill, 1893.

Chadwick, Edwin. THE HEALTH OF NATIONS. A REVIEW OF THE WORKS OF EDWIN CHADWICK WITH A BIOGRAPHICAL DISSERTATION BY BENJAMIN WARD RICHARDSON. 1887. Reprint. London: Dawsons, 1965.

Clyde, D.F. HISTORY OF THE MEDICAL SERVICES OF TANGANYIKA. Dar es Salaam, Tanzania: Government printer, 1962.

Crozier, R.C. TRADITIONAL MEDICINE IN MODERN CHINA. Cambridge, Mass.: Harvard Univ. Press, 1968. Refs., index.

Traces development of medical care in modern China. Reviews impact in terms of events in three historical periods: nineteenth-century exposure to modern medicine; early twentieth-century controversies of the republican period; and contemporary Communist experience.

Dublin, Louis I. HEALTH AND WEALTH: A SURVEY OF THE ECONOMICS OF WORLD HEALTH. New York: Harper Brothers, 1928.

Eckstein, Harry E. "Rational Direction in the British Health Service." Ph.D. dissertation, Harvard Univ., 1957.

Examines the development and current struggles of the NHS in political economic terms and discounts the purely "rational" development of a health system.

Evang, Karl. HEALTH SERVICE, SOCIETY AND MEDICINE. London: Oxford Univ. Press, 1960. Refs., tables, figures, index.

A clear and forceful statement by one of the four guiding spirits in the founding of WHO of the embeddedness of health levels and health care in the socioeconomic, political, cultural, and epidemiologic contexts of different societies.

_____. "Medical Care in Europe." In MEDICAL CARE IN TRANSITION, vol. 2, pp. 15-21. Washington, D.C.: US Pub. H. Service, 1964. Reprinted from AJPH 48 (April 1958): 427-33.

Summary of arrangements for the organization and financing of medical care in Western and Eastern Europe.

Falk, Isidore S. SECURITY AGAINST SICKNESS -- A STUDY OF HEALTH INSURANCE. New York: Doubleday, Doran & Co., 1936.

A discussion of international experiences in costs of sickness and payment for medical care in the 1930s. Gives descriptions and comparative analysis of NHI systems in four countries of Western Europe, with projections for the United States.

Farman, C.H. HEALTH AND MATERNITY INSURANCE THROUGHOUT THE WORLD. Washington, D.C.: Social Security Administration, DHEW, February 1954.

A country-by-country description of principal legislative provisions relating to health and maternity insurance in forty-eight national social security programs, including data on both wage loss indemnity and medical care benefits for insured persons.

General Works

Gantt, W. Horsley. A MEDICAL REVIEW OF RUSSIA. London: British Med. Assn., 1928.

> Mainly of historical interest, but fascinating as a report to a highly curious, somewhat fearful group of outside physicians looking at a totally new sort of system--not entirely unsympathetically.

Goldman, Franz. "Foreign Programs of Medical Care and Their Lessons." NEJM 234 (1946): 155-60.

> Comparative description of the organization and financing of medical care programs in various countries following World War II, with critical discussion of quality and effectiveness according to accepted professional standards of good care.

_____. "Methods of Payment for Physicians' Services in Medical Care Programs." AJPH 42 (February 1952): 134-41.

> Early look at a variety of systems (fee-for-service, flat rate, and salary) suggesting greater service and responsibility from physicians paid on a salary basis. Illustrations drawn from UK, Sweden, and Denmark, but the focus is on bringing about change in the United States.

_____. "Public Medical Care in Great Britain and the Scandinavian Countries." NEJM 243 (1950): 243-68.

> Description and critical discussion of programs using general tax funds for the support of medical care services and the use of public agencies in the administration of tax-supported facilities in Great Britain, Sweden, Norway, and Denmark, as observed in 1949.

Grant, John B. HEALTH CARE FOR THE COMMUNITY, SELECTED PAPERS OF DR. JOHN B. GRANT. Edited by Conrad Seipp. Baltimore: Johns Hopkins Univ. Press, 1963.

_____. "International Trends in Health Care." AJPH 38 (1948): 381-97.

> Summary and appraisal of worldwide trends in the development of health services in the 1940s, with emphasis upon social factors influencing health needs and demands.

Haines, Anna J. HEALTH WORK IN SOVIET RUSSIA. New York: Vanguard Press, 1928.

> A work of primarily historical interest indicating the great need and major efforts undertaken following the success of the revolution in October 1917.

Hodgkinson, Ruth G. THE ORIGINS OF THE NATIONAL HEALTH SERVICE: THE MEDICAL SERVICES OF THE NEW POOR LAW, 1834-1951. Berkeley and Los Angeles: Univ. of California Press, 1967.

Honingbaum, Frank. "Unity in British Public Health Administration: the Failure of Reform, 1926-1929." MED. HISTORY 12 (April 1968): 109-21.

Lewis, Milton James. "'Populate or Perish', Aspects of Infant and Maternal Health in Sydney, 1870-1939." Ph.D. thesis, Australian National University, December 1976.

> "In a capitalist society, where the polarization of human qualities between those defined as 'feminine' and those as 'masculine' was extreme,[27] and at a time when national rivalry was intensifying, it is hardly surprising that organized infant welfare work was motivated at least as much by the desire to advance national power and development as by compassion and the urge to nurture. Indeed, it was considerations of power and development which elevated the question of infant welfare to the level of public debate as the fear of population decline expanded" (p. 321). Note 27: "Feminine qualities would be, for example, compassion, nurturance, receptiveness, while masculine ones would be aggressiveness, initiative, and adventurousness."

Means, James Howard. DOCTORS, PEOPLE AND GOVERNMENT. Boston: Little, Brown and Co., 1953.

> While the bulk of this work examines the relations between government, organized medicine, and the unmet health and medical care needs of the people in the United States, it includes a chapter entitled "Britain's Venture in Government Medicine" (pp. 89-106). Noting that the NHS "went into action on July 5, 1948," the author provides the background for this development, noting that the NHS is "an integral part of the whole British social organism." He exposes the way in which American organized medicine falsely propagandized against the NHS in their struggle against government involvement in medicine in the United States. This chapter is particularly valuable in taking up the issues of that time about the NHS as viewed by American organized medicine: free choice by patients, freedom of practice by physicians, waste of services and money if the services are "free," and so forth. He concludes that after five years the NHS has justified itself in the minds of the people and a majority of the medical profession in Great Britain.

Mountain, Joseph W., and Perrott, George St. J. "Health Insurance Programs and Plans of Western Europe." PUB. H. REPORTS 62 (March 14, 1947): 369-99.

> Description and comparative analysis of organization, scope of benefits, and financial arrangements characterizing the health insurance systems of six countries of Western Europe as observed in 1946, with basic operational data.

Nathan, Carl F. PLAGUE PREVENTION AND POLITICS IN MANCHURIA, 1910-1931. Cambridge, Mass.: Harvard East Asia Monographs, 1967.

Newsholme, Arthur. INTERNATIONAL STUDIES ON THE RELATION BETWEEN THE PRIVATE AND OFFICIAL PRACTICE OF MEDICINE, WITH SPECIAL REF-ERENCE TO THE PREVENTION OF DISEASE. 3 vols. London: George Allen and Unwin, 1931.

> Critical observations and program descriptions of private and public health service programs throughout the world prior to 1930, with major reference to the preventive function usually associated with official departments of health. Conducted for the Milbank Fund. Volume 1: The Netherlands, Scandinavia, Germany, Austria, Switzerland. Volume 2: Belgium, France, Italy, Yugoslavia, Hungary, Poland, Czechoslovakia. Volume 3: England and Wales, Scotland, Ireland.

_____. MEDICINE AND THE STATE. London: George Allen and Unwin, 1932. Index.

> Examines developments, agencies, and sources of friction among those engaged in the private and official practice of medicine in the UK. Discusses general components for prevention and treat-ment of disease within a system of health care delivery, including costs and financing. Surveys obstacles to future developments in existing relationships between general medical practice and state medical services. Offers proposals for improved coordination and delivery of care within the NHS.

Newsholme, Arthur, and Kingsbury, John Adams. RED MEDICINE: SOCIALIZED HEALTH IN SOVIET RUSSIA. Garden City, N.Y.: Doubleday, Doran & Co., 1933.

> An early, cautious but generally sympathetic overview of the de-velopment of medicine and public health in Soviet Russia. Among other interesting facts it is reported that 30 percent of the medical officers in the Georgian Soviet Socialist Republic belonged to the Communist party in the early 1930s, whereas only some 5-10 percent of the population as a whole were in the party (p. 198).

New Zealand Social Security Department. THE GROWTH AND DEVELOPMENT OF SOCIAL SECURITY IN NEW ZEALAND. Wellington: R.E. Owen, 1950. Tables, charts, appendixes, index.

> Examines growth of social security in New Zealand during the period 1898-1949. Analyzes effects of such development in terms of cash benefits and provision of health services. Provides brief profile of New Zealand demographic background. Explores legis-lation, benefits, and resource administration as manifestations of financial gains related to development of social security in New Zealand. Concludes with recommendations for future methods of health services financing.

Orr, Douglass W. HEALTH INSURANCE WITH MEDICAL CARE: THE BRITISH EXPERIENCE. New York: Macmillan Co., 1938.

Palvi, Melchios. COMPULSORY MEDICAL CARE AND THE WELFARE STATE: AN ANALYSIS BASED ON A SPECIAL STUDY OF GOVERNMENTAL MEDICAL CARE SYSTEMS ON THE CONTINENT OF EUROPE AND ENGLAND. Chicago: National Institutes of Professional Services, 1950.

> A broad overview of a number of systems. Largely descriptive, but valuable for marking change from an earlier period until the present. The study was conducted in an attempt to furnish ammunition to US private practitioners and organized medicine in their battle against the adoption of any form of NHI in the United States.

Roemer, Milton I. "Health Service Organization in Western Europe." MILBANK MEM. FUND Q. 29 (1951): 139-64.

> Report of observations of a group of health professionals visiting four countries of Western Europe in 1950, with emphasis upon the sociopolitical background, the interplay of public health and medical care activities, and with critical discussion of the adequacy of observed programs and projection of future trends.

_____. "Medical Care Programs in Other Countries: Henry Sigerist and International Medicine." AJPH 48 (April 1958): 425-27.

_____. "Rural Health Programs in Different Nations." MILBANK MEM. FUND Q. 26 (1948): 58-89.

> An early example of CNSHS focusing on rural health care in seven widely scattered countries. Author applies public health standards of the period in the comparisons.

_____. "World Trends in Medical Care Organization." SOCIAL RESEARCH 26 (Autumn 1959): 283-310.

> Review article on the social organization of health services in varying political and economic situations. Truly international in scope, it touches upon many attempted solutions to health problems, and directions for the future toward the goal of "positive health." Notes that the United States is the last industrialized nation to adopt some form of national compulsory health insurance.

Rorem, C. Rufus. THE MUNICIPAL DOCTOR SYSTEM IN RURAL SASKATCHEWAN. Committee on the Costs of Medical Care, vol. 2. Chicago: Univ. of Chicago Press, 1931.

Rosen, George. FROM MEDICAL POLICE TO SOCIAL MEDICINE: ESSAYS ON THE HISTORY OF HEALTH CARE. New York: Science History Publications, 1974.

> For those who study health services in the context of political philosophy, economic institutions, and technological change, these essays are a rich resource. As Rosen notes, few have stated the importance of historical studies better than F.W. Maitland: "Today we study the day before yesterday, in order that yesterday may not paralyse today, and today may not paralyse tomorrow."

Ross, James S. THE NATIONAL HEALTH SERVICE IN GREAT BRITAIN: AN HISTORICAL AND DESCRIPTIVE STUDY. London: Oxford Univ. Press, 1952.

Sand, René. THE ADVANCE TO SOCIAL MEDICINE. London and New York: Staples Press, 1952. Refs.

> By the renowned Belgian professor of social medicine, one of the four founders of WHO. A classic treatise on the history, theory, and content of health care as a social service, with a valuable description of systems of social medicine in over twenty countries distributed among all continents. Analyzes social characteristics of medicine through study of various factors converging to form the discipline of social medicine. Describes the evolution of components of medical practice including hospitals, programs of personal and social hygiene, industrial medicine, philanthropic as well as public assistance services, and public health activities. Combines problems of health and social economy into one issue, noting the status of medicine as the main ameliorative social service. Emphasizes the necessarily social nature of medicine by virtue of its complex human subject and inextricable relation with all phases of life.

Sigerist, Henry E. CIVILIZATION AND DISEASE. Chicago: Univ. of Chicago Press, 1943. Index.

> Describes complex relationships between civilization and disease. Expresses contact between peoples in terms other than infection and other biologic effects. Stresses that disease, in its effects on man, necessarily influences his civilization. Indicates ways in which humans confront disease through their religious, economic, and other institutions. Describes function of civilization in the genesis as well as resolution of health problems.

_____. "From Bismark to Beveridge: Developments and Trends in Social Security Legislation." BUL. OF THE HISTORY OF MED. 13 (April 1943): 365-88.

> Historical development of national health programs in selected countries in many parts of the world, with special emphasis on the role of political forces in influencing health care systems.

_____. MEDICINE AND HEALTH IN THE SOVIET UNION. Binghampton, N.Y.: Vail-Ballon Press, 1947.

A revised version of Sigerist's SOCIALIZED MEDICINE IN THE SOVIET UNION published in 1937. Mark Field characterizes this work as "well intentioned, sympathetic, but rather uncritical," and goes on to say that Sigerist was influenced by his general favor for socialized medicine and confused the USSR plans, statements of programs, and declarations with realities. Others know Sigerist as a thorough scholar and sharp observer.

_____. "Socialized Medicine." YALE REV. 27 (Spring 1938): 463-81. Reprinted in NATIONAL HEALTH CARE, ISSUES AND PROBLEMS IN SOCIAL-IZED MEDICINE, edited by Ray H. Elling, pp. 21-37. New York: Aldine, 1973.

A penetrating statement by the outstanding historian and professor of social medicine. Recognizes the state system of medicine in revolutionary Russia as an outgrowth of the Zemstvo system of tax-financed state medicine under the czar's introduction in 1864 in restless rural districts. Recalls that the first system of compulsory health insurance was set up in 1883 in Germany under arch conservative Bismark to undercut the growing strength of socialist labor. The lesson is that people will not forever sit idly by in the face of preventable and curable hazards, and health systems develop as a result of political pressures. "There are people today--their number is increasing--who think that man has a right to health. The chief cause of disease is poverty. If we are unable to provide work for everybody and to guarantee a decent standard of living to every individual willing to work, whatever his intelligence may be, we are collectively responsible for the chief cause of disease. The least we can do is to make provisions for the protection and restoration of the people's health. They have an undeniable right to such provisions."

Stampar, Andrija. SELECTED PAPERS OF ANDRIJA STAMPAR. Edited by M. D. Grmek. Zagreb, Yugoslavia: Andrija Stampar School of Pub. H., Univ. of Zagreb, 1966.

Selected works on public health by one of the four founders of WHO. Focuses on themes of social medicine, public health, medical education, and international collaboration, emphasizing sociomedical ideals pursued by Stampar as well as his views on social and economic significance of public health activities. Includes his writings on the progress of public health efforts in diverse national settings, as well as medical and public health education. Presents a biography of Stampar and his contribution to promotion of public health programs throughout the world.

Taylor, M.R. "The Saskatchewan Hospital Services Plan: A Study in Compulsory Health Insurance." Ph.D. dissertation, Univ. of California, 1949.

> One of the earliest studies of the first compulsory health insurance plan adopted in North America.

Timmer, M., and Hansma, J. SOCIAL MEDICINE IN WESTERN EUROPE 1848-1972. Supplemental vol. of TIJDSCHRIFT VOOR SOCIALE GENEESKUNDE (Oegstgeest, Netherlands) 53, no. 3 (1975).

U.S. Social Security Administration. SOCIAL SECURITY PROGRAMS THROUGHOUT THE WORLD, 1967. Washington, D.C.: Government Printing Office, 1967.

> A compendium of data on the organization, financing, benefit schedules, and legislative status of social insurance programs throughout the world.

Weinerman, E. Richard. "Social Medicine in Western Europe." Univ. of California School of Pub. H., Berkeley, June 1951. Reproduced.

> Report of a WHO traveling fellowship to seven countries of Western Europe, with descriptive and critical commentary concerning the organization of health services and the activities of university departments of social medicine in 1950.

Wilson, Charles M. ONE HALF THE PEOPLE: DOCTORS AND THE CRISIS OF WORLD HEALTH. New York: William Sloane Associates, 1949.

Winslow, C.E.A. THE COST OF SICKNESS AND THE PRICE OF HEALTH. WHO Monograph Series, no. 7. Geneva: WHO, 1951.

World Health Organization. THIRD REPORT OF THE WORLD HEALTH SITUATION. Geneva, 1966.

> Detailed information on health status and health service systems as submitted by most member states.

3.2 DEVELOPED COUNTRIES

Abel-Smith, Brian. "Major Patterns of Financing and Organization of Medical Care in Countries Other than the U.S." In SOCIAL POLICY FOR HEALTH CARE, pp. 13-33. New York: New York Academy of Med., 1969.

> Based on the author's survey entitled AN INTERNATIONAL STUDY OF HEALTH EXPENDITURE . . . carried out under WHO auspices (see chapter 3.4).

_____. "The Major Patterns of Financing and Organization of Medical Services That Have Emerged in Other Countries." MED. CARE 3 (January–March 1965): 33–40.

> Review of health insurance movement and medical care financing systems in several countries. Three regional patterns are delineated (among affluent nations): American, West European, and East European.

Anderson, Odin W. "Health Service Systems in the United States and Other Countries--Critical Comparisons." NEJM 269 (October 17 and 24, 1963): 839–43, 896–900.

> Two valuable overview articles by one of the major scholars in the CNSHS field.

Askey, Donald E., ed. "Health: A Major Issue." SCANDINAVIAN REV. 63 (September 1975): entire issue. Reissued as HEALTH CARE IN SCANDINAVIA. Bethesda, Md.: NIH, John E. Fogarty Center for Advanced Study in Med. Science, 1976.

> A survey of health care problems and resources in Denmark, Finland, Iceland, Norway, and Sweden and a comparison with and suggestions for the U.S. health system. An especially important contribution is the piece by Holst and Wagner (cited in chapter 5) on administrative arrangements and motivations which keep primary care practitioners where they are needed in Denmark. Contents: "What can the U.S. Learn from Scandinavia?"; "Health Facts and Figures"; "Doctors and Hospitals in Scandinavia"; "Critical Commentary on Consumerism in Denmark"; "Primary Health Care is the Cornerstone"; "Regional Planning in Sweden: A Social and Medical Problem"; "Iceland Stands a Middle Ground"; "Greenland's Price for Modern Medicine"; "More Reading on Scandinavian Health." This last is a brief annotated review of nine books on Scandinavian health systems.

Charron, K.C. HEALTH SERVICES, HEALTH INSURANCE, AND THEIR INTER-RELATIONSHIP, A STUDY OF SELECTED COUNTRIES. Ottawa, Ontario: Department of National Health and Welfare, 1963. Reproduced.

> In preparation for Canada's adoption of an NHI scheme, the author first collected and read available information, visited ten countries in 1961, then analyzed the information and sought additional information by correspondence. It is a broad but valuable study of the interrelationships between health services and health insurance in (by order of visit) New Zealand, Australia, Great Britain, France, FRG, Norway, Sweden, Denmark, and Holland.

Evang, Karl; Murray, D. Stark; and Lear, W.J. MEDICAL CARE AND FAMILY SECURITY--NORWAY, ENGLAND, U.S.A. Englewood Cliffs, N.J.: Prentice-Hall, 1964. Refs., organization charts.

Analyzes contrasting systems of health insurance and health care delivery in Norway, England, and the United States. Considers historical development, structure, and social goals pursued within each system. Discusses the doctor-patient relationship in the NHS of the UK, operative principles of Norwegian health insurance, and medical care gaps in the United States. The analysis is poorly organized, since a common framework is not utilized. The descriptions of the three systems appear separate and for the most part unrelated.

Eyer, Joseph. "Hypertension As A Disease of Modern Society." INT'L. J. H. SERV. 5 (1975): 539-58. 131 refs.

From the author's summary: "About 50 per cent of people in modern societies have blood pressure sufficiently elevated to result in increased mortality. This proportion is much smaller in undisrupted societies of hunter-gatherers. In most cases the elevated blood pressure in modern societies is associated with physiological changes characteristic of chronic stress." A provocative scholarly exercise in social epidemiology.

Field, Mark G. "The Doctor-Patient Relationship in the Perspective of 'Fee-for-Service' and 'Third-Party' Medicine." J. OF H. AND HUMAN BEHAVIOR 2 (Winter 1961): 252-62.

Offers comparisons between the United States and the Soviet Union.

Follman, Joseph, Jr. "Financing Medical Care in Other Nations." In his MED. CARE AND H. INSURANCE, pp. 10-52. Homewood, Ill.: Richard D. Irwin, 1963.

Fraser, R.D. "Health and General Systems of Financing Health Care." See chapter 7.

An article attempting to explain variance in infant mortality rates among eighteen developed countries by the proportion of health care financing devoted to nonpersonal health services.

Fry, John. "The Place of the General Practitioner in Modern Medical Care--Some International Comparisons." PROCEEDINGS OF THE ROYAL SOCIETY OF MED. 63 (February 1970): 205-9.

Reports the general trend toward lesser emphasis on and prestige for the general practitioner and greater emphasis on specialty and hospital care in many systems but notes measures to ameliorate this trend in socialist and social welfare countries as compared with market-oriented countries. For other works by this author on the US, UK, and the USSR, see chapter 4.

Fulcher, Derick. MEDICAL CARE SYSTEMS, PUBLIC AND PRIVATE HEALTH COVERAGE IN SELECTED INDUSTRIALIZED COUNTRIES. Geneva: ILO, 1974. Ten refs., no index.

A very useful addition to CNSHS. Focuses on the mix of public and private financing and extent of coverage in segments of the population in ten industrialized nations. Finds tremendous variations, but groups the countries into those offering universal and relatively complete coverage (Great Britain, New Zealand, Sweden, and Denmark) and those offering less complete coverage through a mix of simultaneously operating separate health insurance schemes (Australia, Belgium, Japan, FRG, Netherlands, and Switzerland). Outlines the historical background of each system. Shares the failing of nearly all other available works describing a number of systems, namely, the lack of an explicit framework explaining what is described commonly for each system and why. Recognizes the embeddedness of systems in their political, economic, cultural, and historical contexts, and impossibility of transplants from one country to another, but sees value in evaluating other countries' programs.

Glaser, William A. "Controlling Costs through Methods of Paying Doctors: Experiences from Abroad." Prepared for the Conference on Policies for the Containment of Health Care Costs and Expenditures. Bethesda, Md.: NIH, John E. Fogarty International Center for Advanced Study in the Med. Sciences, June 1976.

In an effort to control health care costs, nearly all Western European countries using fee schedules to reimburse physicians under NHI have eventually adopted the schedule as the maximum allowable charge to the patient, rather than a minimum above which the physician could charge what patients of good circumstances would pay. Negotiation structures must be set up to allow schedule changes. Without countervailing forces, the physicians' interests will lead to fees rising faster than the cost of living generally. For a more complete study of modes of physician payment by this researcher, see chapter 3.4.

Hogarth, James. THE PAYMENT OF THE PHYSICIAN. New York: Macmillan Co., 1963. Tables, appendixes, index.

Analyzes social characteristics of medicine through study of Great Britain, Sweden, Norway, France, Germany, Switzerland, Austria, Denmark, Holland, USSR, New Zealand, and Australia. Discusses background payment schemes, existing mechanisms for their operation, and provisions for general medical services within each area. Comments on total cost of physician services, noting attitudes of the patient and physician toward respective finance systems. Observes operation of each system in comparison to the NHS in the UK. Discusses possible recommendations for change in methods of

paying the physician. The main focus is on financing and payment and the work suffers from too limited a scope in terms of
ignoring important variations in sociopolitical contexts.

Hu, T.W., ed. INTERNATIONAL HEALTH COSTS AND EXPENDITURES.
DHEW Pub. no. (NIH) 76-1067. Bethesda, Md.: NIH, John E. Fogarty International Center for Advanced Studies in the Med. Sciences, 1976.

Collection of papers devoted primarily to expenditures and approaches to controlling costs for medical care in developed countries.

International Labour Organization. "Medical Care Protection under Social
Security Schemes: A Statistical Study of Selected Countries." INT'L. LABOR
REV. 89 (June 1964): 570-93.

Kaser, Michael. HEALTH CARE IN THE SOVIET UNION AND EASTERN
EUROPE. Boulder, Colo.: Westview Press; London: Croom Helm, 1976.

A valuable description of each system with extensive data and
references.

Layton, Lee E. "Medical Care and Economic Security: A Study of Selected
Foreign Programs." Ph.d. dissertation, microfilm no. 68-7348. Univ. of
Minnesota, 1967.

Logan, Robert F.L., et al. "Resources and Systems." MILBANK MEM. FUND
Q. 50, pt. 2 (July 1972): 45-56.

One of several papers in this special volume edited by David L.
Rabin with an introduction by George Silver giving a preliminary
overview of the massive international study of utilization (see K.L.
White, et al., this chapter). This paper reports differences studied
in Canada, the United States, Argentina, UK, Finland, Poland,
and Yugoslavia. Although valuable data is presented showing remarkable variations (e.g., the apparent extreme excess of physicians in Buenos Aires) there is not enough presentation and discussion of the political economic systems to allow a full understanding of these variations (e.g., the opening of the medical
schools to classes of 7,000 or more under Peron as a way of seeking popular support).

Lynch, Matthew J., and Raphael, Stanley S. MEDICINE AND THE STATE.
Springfield, Ill.: Charles C Thomas, 1963.

A curious book. For its time, one of the most complete descriptions of the health systems in several industrialized countries with
summary chapters evaluating these countries--Germany and Austria,
USSR, UK, New Zealand, Australia, and Sweden. Although the
authors claim this work is "objective," not "based on emotion,

idealism, or political theories," they say the medical professions
in North America will soon be in "the front line of the ideological
battle between the planned and the free societies. We would consider our purpose well served if we could feel that our efforts had
strengthened the conviction, the resolve and the dedication of the
free." In fact, the book is one of the most biased and ideo-
logically oriented works in the literature written from the stance
of private practice entrepreneurial medicine. There is considerable
worrying about "malingering" under "socialized" medicine--what
today might be spoken of as unnecessary utilization, some of it
caused by physicians seeking reimbursement under health insurance
or seeking convenience in hospitalizing a patient. The major conclusion of the book is that the state interferes with the doctor-
patient relationship under socialized medicine. If one can "read
around" this bias, the work is very valuable in the wealth of descriptive information it provides on each of these systems.

Maxwell, Robert. HEALTH CARE, THE GROWING DILEMMA: NEEDS VERSUS
RESOURCES IN WESTERN EUROPE, THE U.S. AND THE U.S.S.R. Foreword
by Sir George Godber. New York: McKinsey and Co., 1974. Graphs,
charts, tables.

One of the major resource works in the CNSHS field. Increasing
costs and demands of population for health care are often due to
medical advances, but some problems are not susceptible to a
medical approach. Countries need information and incentives to
stop waste, as well as coordination of services and assignment of
responsibilities to meet the changing needs of the population. Very
good for its policy relevance and as a source of comparable data
on European, US, and USSR systems. Countries for which most
data sets are provided include the United States, England and
Wales, Sweden, Italy, Portugal, Netherlands, France, and FRG.
The USSR also receives special attention. Selected data are presented in a valuable set of nineteen tables on nineteen countries.

Maynard, Alan. HEALTH CARE IN THE EUROPEAN COMMUNITY. Pittsburgh:
Univ. of Pittsburgh Press, 1975.

A valuable description of EEC countries: FRG, the Netherlands,
Belgium, France, Luxembourg, Italy, UK, Ireland, and Denmark.
Includes some comparisons and an overview.

Montague, Joel B., Jr. "Professionalism among American, Australian, and
English Physicians." J. OF H. AND HUMAN BEHAVIOR 7 (Winter 1966):
284-89.

Explores "professional" organization and orientations of organized
medicine toward government financing and control of medical care
services.

"National Health Programs in Other Countries." In TOWARDS A NATIONAL HEALTH PROGRAM, 1971 HEALTH CONFERENCE, edited by J. Post, pp. 58-119. BUL. N.Y. ACAD. MED. 48 (1972).

> Articles in this international section of the conference include "Trends in the British National Health Service," "Toward a National Health Program: Canadian Experience," "Taming a Profession: Early Phases of Soviet Socialized Medicine," "Social Insurance as Leverage for Changing Health Care Systems: International Experience," "Introduction to the Presentation of Lord Ritchie-Calder," and "Health, Humanism, and Human Rights."

Orzack, Louis H. "The Cross-National Analysis of Professionalization." Paper presented at the ASA meetings, Montreal, August 1974.

> Examines the history of opening medical practice privileges in any EEC country to physicians trained in other EEC countries.

Pharmaceutical Manufacturers Association. NATIONAL HEALTH PROGRAM SURVEY OF EIGHT EUROPEAN COUNTRIES. Washington, D.C., 1970.

> With an eye on the likely further development of some form of general compulsory national health insurance in the United States (Medicare came in 1965), this report examines the legal, financial, and administrative structures of eight European systems and their effects upon and implications for the pharmaceutical industry.

Quaethoven, P. "Het financieel statuut van de ziekenhuisgeneesheer in Duitsland, Frankrijk en Nederland" [Pay regulations for hospital doctors in Germany, France and the Netherlands]. ACTA HOSPITALIA 9 (1969): 122-63.

> The different systems in force in FRG, France, and the Netherlands for the payment of hospital medical staff are of particular interest within the EEC. They will serve as models for the other member nations. This article gives full details of the current methods of payment in each of the three countries. In the main, France, and, to a lesser degree, FRG, have opted for the payment of salaries while the Netherlands retains a system of fees. However, the profession seems to be losing its characteristic economic autonomy, the hospital becoming more and more an employer.

Rabin, D.L. "International Comparisons of Medical Care." Supplemental issue of MILBANK MEM. FUND Q. 50, pt. 2 (July 1972).

> Introduction by George Silver presents international comparative studies for selected communities in Canada, the United States, Argentina, UK, Finland, Poland, and Yugoslavia dealing with determinants of use, organization, and role of physician. Gives research methods and data collection procedures used in this important comparative study. Presents a path analysis model of causality in the variations in utilization of health services. An early report from the most extensive study ever conducted of this facet of several health systems.

Roemer, Milton. "Hospital Utilization and the Health Care System." AJPH 66 (1976): 953-55. 22 refs.

A brief but well-documented editorial describing the need for and growing tendency toward governmental regulation of medical care in an effort to control costs and assure quality. The double rate of operations and ratio of surgeons in the United States as compared with England is noted. The author also states, "The Canadian government has recently decided to restrict the immigration of foreign physicians, less because the nation is considered to be well supplied with doctors everywhere than because of an estimate that each new doctor admitted costs the Canadian population $150,000 a year; this is referrable to $70,000 for the doctor's gross earnings plus $80,000 for the secondary costs (in hospitalization, prescribed drugs, X-ray examinations, etc.) that he generates" (p. 954).

Roemer, Ruth. "Legal Systems Regulating Health Personnel, A Comparative Analysis." In POLITICS AND LAW IN HEALTH CARE POLICY, A SELECTION OF ARTICLES FROM THE MILBANK MEMORIAL FUND QUARTERLY, edited by John B. McKinlay, pp. 233-73. New York: Prodist, 1973. Reprinted from vol. 46 (October 1968): 431-71. 152 refs.

An international comparison is made of legislation governing licensure of health personnel. Licensure processes affect health personnel, development of educational programs, and development of occupational groups. Examples are taken from Sweden, Japan, Colombia, UK, FRG, Poland, France, and the United States. In all but the United States a national health agency plays an important role in licensure.

Schoeck, Helmut. FINANCING MEDICAL CARE. Caldwell, Idaho: Caxton Printers, 1962. Refs., tables.

From the conservative (antigovernmental) stance of a work commissioned by the AMA; critically examines operation of and attitudes toward compulsory health insurance. Confines study to seven medical care systems (in UK, France, FRG, Austria, Sweden, Switzerland, and Australia) performing under conditions presumed comparable to those in the United States. Establishes perspective on compulsory health insurance through discussion of these various national adaptations. Reports on problems of compulsory as opposed to voluntary health insurance, noting dilemmas in expanding services, overcoming political dilemmas, and meeting unexpected effects of a national health system.

Seham, Max. "An American Doctor Looks at Eleven Foreign Health Systems." SOC. SCI. MED. 3 (1969): 65-82.

This paper compares efficiency of medical care systems of eleven countries, noting the importance of relating the practice of medicine to the prevailing social conditions. The countries studies are UK, Sweden, Norway, France, FRG, Switzerland, Austria, Denmark, Holland, New Zealand, Australia. A useful chart is provided giving for each country a descriptive label or set of figures on (1) type of health system (whether compulsory insurance and extent of reimbursement); (2) type of government; (3) population density; (4) physician to population ratios; (5) organizations administering the health system; (6) income of GPs; (7) hospitals (ownership and bed/population ratios); (8) funding methods; (9) population coverage; and (10) health services covered. The study would have been improved by more sharply defining these common points of concern and spelling out the methods of measurement used.

Selby, Philip. HEALTH IN 1980-1990. Basel, Switzerland: S. Karger, 1974.

A futurist research carried out by the Delphi method (in this case asking physicians to imagine what medical practice will be like in the years indicated). The increasing use of high technology (including bio-engineering) and rising costs along with a greater government role in control and organization was generally forseen. Includes many other provocative views.

Sidel, Victor W., and Sidel, Ruth. A HEALTHY STATE. New York: Pantheon, 1977.

An important book placing the present US health system and its future prospects in the context of experience in other countries. Characterizes the systems studied in this way: Sweden--planned pluralism; Great Britain--equitable entitlement; the Soviet Union--centralized socialism; the PRC--mass mobilization. For each country, the authors describe the setting, give the central idea of the health system, a brief description of one of the central features, an overview of historical roots, and a summary of strengths and remaining problems.

Somers, Anne R. "The Rationalization of Health Services: A Universal Priority." INQUIRY 8 (March 1971): 48-60.

Compares the responses of Sweden, Denmark, and UK to the fragmentation of care, increase in costs, and the dangers of over-bureaucratization. Their approaches to regionalization are discussed, and the essential need for cost and quality control is noted. The strain toward rationalization of services in the face of rising costs and demands is seen as worldwide.

Szameitat, K. "Was Kostet die Gesundheit? Zahlen and Kritische Aspekte." [What does health cost? Figures and critical aspects]. OEFFENTLICHES GESUND-HEITSWESEN [Public Health] 32 (1970): 672-90.

A valuable examination of rising costs in different developed countries including consideration of competing demands of other economic sectors.

Timmer, M., and Hansma, J. SOCIAL MEDICINE IN WESTERN EUROPE 1848-1972. Supplemental vol. of TIJDSCHRIFT VOOR SOCIALE GENEESKUNDE (Oegstgeest, Netherlands) 53, no. 3 (1975). Refs.

Valuable examination of teaching, research, and conceptions of social medicine based importantly on responses by professors of social medicine to a mail questionnaire, but also includes historical conceptions of the great figures of the field. Responses are quoted for certain questions, such as those concerning purposes of the field and directions toward which research ought to be encouraged. The disciplines of social medicine and relations of the field to others are also discussed. Replies were received from professors at major teaching-research centers in Belgium, France, FRG, the Netherlands, Norway, Sweden, Switzerland, and the UK. The questionnaire is included as annex 1.

U.S. Department of Health, Education and Welfare. TASK FORCE ON PRESCRIPTION DRUGS: CURRENT AMERICAN AND FOREIGN PROGRAMS. Washington, D.C.: Government Printing Office, 1968.

White, Kerr L., et al. "Health Care: An International Comparison of Perceived Morbidity, Health Services Resources and Use." INT'L. J. H. SERV. 6 (1976): 199-218.

From the author's summary: "Selected summary findings from the World Health Organization/International Collaborative Study of Medical Care Utilization are presented, based on data collected during a twelve-month period in 1968-1969 in twelve study areas in seven countries in the Americas and Europe. A household interview survey of almost 48,000 persons, representing a total population of about 15 million, elicited information on demographic characteristics, on perceptions of illness, its severity and character, and on attitudes toward and use of major components of health services. Information was also collected on the prevailing health care systems and resources available to the study population, as well as socio-economic characteristics of the study areas. . . . Wide differences are observed between the extremes of the measures of need, resources, and use employed in the study, raising questions about the ways in which resources are organized to provide services and about the effectiveness and efficiency of these services." Valuable summary report from the most ambitious CNSHS ever undertaken. The twelve study areas were located in the following seven countries: Argentina, Canada, Finland, Poland, UK, United States, and Yugoslavia.

3.3 UNDERDEVELOPED COUNTRIES

Akhtar, Shahid. LOW-COST RURAL HEALTH CARE AND HEALTH MANPOWER TRAINING: AN ANNOTATED BIBLIOGRAPHY WITH SPECIAL EMPHASIS ON DEVELOPING COUNTRIES. See chapter 9.

> A very valuable annotated bibliography. First in a series of two volumes. See Delaney below.

Bader, Michael B. "The International Transfer of Medical Technology--An Analysis and A Proposal for Effective Monitoring." INT'L. J. H. SERV. 7 (1977): 443-58.

> The international transfer of medical technology to the developing countries occurs at four levels: (1) medical education, research, and missions; (2) multinational corporate transactions; (3) technical assistance projects sponsored by WHO; and (4) bilateral foreign aid programs. This article proposes effective monitoring of international medical technology transfer through political and legal means, including a specific code of conduct for corporations engaged in medical technology transfer. Discusses the development of "intermediate health technologies" along the lines suggested by E.F. Schumacher, and the advantages of such an innovation in terms of population issues and economic development.

Banerji, D. "Health Economics in Developing Countries." J. OF THE INDIAN MED. ASSN. 49 (January 11, 1967): 417-21.

> Especially valuable for its consideration of national political dimensions in different countries, particularly the degree of democratization and extension of adequate health care to rural and "lower" classes. While the focus is on India, lessons are drawn from a range of other countries.

Beckford, George L. PERSISTANT POVERTY: UNDERDEVELOPMENT IN PLANTATION REGIONS OF THE THIRD WORLD. New York: Oxford Univ. Press, 1972.

Board, L.M. "Problems and Priorities in Combatting Air, Water, and Soil Pollution in Developing Countries." ARCHIVES OF ENVIRONMENTAL HEALTH 18 (February 1969): 260-64.

> The so-called third world suffers now and will suffer more from the mythology encouraged by exploitative external as well as internal economic interests that the environments of these countries are far from saturation and are relatively "unburdened" by pollution. As Commoner points out in THE CLOSING CIRCLE (see chapter 2) we are first of all dealing with a single world ecology and the biological damage is often unrecoupable.

Bryant, John. HEALTH AND THE DEVELOPING WORLD. Ithaca, N.Y.: Cornell Univ. Press, 1969. Charts.

Perhaps the best known book in the field. Discusses the demand for services, rising expectations, and predominant diseases in developing countries. Proposes the health team concept for the division of tasks to correspond to the constellation of health problems encountered. A fine overview of health and resources problems in UDCs. Probably places undue emphasis on redirection of medical education as the way to solve the rather mammoth problems of this part of the world, and gives no serious attention to political economies. Includes useful data delineating the marked differences in disease patterns and health resources in underdeveloped and developed countries. The former have few modern services and predominantly infectious, parasitic, and nutritional diseases, while the latter have more modern services and predominantly chronic and degenerative diseases. The first seventeen papers give case vignettes of care patterns in a variety of UDCs.

Candau, Marcolino G. "Keynote Address: Knowledge, the Bridge to Achievement." ISRAEL J. OF MED. SCIENCES (Jerusalem) 4 (May-June 1968): 343-49.

From the Fourth Rehovoth Conference on Health Problems in Developing States, Rehovoth, Israel, August 15-23, 1967. This keynote address by the then-director-general of WHO stresses that health problems in developing countries are complex and varied and that innovative solutions are required. An "ecological" approach of an interdisciplinary nature must be used to solve health problems. Developmental projects do not solve problems in isolation from one another, but require coordinated planning so that solutions to one problem do not create new hazards.

Christian Medical Commission. ANNUAL REPORT. Geneva, 1973.

One of an annual series of valuable statements reviewing problems and work of the Christian Medical Commission, especially in UDCs. Some inventive approaches have been taken through the projects sponsored by this body, an arm of the World Council of Churches.

Delaney, Frances. LOW-COST RURAL HEALTH CARE AND HEALTH MANPOWER TRAINING: AN ANNOTATED BIBLIOGRAPHY WITH SPECIAL EMPHASIS ON DEVELOPING COUNTRIES. See chapter 9.

Second volume in a series of annotated bibliographies on low-cost rural health care.

Djukanovic, V., and Mach, E.P., eds. ALTERNATIVE APPROACHES TO MEETING BASIC HEALTH NEEDS OF POPULATIONS IN DEVELOPING COUNTRIES, A JOINT UNICEF/WHO STUDY. Geneva: WHO, 1975. Appendixes.

One of the most important general works in this field. Presents general lessons drawn from in-depth case studies of a number of "promising" approaches. These general lessons and some of the guiding framework for this important study could contribute to developing a more adequate framework for comparing health systems. Unfortunately does not include negative cases to contrast with promising ones. Cases are included in the appendixes which describe and to some extent analyze (but sometimes too uncritically) each approach. Among these are China, Cuba, Tanzania, the Jamshed project in India, Ayurvedic medicine in India, a simplified medicine project in Venezuela, a two-way radio system in Nigeria, and a comprehensive care and citizen-involvement approach in a rural area of Yugoslavia.

Dorozynski, Alexander. DOCTORS AND HEALERS. Ottawa, Ontario: IDRC, 1975.

A photographic study with text showing the exciting range of alternative kinds of health care in developing countries whose short resources force them to seek their own ways.

Elliott, Katherine. "Meeting World Health Needs: The Doctor and the Medical Auxiliary." WORLD HOSPITALS 9 (1973): 94-97.

A clear and forceful statement of the impossibility of meeting health needs in poor countries through the "modern" or, so-called western model. Notes the variety of new types of health personnel developing in different parts of the world, reports favorably on this experience, and encourages its further development.

Fendall, N.R.E. "Auxiliary Health Personnel; Training and Use." PUB. H. REPORTS 82 (June 6, 1967): 471-79.

Comprehensive medicine is beyond the present reach of developing countries, but integrated medicine--that is, a balanced program of curative, preventive, and promotional medicine--is not. The use of auxiliary health workers offers a means of achieving integrated medicine. This paper reviews the main types of auxiliary health workers (single-purpose, multipurpose, and all-purpose), their selection, training, and function.

_____. "Organization of Health Services in Emerging Countries." LANCET 2 (July 11, 1964): 53-56.

_____. "Primary Medical Care in Developing Countries." INT'L. J. H. SERV. 2 (1972): 297-315.

A classic article in the field. From the author's summary: "Common to all developing nations are lack of financial resources and a trained manpower, illiteracy, high fertility, a traditional society based on the soil, and diseases related to undernutrition, infections, and vector-borne illnesses. . . . The distribution of scarce physician resources is poor. Most seek to live and work in capital cities and not in the rural areas where most of the people live. There are too few paramedical workers to support the physicians. The growth of the population constantly exceeds the growth of new physicians, some of whom are lost through the brain drain to more developed countries. . . . The only hope lies in greater use of nonprofessional workers operating from planned centers. . . ."

Feuerstein, Marie-Therese. "Comprehensive Community Approach to Rural Health Problems in Developing Countries." INT'L. NURSING REV. 23, no. 6, (November-December 1976): 174-82.

An eleven-point statement on community involvement, development, and health education, citing works by WHO, John Bryant, Halfdan Mahler, Karefa Smart, Benjamin Paul, George Foster, and others.

Frankenhoff, Charles A. "Meeting the Health Needs of the Urban Poor in Developing Countries." Paper presented at the 105th annual meeting of the APHA, Washington, D.C., October 30-November 3, 1977.

A useful paper calling attention to the often ignored but gross problems of people in the rapidly growing urban and peri-urban slums of most poor countries. Available through the APHA, Washington, D.C.

Garlick, J.P., and Keay, R.W.J., eds. HUMAN ECOLOGY IN THE TROPICS. New York: Halsted Press, a division of John Wiley, 1976.

The emphasis of these papers is on the interaction of man with the natural environment. Included are papers on man's efforts to obtain food through agriculture, forests, the development of tropical countries, disease organisms and their vectors, and the problems of health in the tropics. A final paper underlines the importance of sociological factors and their interrelation to ecological factors.

Gilles, H.M. "The Ecology of Disease in the Tropics." BUL. N.Y. ACAD. MED. 51 (May 1975): 621-30.

Brief but good basic treatment of the subject showing the interwoven character of disease, sanitation, nutrition, and economy. There has developed a growing awareness among world health experts that it is not tropical climate but poverty which is central to the ecology of infectious parasitic and nutritional diseases.

Gish, Oscar. "Resource Allocation, Equality of Access, and Health." INT'L. J. H. SERV. 3 (1973): 399-412. Refs.

Based upon the experience of Tanzania, this paper relates resource

allocation in the health sector to the output of health, by contrasting access to and utilization of available health services by
urban and rural populations. Increased expenditures alone cannot
yield an efficient health care return unless the additional expenditure is spread thinly, in keeping with the population distribution,
transport possibilities, and disease patterns in most poor countries.
Because medical referral systems function only marginally, further
building of large hospitals is not justified in most poor countries.
The author concludes that the major obstacles to change are not
shortages of resources or technologic ignorance but social systems
that do not place high value upon the health care needs of rural
peasants.

_____, ed. HEALTH MANPOWER AND THE MEDICAL AUXILIARY: SOME
NOTES AND AN ANNOTATED BIBLIOGRAPHY. London: Intermediate Technology Group, 1971.

This publication arises from the Intermediate Technology Development Group's discussions about rural health. It is intended as a
guide for those who plan and administer health programs in developing countries. Included are chapters on health planning in
developing countries, the use of intermediary medical personnel,
and medical auxiliaries as physician substitutes. There is also an
annotated bibliography (134 entries) presenting most of the significant material published from 1960 to 1970 that is concerned with
medical manpower and particularly medical auxiliaries. In the
chapter by Gish, "Towards an Appropriate Health Care Technology,"
three reasons are noted why health care must be basically different
in UDCs: (1) fewer resources (money and skilled manpower); (2)
different population structures (younger and more rural); and (3)
drastically different disease patterns.

Gonzales, C.L. MASS CAMPAIGNS AND GENERAL HEALTH SERVICES. Public
Health Papers, no. 29. Geneva: WHO, 1965.

Two possible approaches to the problem of health in developing
countries are discussed: (1) building up a framework of general
health services able to deal in due course with the prevalent diseases, or (2) attacking the principal diseases by mass campaigns.
The role of general health services in mass campaigns, and suggested approaches to conducting mass campaigns are considered.
Specific examples from India, Taiwan, Togo, and Thailand.

King, Maurice, ed. MEDICAL CARE IN DEVELOPING COUNTRIES. Nairobi,
Kenya: Oxford Univ. Press, 1966. Appendixes, index, tables, figures.

Although it presents a primarily managerial-technological perspective
and fails to recognize human action in political-economic terms,
this is an early ground-breaking statement from the point of view
of the medical establishment. Reports proceedings of a conference

on provision of medical care in UDCs. A major, valuable attempt
to demystify modern medical knowledge and put portions of it most
relevant for UDCs into how-to terms so new types of health manpower and delivery systems can put it into practice where it is
sorely needed. As a "primer on the medicine of poverty," reviews
practical and theoretical aspects of the organization of an effective
health services system. Examines structure of service components
including health education, hospital management, and basic clinical
services. Discusses role of family planning and other supportive
services necessary to the health services system of a developing
nation.

Leeson, Joyce. "Social Science and Health Policy in Preindustrial Society."
INT'L. J. H. SERV. 4 (1974): 429-40. 40 refs.

The author points out that social scientists in the health field in
the third world could make an important contribution by examining
why "rational solutions" are not applied to the multitude of problems that exist. This would require analyzing the status and roles
of health personnel, and recognizing the contradictions between
the interests of the metropolitan countries and the urban elites of
the third world on the one hand, and the rural masses on the other.
The principles guiding the health services of the PRC have led to
very different and apparently more appropriate services, but it
seems unlikely that these will be applied elsewhere under present
circumstances. The article offers an excellent coverage of relevant
literature. Also provides brief historical view of the ways in
which social science, particularly anthropology, has functioned,
often unwittingly, as an informant on behalf of colonialist powers
seeking firmer or more effective control over natives.

Leslie, Charles, ed. ASIAN MEDICAL SYSTEMS. Berkeley, Los Angeles, and
London: Univ. of California Press, 1976. Refs., index.

By emphasizing traditional and historically great systems of health
care, underlines clearly that medical systems are pluralistic structures of different kinds of practitioners and institutional norms. As
the editor notes, "Even in the United States the medical system is
composed of physicians, dentists, druggists, clinical psychologists,
chiropractors, social workers, health food experts, masseurs, yoga
teachers, spirit curers, Chinese herbalists, and so on" (p. 9).
Chapters: "The Practice of Medicine in Ancient and Medieval
India"; "Secular and Religious Features of Medieval Arabic Medicine"; "The Intellectual and Social Impulses behind the Evolution
of Traditional Chinese Medicine"; "The Modern Medical System:
The Soviet Variant"; "The Sociology of Modern Medical Research";
"Disease, Morbidity and Mortality in China, India, and the Arab
World"; "Traditional Asian Medicine and Cosmopolitan Medicine
as Adaptive Systems"; "The Cultural and Interpersonal Context of
Everyday Health and Illness in Japan and America"; "Strategies of

Resort to Curers in South India"; "The Impact of Ayurvedic Ideas on the Culture and the Individual in Sri Lanka"; "The Social Organization of Indigenous and Modern Medical Practices in Southwest Sumatra"; "Chinese Traditional Etiology and Methods of Cure in Hong Kong"; "Systems and the Medical Practitioners of a Tamil Town"; "The Place of Indigenous Medical Practitioners in the Modernization of Health Services"; "The Social Organization and Ecology of Medical Practice in Taiwan"; "The Ideology of Medical Revivalism in Modern China"; "The Ambiguities of Medical Revivalism in Modern Nineteenth- and Twentieth-Century Bengal"; "World-Views and Asian Medical Systems: Some Suggestions for Further Study."

McGilvray, J.C. "Health Services and Health Manpower for the Developing Countries." WORLD HOSPITALS 6 (1970): 1-4.

Malenbaum, W. "Health and Economic Expansion in Poor Lands." INT'L. J. H. SERV. 3 (1973): 161-76.

An important conceptual article. Economic progress in poor lands remains a major goal as the income gap between poor lands and the rich world continues to widen. Effective solutions require new approaches in three areas: (1) the process of economic development, (2) the dynamics of population growth, and (3) the function of the health of man. This article appraises the theory and the historical and current evidence in all three areas. Against this assessment it offers a research prospectus for further analysis of the interdependence of health, demographic, and economic progress in poor lands.

Masters, D. "Is Your Talent Being Wasted?" SAVING HEALTH (London) 12 (June 2, 1973): 26-28.

An appeal is made from a religious, missionary perspective to Western medical workers to help care for the urgent health needs of the developing world. Advantages of the experience are described. In Zaire, Africa, a state-recognized school trains auxiliary nurses but, although missionary nurses are on hand to train students, the school may close because the law requires the presence of a doctor. This is one example of an urgent need. Details of the kinds of problems expatriate physicians and health personnel face in translating their previous training to local health problem solving is illustrated several times.

Mendia, L. "Environmental Health in Developing Countries." ISRAEL J. OF MED. SCIENCES (Jerusalem) 4 (May-June 1968): 415-24.

English paper presented at the Fourth Rehovoth Conference on Health Problems in Developing States, Rehovoth, Israel, August 15-23, 1967. Problems common to all human environments are

water supply, sewage disposal, solid waste disposal, and housing.
These are interrelated; it is not possible to set a single priority
in attempting a solution to these multiple, interwoven problems.
Nevertheless, education in environmental hazards is often ignored,
so special attention should be given to this field of concern.
Often religious and traditional beliefs must be overcome to make
progress in this field.

Morley, David. PAEDIATRIC PRIORITIES IN THE DEVELOPING WORLD. Foreword by Otto Wolff. London: Butterworth, 1973.

This book grows out of the author's work with Margaret Woodland
and others in the village of Imesi on the edge of the Ekiti hills
in the western state of Nigeria. There, a medical-health team
helped to cut sharply the infant mortality in a three-year period,
established a special clinic for under-fives, and designed a weight
chart to aid in preventing malnutrition. The foreword frames the
problem by noting that while there are 625 deaths per year per
million children under five in developed countries, in UDCs this
figure is around 48,000. The first few chapters are especially
valuable for drawing out the major disease and resource differences
between so-called developed and developing countries and in urg-
ing a rural, primary-preventive care orientation especially in developing countries (for a critical view of the term "developing,"
see chapter 2 and some of the works annotated there). Much of
the rest of the book is devoted to technical medical information
on prevention and treatment of childhood disease as these are
found in poorer, rural-based countries with emphasis on doing
things in simplified, less costly ways. Very valuable contribution
to world health.

Newell, Kenneth W., ed. HEALTH BY THE PEOPLE. Geneva: WHO, 1975.

A collection of descriptions of health services development efforts
involving the citizenry in a variety of ways in a number of UDCs
including the exciting experience in China and Cuba and the plans
of Tanzania. The simplified medicine project of Venezuela is included. The chapter on Iran illustrates a shortcoming of the book:
stemming from the official auspices it does, there is a lack of
frankness as to the depth of problems faced by the people in a
country like Iran where power is elitist and highly centralized and
disparities great. Nevertheless, tone and thrust of the book are
good.

New York Academy of Medicine. "Symposium on Medicine and Diplomacy in
the Tropics." BUL. N.Y. ACAD. MED. 46 (May 1970): entire issue.

An interesting collection of views more openly and frankly placing
health aid in the context of diplomacy and international relations
than is usually admitted. For example, one of the articles is entitled "A War We Can Win: Health as a Vector of Foreign Policy."

Prywes, M., and Davies, A.M., eds. "Proceedings of the Fourth Rehovoth Conference on Health Problems in Developing States." ISRAEL J. OF MED. SCIENCES (Jerusalem) 4 (May–June 1968): 326–778. (entire issue).

> Seventy-one delegates participated in the Fourth Rehovoth Conference on Health Problems in Developing States, held in Rehovoth, Israel, in August 1967. The keynote address by Dr. M.G. Candau is annotated above, this chapter. Of the thirty-two papers presented, most are related to issues of health care delivery in developing countries.

Read, Margaret. CULTURE, HEALTH, AND DISEASE: SOCIAL AND CULTURAL INFLUENCES ON HEALTH PROGRAMMES IN DEVELOPING COUNTRIES. London: Tavistock Publications; Philadelphia: J.B. Lippincott, 1966. Refs., figures, index.

> Examines rural areas of developing countries in terms of problems in health and disease control. Studies social and cultural influences on public health and manpower training programs. Identifies public health as a social and cultural effort. Calls for agency recognition of the singular nature of rural life in order for modern health programs to prove successful. Examines traditional cultural and religious aspects of health care as determinants of rural health. Emphasizes dependence of manpower training programs on awareness of problems in social change and in indigenous populations' response to modern health efforts.

Rifkin, S.B. PROPOSAL FOR THE INVESTIGATION OF RURAL HEALTH SERVICES IN CHINA. Brighton: Univ. of Sussex, Science Policy Research Unit, n.d.

> Development strategy goals set by the PRC include (1) closing of the urban-rural gap, (2) building of both industry and agriculture, (3) eliminating distinctions between manual and mental work, and (4) self-reliance. In this article (an expanded outline for research proposals) the rural health policies of China are used to argue that China should be classified as an important developing country, and that Chinese strategies and tactics for development may be applicable to other developing nations. Research is proposed that will outline some major problems of creating adequate health services in developing countries, and to examine the PRC's approaches in solving these problems.

Ritchie-Calder, Lord. "World Health: An Ethical-Economic Perspective." BUL. N.Y. ACAD. MED. 51 (1975): 608–20.

> Although raising the Malthusian specter of population outrunning food (in large part, as he sees it, because of medical-public health interventions such as germ-specific sulfa drugs), the main thrust is to illustrate the interweaving of socioeconomic and political and ethical changes and changing health conditions in UDCs.

Provides a set of beautifully stated examples ranging from involvement of royal princesses in health clinic functions and women's
liberation in Afghanistan to malaria control through efforts of a
tough-minded public health nurse acting among two female-dominated
tribes (the Tharus and Bhukes) of Uttar-Pradesh in Northern India.
One of the main messages is that people have to do things for
themselves in their own way and the world is intertwined. "There
is no 'we' and 'they'--just 'we' in a world which has shrunk to a
neighborhood."

Roemer, Milton I. "Social Security for Medical Care: Is It Justified in Developing Countries?" INT'L. J. H. SERV. 1 (1971): 354-61. 21 refs.

Social insurance spread from Europe to the developing countries,
especially in Latin America, after World War I. In these countries, however, the percentage of persons insured is typically
small, so the "inequities" are created relative to the larger non-
insured populations. Nevertheless, the social insurance device is
justified because of its effects in upgrading the overall health service resources and promoting the general economic development of
the predominantly agricultural countries. Moreover, social security
programs are in the long run not obstructive to but promotive of
ministries of health and their services.

Sicault, Georges, et al. POLITIQUES ET PLANIFICATIONS DE LA SANTÉ
DANS LES PAYS EN VOIE DE DÉVELOPPEMENT [Politics and planning of
health in developing countries]. REVUE TIERS-MONDE 14, no. 53 (January-
March 1973): entire issue. Paris: Presses Universitaires de France. In French.

Partial contents (French titles translated here): "The different
orientations to the politics of health"; "Health planning--introductory
questions"; "The health variables of a politics of health planning";
"The development of health personnel in third-world countries in
Africa"; "The place of pediatrics in the health services of third-
world countries"; "Demographic control"; "Nutrition and planning";
"Toward a questioning of the politics of public health in West and
Central Africa"; "Prevention of births and demographic perspectives
in Asia"; "The politics of health in North Vietnam"; "The rural
health service in PRC"; "Health and development in a rural setting:
the Niger experience in the department of Maradi"; "Selected
bibliography on the economics of health assembled by the secre-
tariat of WHO/EURO." A statement by Kane and Mandl is particularly useful and potent in its critique of misguided development
efforts and their effect, particularly on the health of mothers, infants, and children.

Sorking, Alan L. HEALTH ECONOMICS IN DEVELOPING COUNTRIES. Lex-
ington, Mass.: D.C. Heath, 1976.

"Symposium on Health and Development." BUL. N.Y. ACAD. MED. 51 (May 1975): 569-654 (entire issue).

SYNCRISIS: THE DYNAMICS OF HEALTH: AN ANALYTIC SERIES ON THE INTERACTION OF HEALTH AND SOCIOECONOMIC DEVELOPMENT. Washington, D.C.: U.S. HEW Division of Planning and Evaluation, June 1972. Ongoing.

> A series of descriptions (usually published as separate volumes) of health systems in UDCs put together through a combination of field visits and document studies. Some twenty volumes had been produced as of the end of 1976. Most recent were BANGLADESH by Scott A. Loomis (vol. 17), PAKISTAN by Arthur H. Furnia (vol. 18), and SENEGAL by Robin J. Menes (Vol. 19). More recently available: EGYPT; JORDAN; and SYRIA.

Taylor, Carl E. "The Doctor's Role in Rural Health Care." INT'L. J. H. SERV. 6 (1976): 219-30. 13 refs.

> Author's summary: "A new pattern of health care in developing countries promises to meet the needs of rural people and still provide reasonable gratification for health workers. The service must have mutually strengthening linkages between all levels of the health care system. Reallocating roles in the health team requires turning routine medical care over to auxiliaries so that professionals can concentrate on more complex problems, such as community diagnosis and therapy. Young doctors are reasonable and willing to undertake a rural rotation early in their medical careers. This will help to identify those few who will provide leadership in improving rural services."

World Bank. HEALTH SECTOR POLICY PAPER. See chapter 2.

World Health Organization. EPIDEMIOLOGY AND CONTROL OF SCHISTOSOMIASIS, REPORT OF A WHO EXPERT COMMITTEE. Technical Report Series, no. 372. Geneva, 1967.

> Recognizes cultural, health service organization, and economic planning elements in the successful control of this widespread parasitic disease.

3.4 GENERAL

Association of American Medical Colleges. AN INTRODUCTION TO INTERNATIONAL HEALTH: PRINCIPLES OF A CROSS-CULTURAL AND COMPARATIVE APPROACH TO HEALTH PROBLEMS. Washington, D.C., 1977. Also published as INTERNATIONAL HEALTH PERSPECTIVES, AN INTRODUCTION IN FIVE VOLUMES. 5 vols. New York: Springer, 1977.

An approximately thirty-unit, fifty-hour self-study course in the
form of booklets covering units within categories as indicated below. The course was developed under the general editorial assistance of Emanuel Sutter and Wendy Waddell with support from
the John E. Fogarty International Center for Advanced Study in
the Health Sciences, NIH, coordinated through Donald Pitcairn.
Russell Mills chaired the advisory group and Robert Perlioni provided educational consultation. Course developers are indicated
in relation to content areas: Category 1, Introduction (5 units),
Dieter Koch-Weser and Stephen Joseph, Harvard University. Category 2, Assessment of Health Status and Needs (2 units), Timothy
Baker, Johns Hopkins University. Category 3, Ecologic Determi-
nants of Health Problems (9 units), Michael Stewart, Columbia
University. Category 4, Sociocultural Influences on Health and
Health Care (6 units), Ray Elling, University of Connecticut.
Category 5, Systems of Health Care (9 units), Milton Roemer,
University of California, Los Angeles.

Abel-Smith, Brian. AN INTERNATIONAL STUDY OF HEALTH EXPENDITURE
AND ITS RELEVANCE FOR HEALTH PLANNING. Public Health Papers, no.
32. Geneva: WHO, 1967.

A careful study which broke new ground in attempting to obtain
and analyze relatively standard and dependable data on health expenditures in total and by selected subcategories in relation to
national accounts (e.g., GNP) in thirty-three countries. Data
were obtained through a variety of sources including a questionnaire sent to each country through WHO. The "Sources and
Methods" chapter and the questionnaire included as an annex explain the data gathering fully. After a special look at nine high-
income countries, the author observes, "In all high-income countries there has been a secular trend for expenditure on health services to increase as a proportion of national income or national
product. The only exception is the United Kingdom, where there
was no increase between 1949 and 1964. Moreover, it appears
that in all countries for which data are available, an increasing
proportion of total health expenditures has been devoted to hospitals. . . . Before the end of the century, if present trends
continue, there will be countries in which more than 10% of the
gross national product will be devoted to health services" (p. 92).

Bourmer, Horst. "Das Gesundheitswesen als 'integrierter Bestandteil' der so-
zialistichen Gesellschaftsordnung." [The health system as "integrierter component" of the socialist social structure] DEUTSCHES AERZTEBLATT--AERZTLICHE
MITTEILUNGEN 72 (April 10, 1975): 1-10. No refs.

Based on a symposium devoted to pulling together impressions from
study trips conducted mainly by West German private physicians
to a number of "eastern" countries. Support for the travel and
symposium was provided by the foundation of German physicians,

the Thieding Stiftung of the Hartmannbund. No systematic studies
were made nor is there a listing of countries visited, but examples
of strengths and (mostly) weaknesses are given for Bulgaria, China,
GDR, Hungary, Poland, and USSR. The article evidences bias
against any form of state-controlled medicine. "We doctors reject
a nationalization (Verstaatlichung) of the health system, because
in such a system much freedom for patients and doctors must be
sacrificed, without realising the saving of expenditures hoped for
the defenders of nationalization" (p. 2). Still this is a valuable
article for identifying some of those elements of so-called socialist
state medical systems which are seen as strengths and weaknesses
by Western private practitioners. For example, strengths are found
in the broader mandate of industrial physicians, health education
for the public especially in the schools, required periodic continuing education for physicians, and strong discipline in the universities so that the business of learning to be a physician is taken
seriously. Weaknesses (some resembling problems in Western countries) are urban-rural maldistribution of physicians, long waiting
times in polyclinics and other service settings (though data were
unscientifically obtained), and relative lack of a confidential
doctor-patient relationship. The most extreme example given,
about which the author seems outraged, was a large board showing
quite publicly the birth control means used by each couple in a
Chinese barefoot doctor's area.

Bowers, John Z. "Women in Medicine--An International Study." NEJM 275
(August 18, 1966): 362-65.

Shows the United States and a few other countries to be peculiarly
low in the proportion of women physicians, while the USSR and
certain other countries have much higher proportions of women in
medicine.

Brockington, Fraser. WORLD HEALTH. 2d ed. London: J. and A. Churchill,
1967. Refs., figures, appendixes, index.

Examines national commitments to public health activities throughout the world in light of such factors as geography, customs, hospitals, and industrialization. Discusses current methods used to
support public health efforts. Stresses need for statistically accurate measurement of health levels by methods of standardization of
recording, appropriate data collection, and measurement of morbidity.

Bryant, John H., and Jenkins, David E. "Health Care and Justice." In SIXTH
ANNUAL MEETING REPORT, ECUMENICAL INSTITUTE. Bossey (Geneva):
Christian Medical Commission, July 2-6, 1973.

Reflects on the meaning of the world's gross disparities in life expectancy, health, and health services in relation to the Christian
ethic, and considers courses of action.

Btesh, Simon. "International Research in the Organization of Medical Care." MED. CARE 3 (January-March 1965): 41-46. 10 refs.

> All countries can benefit from studying medical care organization in other countries. A methodology is needed. Performance, economy, and effectiveness should be concerns. At present no direct measure of quality is available. Provides some comparative data from Czechoslovakia, Denmark, Finland, Israel, Italy, Portugal, United States, USSR, and Yugoslavia. Written when the author was director, Office of Research Planning and Coordination, WHO, Geneva.

Candau, Marcolino G. "Problems in Developing Public Health Programs." In PUBLIC HEALTH IS ONE WORLD, pp. 3-7. Supplemental vol. to AJPH 50 (June 1960).

> Statement by the then-director-general of WHO who retired in 1973 after twenty years of service in that position. Reflects on the international character of some diseases and disease control procedures in relation to national sovereignty, among other issues.

Coppini, Mario A., and Illuminati, G. "Relations between Social Security Institutions and the Medical Profession." INT'L. SOCIAL SECURITY REV. (Geneva) 18, no. 2 (1968): whole issue.

Doan, Bui-Dang-Ha. "World Health Trends in Health Manpower." Paper presented at the Eighth Int'l. Scientific Meetings of the IEA, Puerto Rico, September 17-23, 1977.

> In the industrial countries, decrease in general practice among medical doctors, urbanization of all the health workers are main factors of gaps between supply and demand in primary health care. Meanwhile, technological innovation and job parcelling contribute to the emergence of new categories of personnel. In almost developed countries, the population/health personnel ratio is growing, but the pace of increase in health services demand is often faster. Assesses personnel shortage and the ever-growing financial burden for health care in many countries. The developed world is now facing a dramatic choice: more resources for health or zero growth in health services demand. In the developing countries, many factors are contributing to poor health services supply; population growth, lack of financial assets of the people, poor management, urbanization and out-migration of health workers. Meanwhile, health services demand is sharply increasing, partly under the demonstration effect of the Western way of life. Available through the IEA.

Douglas-Wilson, I., and McLachlan, G., eds. HEALTH SERVICES PROSPECTS, AN INTERNATIONAL SURVEY. Boston: Little, Brown and Co., 1973. Refs., index.

Perhaps the best collection of descriptions of a number of national health and medical care systems. Concentrates on industrialized countries but includes some UDCs. Includes an overview chapter on EEC countries. The studies are weakened by the authors' use of unstated, probably differing frameworks for selecting the aspects of systems they describe. Chapter titles: "United Kingdom"; "EEC: The Founding Six"; "France"; "German Federal Republic"; "Ghana"; "Sweden"; "Cuba"; "India"; "Japan"; "Union of Soviet Socialist Republics"; "China"; "Introduction"; "Medical and Health Work"; "Medical Care in the Countryside"; "Peking Teams Serving Minority Areas"; "United States of America: The Setting, and Present and Future"; "Health in America."

Elling, Ray H., ed. COMPARATIVE HEALTH SYSTEMS. Supplemental issue of INQUIRY 12 (June 1975). Notes, refs.

Based primarily on papers prepared for a session by the same title at the eighth World Congress of Sociology. The session was organized under the auspices of the Medical Sociology Research Committee of the International Sociological Association, August 23, 1974, Toronto. Contents are as follows: "Foreword"; "Introduction"; Part 1, Framework and Methods: "A Framework and Approach for the Study of National Health Systems"; "Selection of Contrasting National Health Systems for In-depth Study." Part 2, System Descriptions and Analysis: "Developed" Countries: "The Health and Medical System in Japan"; "Health Services System in Hong Kong: Professional Stratification in a Modernizing Society"; "Health Services in the German Democratic Republic Compared to the Federal Republic of Germany." Part 3, System Descriptions and Analyses: "Underdeveloped" Countries: "Social and Cultural Foundations of the Health Services Systems of India"; "The Cuban Health Area and Polyclinic: Organizational Focus in An Emerging System"; "Health Care in the People's Republic of China: The Barefoot Doctor." Part 4, Specific Studies in Several Countries: "Changes in Response to Symptoms of Illness in the United States and Sweden"; "Hospital Staffing Ratios in the United States and Sweden"; "A Family Practice in England: Challenge to the Conventional Order"; "Community Involvement in Solving Local Health Problems in Ghana."

_____. "Regionalization of Health Services: Sociological Blocks to Realization of an Ideal." See chapter 6.

Evang, Karl. HEALTH SERVICE, SOCIETY, AND MEDICINE. London: Oxford Univ. Press, 1960. Refs., tables, figures, index.

Analyzes modern medical practice in terms of its role as a service organization. Establishes four categories of health services systems (Western European, American, Soviet Russia, and technically underdeveloped nations). Discusses basic structure within each system, emphasizing respective roles of the hospital, general practitioner, drugs, and public health services.

_____. "The Politics of Developing A National Health Policy." INT'L. J. H. SERV. 3 (1973): 331-40.

Author's summary: "Since national health policy is developed through the political instruments and modalities of a given country, it would be unrealistic to prescribe a solution applicable everywhere. Health matters are 'in' in the political world, due partly to the rapidly rising cost of medical care and related social services, and partly to pressure groups which have become aware of the potentialities of health services in the population. Also, the 'man-consuming' sector of society, industry and war machines, can use man as he is produced by nature only to a limited extent; more must, therefore be invested in his health. The emergency period in health protection and promotion is over in the richer parts of the world. However, few countries have yet produced a national health policy. The difficulties encountered in this process are discussed, and it is suggested that a great deal can be learned from the initiative, made in the 1920s, of a recommendation by the Health Section of the League of Nations that every country develop a national food policy. It is argued that it is time for the World Health Organization to urge its members states to develop and introduce a national health policy."

Evang, Karl; Stark, Murray D.; and Lear, Walter J. MEDICAL CARE AND FAMILY SECURITY--NORWAY, ENGLAND, U.S.A. Englewood Cliffs, N.J.: Prentice-Hall, 1963.

An important work drawing on the experiences of Norway, Sweden, UK, and other countries to offer a thorough and clear presentation of the "socialized medicine" perspective. As Dr. Evang put it for Norway: "Money has, as we know, no value in itself. It is a convenient yardstick for a large number of material values. But the health and life of an individual, as well as the health of the nation, cannot be measured by that yardstick. If we, entrusted with protecting and defending the health of the population, give in to a salesman's scale of values, we are lost."

Farvar, M. Taghi. "Alternatives to Health: An Eco-societal Approach." DEVELOPMENT DIALOGUE (Sweden), Summer 1975, special issue.

Paper prepared for the 1975 Dag Hammarskjold Project, referred to in appendix to What Now? The 1975 Dag Hammarskjold Report.

First International Congress on Group Medicine. NEW HORIZONS IN HEALTH CARE. Winnipeg, Manitoba, 1970. Refs., tables, figures, index.

Assembles presentations by international representatives of public, private, and health professional groups in developing an international perspective on issues in the provision of health services. While seeking to establish the role of group medicine in health care delivery, also discusses general organization and operation of a health care system. Includes sessions on socioeconomic philosophies

of health care, utilization of allied health personnel, data processing, research, education, and questions related to development
of group practice in various national settings (Australia, Brazil,
Canada, France, Germany, India, Japan, Scandinavia, and UK).

Fraser, R.D. "An International Study of Health and General Systems of Financing Health Care." INT'L. J. H. SERV. 3 (1973): 369-97. Refs.

The author explores the linear relationship between infant mortality
and real gross domestic product per capita, the number of physicians per 10,000 persons, and the number of hospitals per 1,000
persons. Fraser here expands and updates a previous study for a
current total twenty-five countries. In addition, the present study
adds several variables and includes data for 1965 so that the data
set now covers 1955, 1960, and 1965. The results show that the
percentage of health services financed or directly controlled by
governments, and the relative size of the health sector, are apparently not important determinants of levels of health. On the
other hand, the proportion of health care resources devoted to the
provision of nonpersonal public health care does appear to be a
significant determinant and therefore the role of nonpersonal public
health warrants further study.

Fry, John, and Farndale, W.A.J. INTERNATIONAL MEDICAL CARE AND
EVALUATION: A COMPARISON OF MEDICAL CARE SERVICES THROUGHOUT
THE WORLD. Wallingford, Pa.: Washington Square East Publishers, 1972.

No common framework is employed. Authors use their own implicit
ones in describing different systems. The book does not offer as
much as the subtitle promises. Chapters: "Medicine and the Society of Man"; "International Trends in Medical Care Organization
and Research"; "Medical Care in Europe"; "Medical Care in the
United Kingdom"; "Medical Care in the United States"; "Medical
Care in Canada"; "Medical Care in the U.S.S.R."; "Medical Care
in the Developing Nations"; "Medical Care in Australia"; "The
Status of Medical Care in America"; "Government and Medical
Care"; "Health Planning--A View from the Top with Specific Ref-
erence to the U.S.A."; "The World Medical Association and
Medical Care"; "Comparisons, Implications and Applications."

Glaser, William A. PAYING THE DOCTOR--SYSTEMS OF REMUNERATIONS
AND THEIR EFFECTS. Baltimore: Johns Hopkins Univ. Press, 1970. Refs.,
tables, appendixes, index.

Analyzes principal methods of physician remuneration in sixteen
countries of European and the eastern Mediterranean region. Examines dynamics of these systems, their development, and administrative structures. Summarizes evidence pertaining to effects of
payment systems on medical care and the medical profession. Calls
attention to processes of establishing payment systems, determining

operational forms, and analyzing consequences of mode of payment. Fits in with convergence theorists (Field, Mechanic) in suggesting that almost regardless of the form of the system, physicians maintain considerable bargaining power and "once the procedures and levels of pay suffice, and if the nonpecuniary rewards are protected, doctors will adjust to any system of compensation. In practice, the most familiar system usually arouses the least protest." Suffers somewhat from too limited a scope--that is, in relation to sociopolitical contexts. A revised, second edition was issued in July 1976 in paperback through the Bureau of Applied Social Research, Columbia University, New York. This was based on NHI systems--France, the Netherlands, FRG, Switzerland, and Canada-- and was titled PAYING THE DOCTOR UNDER NATIONAL HEALTH INSURANCE: FOREIGN LESSONS FOR THE UNITED STATES.

Harwood, Grace, ed. "Medicine and Torture." Special section of MATCHBOX, AN INT'L. J. ON HUMAN RIGHTS 1 (Fall 1974).

The journal is published by Amnesty International of the United States. Describes for very many countries the way unprincipled physicians have cooperated with and advised police and other officials in the torture of political prisoners.

Illich, Ivan. MEDICAL NEMESIS: THE EXPROPRIATION OF HEALTH. London: Calder and Boyors, 1975.

Describes, examines and decries the worldwide technologization, bureaucratization, depersonalization of health care, and the medical appropriation of human problems, and builds a strong case for raising the question as to whether modern medical care does more iatrogenic harm than good. Has been critically reviewed by, among others, Navarro, who sees Illich throwing the baby out with the bath water and ignoring the more humane and effective functioning of modern medicine in countries with a democratic socialist form of political economy (see Navarro, this chapter).

Ingman, Stanley, and Thomas, Anthony, eds. TOPIAS AND UTOPIAS IN HEALTH: POLICY STUDIES. The Hague: Mouton; Chicago: Aldine, 1975.

Analyzes and criticizes the processes of health systems and their components. Offers experimental and innovative approaches to health systems in a range of developed and underdeveloped countries. Analyzes the problems of continuity and change, and of social science research aimed at solving health problems. A major work in the field.

INTERNATIONAL CONFERENCE ON WOMEN IN HEALTH, WASHINGTON, D.C., 1975. DHEW Pub. No. (HRA) 76-51. Washington, D.C.: Government Printing Office, 1976.

Includes bibliographies.

International Labour Organization (ILO), MONOGRAPHS ON THE ORGANI-
ZATION OF MEDICAL CARE WITHIN THE FRAMEWORK OF SOCIAL SECURITY.
Geneva, 1968.

> Reports findings of series of studies investigating nature of medical
> care within framework of social security. Describes personal health
> services, methods of remuneration, and attitudes of involved parties.
> Summarizes statutory provisions and actual practice in countries in-
> cluding Belgium, Canada, Ecuador, India, Poland, Tunisia, and
> the UK. Provides much of the data base for Roemer's work (see
> chapter 4).

Kent, Peter, ed. INTERNATIONAL ASPECTS OF THE PROVISION OF MEDICAL
CARE. Stocksfield, London, Henley on Thames, and Boston: Oriel Press,
1976. Index.

> Oriented toward European countries with a chapter on USSR, two
> on the United States, two on Canada, one each on Australia and
> China. France and the FRG are given most attention, though
> there are chapters on Scandinavian countries. A fair portion of
> the book is concerned with the education of health personnel, es-
> pecially physicians and the effects of the hospital environment
> on this education versus more involvement in delivery of care in
> the community. Overall, this work repeats many things stated
> elsewhere but does not move the field forward, although there are
> some strong parts like the opening chapter by McKeown which is
> a truly provocative statement examining the limits of medical care
> systems and their seemingly everchanging internal dynamics in such
> fundamental matters as the division of labor. The chapter by
> Saward on the United States is also good as that by Evans on
> physician manpower in Canada.

Klarman, Herbert. "Economic Determinants of Health Care Expenditures: Comparisons over Time and among Nations." Paper presented at the symposium,
Health Care Costs Explosion: Which Way Now? WHO, Geneva, October 14-
16, 1974.

> A valuable overview and assessment by a noted medical economist
> in the United States, of forces leading to increased health care
> costs in all countries with comparisons showing differences which
> are discussed in relation to system organization, controls, and
> public expectations.

Lathem, Willoughby, and Newbery, Anne, eds. COMMUNITY MEDICINE;
TEACHING, RESEARCH AND HEALTH CARE. New York: Appleton-Century-
Crofts, 1970.

> Records a conference on community medicine, at which medical
> educators, health administrators, government officials, and founda-
> tion executives from five continents discussed health needs, health
> systems, educational institutions, and the development of community

medicine in their respective countries. Programs in community
medicine at six universities in developing countries are described.
The following aspects of community medicine are examined in detail: objectives; development of improved health care systems;
education, training, and utilization of health personnel; influence
of cultural attitudes; relationships between universities and governments. Includes chapters as follows: by G. Velazquez on the program at the Universidad de Valle in Columbia; by A. Aguirre on
the history of the program; by L.R. Allen on the community health
care demonstration and teaching through the All India Institute of
Medical Sciences; by P. Buri on physician education in community
medicine; by the same author on a program in Thailand; by P.C.
Campos describing community medicine practice and teaching at
the University of the Phillipines; by A.O. Lucas on the program
at the University of Ibadan, Nigeria; and by J.S. Lutwama on
the program at Makerere Medical School at Kasongoti, Kampala,
in Uganda, East Africa.

Lawson, Ian R. "Health: A Demystification of Medical Technology." LANCET
1 (February 28, 1976): 481-82.

A reply to Dr. Francis D. Moore, surgeon at Harvard who attacked an
article by Dr. Mahler (director general, WHO). Mahler had recom-
mended public health over high-powered medicine. Lawson says
neither is doing well in the United States. (Moore's letter, LANCET,
January 10, 1976, p. 83.)

Logan, Robert F.L. "International Studies of Illness and Health Services."
MILBANK MEM. FUND Q. 46, pt. 2 (April 1968): 126-40.

Noting that all countries face the problem of rising health costs
and competition from other sectors of their economies, the author
presents data from several countries (mainly Sweden, UK, and
the United States, but also selected data on hospital beds and
health personnel from fifteen countries, some underdeveloped and
some developed) showing remarkable variations in levels and mixes
of health services resources. This study points out the utility of
cross-national comparisons for learning what ranges and concentra-
tions there are to inform efforts at rational planning such as in the
health manpower planning project in Columbia.

McNeur, Ronald W., ed. THE CHANGING ROLES AND EDUCATION OF
HEALTH CARE PERSONNEL WORLDWIDE IN VIEW OF THE INCREASE OF BASIC
HEALTH SERVICES. Philadelphia: Society for Health and Human Values, 1978.

Paper from a consultation sponsored by the Society for Health and
Humane Value at Rockefeller Foundation Study and Conference
Center, Villa Serbelloni, Bellagio, Italy, May 2-7, 1977. A
valuable collection on experiences and concepts involved in spreading the medical and public health work to new hands in many parts
of the world.

Mahler, Halfdan T. "The Health of the Family, Keynote Address." In HEALTH OF THE FAMILY, pp. 4-7. Reston, Va., and Washington, D.C.: National Council for Int'l. Health, ca. 1975.

> Paper presented at a conference sponsored by the National Council for International Health, October 16-18, 1974. Forceful, clear statement by the man who assumed the position of director general of WHO in 1973. Identifies in potent language the rising demands and costs of modern medical care at the same time as it becomes increasingly directed toward expensive, specialized care for the few rather than adequate general and preventive care for the many. Speaks of hospitals as "disease palaces" wherein the interests of superspecialty medicine are pursued.

_____. "Social Perspectives in Health: A Fairer Sharing of Health Resources is Needed." INT'L. J. H. ED. 19 (1976): 74-76.

> A ringing editorial-type statement abstracted from an address to the twenty-ninth World Health Assembly by the director general of WHO urging that priority be given to coverage for the total population with essential care rather than exotic, expensive care for the privileged few. The achievement of more equitable distribution is seen not as a technical problem but as a social problem. "Conditions appear to be ripe for a truly critical re-evaluation in social terms of the means for attaining health. Perhaps such a revolution in our approach to health development has more chance than any other kind of social revolution to become truly universal in the near future." The author does not, however, define the social approach which he somehow distinguishes from other key sets of factors classed as technical, economic, and political.

Mechanic, D. "Ideology, Medical Technology and Health Care Organization in Modern Nations." AJPH 65 (March 1975): 241-47. 26 refs.

> Nations dealing with common health services problems become similar in effective means of coping. Sees a movement to government financing of health care as a social and political right. Worldwide convergences of goals are identified: diminish inequality; link service and community needs; integrate health system; emphasize primary medical service; and improve efficiency and effectiveness. Records the glaring disparities between whites and blacks in South Africa. An important statement.

Milio, Nancy. THE CARE OF HEALTH IN COMMUNITIES--ACCESS FOR OUT-CASTS. New York: Macmillan, 1975.

> Describes special service arrangements for special groups in many parts of the world: creches for "urban nomads" in India; hospices for the dying in the UK, and so forth. The first chapter gives an overview of world population, resources, and mortality. Common (though not always comparable) items of information are given for a large number of national health systems in the appendixes.

Murray, D. Stark. "Who Has the Best Health Service?" BRITISH HOSPITAL AND SOCIAL SERV. REV. 80 (October 3, 1970): 1936-37.

The health services of seventeen countries are compared in this article which finds that they can be divided into three groups: (1) those like the NHS which are available to all and free at the time of use; (2) the American 'nonsystem'; and (3) the majority which are based on insurance. In a largely impressionistic way the author tries to "make sense" out of the quality of the systems for most people in the seventeen countries visited. Provides a surprising amount of information and insight in only two pages. Only the Scandinavian systems and that of USSR are seen as providing close to the same generally adequate care as the NHS offers to nearly all persons in the UK. Notes the disparities of the United States in which one finds the anomaly of the richest nation on earth spending 7 percent of its GNP on health (in 1977 it was 8.6 percent) with portions of its population less well served than the average person in Greece or the unsocialized parts of Turkey. Suggests key questions to be asked of different systems.

Murray, Martin J. "The Pharmaceutical Industry: A Study in Corporate Power." INT'L. J. H. SERV. 4 (1974): 625-40. 60 refs.

Author's summary: "Most studies of the pharmaceutical industry have focused on such issues as restrictive patent regulation, ineffective products, duplicative marketing procedures, misrepentative advertising, and the peculiar noncompetitive structure of markets. These investigations have revealed only certain aspects of the structure of the pharmaceutical industry. Three significant trends are investigated in this paper: international expansion, diversification through mergers and acquisitions, and interlocking directorates with financial institutions. The thesis of this paper is that small-scale drug manufacturing firms have been gradually replaced by large-scale multinational conglomerates. Production and sales are no longer dependent on pharmaceutical products. In the typical case, large-scale pharmaceutical producing firms have been increasingly linked to financial institutions through interlocking directorates."

Navarro, Vicente. "The Industrialization of Fetishisms or the Fetishism of Industrialization: A Critique of Ivan Illich." INT'L. J. H. SERV. 5 (1975): 351-71.

Recognizes the importance of Illich's warning (see above, this chapter) against medicalization of too many aspects of life and the iatrogenic effects of modern medicine, but presents a penetrating criticism of (1) Illich's tendency to throw the good of modern medicine out with the bad and (2) his failure to recognize the ways in which a true democratic socialist system, as distinct from market-oriented capitalism or state capitalism, can make proper human use of modern health and medical care.

Pan American Health Organization (PAHO). BASIC REFERENCE DOCUMENT
SUGGESTED TARGETS AND STRATEGIES OF HEALTH FOR THE DECADE 1971-
80. Washington, D.C., 1972.

> Background document developed in preparation for a meeting of
> ministers of health of the Americas in Santiago, Chile, in 1971
> at which a ten-year general health plan was adopted. Conditions
> in each country are discussed, but without reference to the growing
> repression and official terror in a number of countries (Argentina,
> Brazil, Paraguay, Uruguay, etc.). Thus, although problems are
> identified--concentration of resources in urban areas while the
> majority of population is still on the land; growth of periurban
> slums (shack towns) without basic sanitary and other services--there
> is an air of unreality to the document. Nevertheless, this is an
> important resource and gives a good overview of the difficulties
> of achieving adequate general health care for all segments of a
> nation's population within the resource limits of the country.

_____. COORDINATION OF MEDICAL CARE: FINAL REPORT AND WORK-
ING DOCUMENTS OF A STUDY GROUP. Washington, D.C., 1970.

> Examines from several points of view the continuing fractionation
> of services in most countries. The major gap is between public
> and private services. The Cuban exception is not specifically dis-
> cussed in detail.

Peters, R.J., and Kinnaird, J., eds. HEALTH SERVICES ADMINISTRATION.
Edinburgh: E. and S. Livingston, 1965. Refs., tables, index.

> Examines role of administrative functions in the provision of health
> services. Outlines history and trends of health-related activities
> in Great Britain and selected other countries. Discusses general
> administrative theory, systems of health economics, and relevant
> manpower developments. Concludes with discussion of resources
> available for program evaluation, including statistical methods and
> theory.

Quimby, F.H. THE POLITICS OF GLOBAL HEALTH. Washington, D.C.:
Government Printing Office, for the Subcommittee on National Security Policy
and Scientific Developments of the House Committee on Foreign Affairs, May
1971.

> Historical overview of attempts at worldwide cooperation in health,
> the role of persistent political problems in WHO and in some American
> agencies involved in world health programs. Calls for the develop-
> ment of institutional devices for encouraging the sharing and ex-
> changing of knowledge supported by individual nations.

Rabin, David L., and Bush, Patricia J. "The Use of Medicines: Historical
Trends and International Comparisons." INT'L. J. H. SERV. 4 (1974): 61-87.
68 refs.

Reviews the development of current levels of medicine consumption with a literature review of cross-national and limited surveys and national statistics on rates of medicine use. Medicine use has increased worldwide at rates exceeding increases in national incomes in many countries. Problems in the use of data for international comparison of medicine use are discussed.

Roemer, Milton I. "The Expanding Scope of Governmental Regulation of Health Care Delivery." UNIV. OF TOLEDO LAW REV. 6 (Spring 1975): 591-616.

Describes the nearly worldwide concern with rising medical care costs and concern for quality received in relation to money paid. Discusses moves by governments to establish cost and quality controls over hospital utilization and other costly aspects of medical care. Gives examples of control measures from a number of countries.

_____. HEALTH CARE SYSTEMS IN WORLD PERSPECTIVE. Ann Arbor, Mich.: Health Administration Press, 1976.

A valuable collection of the author's previously published articles.

_____. "Health Departments and Medical Care--A World Scanning." AJPH 50 (February 1960): 154-60.

An overview, not a detailed study. Remarks on the peculiar US pattern of health departments having little or nothing to do with personal health services while many other countries merge preventive and personal services through health departments, though this was not true in the UK where general physicians, health departments (under local authorities), and hospitals (nationalized) functioned as three rather separate spheres. Presents a useful scheme for categorizing various national systems of health service organization.

_____. "Medical Care in Relation to Public Health: A Study of Relationships between Preventive and Curative Health Services throughout the World." Geneva: WHO, December 1956.

A consultant's report surveying the world situation on this topic. The general finding is that gaps all too often exist between curative and preventive services with the former receiving the bulk of funding and attention, though this is less true in socialist countries with regionalized systems of care.

_____. "Organized Ambulatory Health Service in International Perspective." INT'L. J. H. SERV. 1 (1971): 18-27.

Historically, health services for the ambulatory patient have been organized throughout the world along several paths: (1) separate dispensaries for treatment of the sick; (2) hospital outpatient departments; (3) specialized preventive clinics under public health agencies, industries or schools; (4) private group medical practice; and (5) health centers of either preventive or integrated preventive-curative scope. All five of these types of organized service continue to expand throughout the world, in relation to a declining importance of private individualistic medical practice. The trend is toward integrated ambulatory service of both preventive and curative services in health centers. The staffing and scope of health centers vary with the economic development of a country and its prevailing political philosophy. Increasing use is being made of paramedical personnel working with doctors in health teams.

Royal Society of Medicine and the Josiah Macy, Jr. Foundation. THE GREATER MEDICAL PROFESSION, REPORT OF A SYMPOSIUM. New York, 1973.

Discusses international as opposed to national responsibilities. In the epilogue (pp. 225-36) Lord Gordon Wolstenholme suggests the concept of a "world medical profession."

Sackler, Arthur M. A STATE OF EMERGENCY IN WORLD HEALTH CARE: REPORT OF THE INTERNATIONAL TASK FORCE ON WORLD HEALTH MAN-POWER OF WHO. Geneva: WHO, 1970.

Critical shortages of health man and woman power are identified for most countries, especially the underdeveloped nations, and the need to find new approaches is recognized. The modern, physician-staffed model is seen as impossible to fulfill in the forseeable future in the poorest two-thirds of the world.

Silverman, Milton. THE DRUGGING OF THE AMERICAS: HOW MULTINA-TIONAL DRUG COMPANIES SAY ONE THING ABOUT THEIR PRODUCTS TO PHYSICIANS IN THE UNITED STATES, AND ANOTHER THING TO PHYSICIANS IN LATIN AMERICA. Berkeley and Los Angeles: Univ. of California Press, 1976.

See annotation for the article based on this book in item following.

_____. "The Epidemiology of Drug Promotion." INT'L. J. H. SERV. 7 (1977): 157-66.

A survey was conducted on the promotion of twenty-eight prescription drugs in the form of forty different products marketed in the United States and Latin America by twenty-three multinational pharmaceutical companies. Striking differences were found in the manner in which the identical drug, marketed by the identical company or its foreign affiliate, was described to physicians in the United States and to physicians in Latin America. In the United States, the listed indications were usually few in number, while the contraindications, warning, and potential adverse reactions were given in extensive detail. In Latin America, the listed in-

dications were far more numerous, while the hazards were usually
minimized, glossed over, or totally ignored. The differences were
not simply between the United States on the one hand and all the
Latin American countries on the other. There were substantial
differences within Latin America, with the same global company
telling one story in Mexico, another in Central America, a third
in Ecuador and Colombia, and yet another in Brazil. This article
is taken primarily from the author's book THE DRUGGING OF
THE AMERICAS (see above). There is an interesting epilogue on
the last page of the article reporting on US congressional hearings
and promises by major multinational drug companies to change their
promotional policies as well as a policy statement from the council
of the International Federation of Pharmaceutical Manufacturers
Associations calling for consistent labeling and advertisement based
upon "the body of scientific and medical evidence pertaining to
that product."

Smith, R.A., and Banta, James E. "Global Community Health--A 'New' Health
Direction." AJPH 59 (September 1969): 1713-19. Refs.

The United States is not isolated from the rest of the world community and the health problems occurring around the globe. Direct
and indirect effects of our overseas activities on the well-being of
Americans are identifiable. The first step in dealing with these
effects is to recognize the areas of greatest impact, such as health
manpower, research, epidemic prevention, and others. The work
of health personnel in the Peace Corps is discussed, as is the
"brain drain" of foreign-trained physicians to the United States.
The article concludes with a section entitled "Health as a Promoter
of American Diplomacy Overseas."

Sokolowska, Magdalena, et al., eds. HEALTH, MEDICINE, SOCIETY. Dordrecht, Netherlands, and Boston: D. Reidel; Warsaw: PWN--Polish Scientific
Publishers, 1976.

A valuable selection of the papers presented at the International
Conference on the Sociology of Medicine, Warsaw (Jablonna),
August 20-25, 1973, organized by the Institute of Philosophy and
Sociology of the Polish Academy of Sciences in collaboration with
the Research Committee on the Sociology of Medicine of the International Sociological Association. Following a fascinating paper
by Sokolowska on the development of medical sociology in Poland,
the book is divided in five parts. The first, "Health in Society"
is made up largely of papers by Polish and other East European
scientists concerned with disease or specific diseases in relation to
societal conditions (social epidemiology). The second part has
papers entirely by Western sociomedical scientists on changing aspects of health interventions. Part 3, "Sociological Insights into
the Health Sciences" has a mix of Eastern and Western papers on
a number of special problem areas. The papers by Elinson and

Pflanz are particularly valuable in terms of methodological considerations for CNSHS. Part 4, "The Health System," has the most
interesting papers from a conceptual point of view for CNSHS:
"The Health System and the Social System"; "The Adaptation Patterns of the Medical System and Social Change"; a paper on health
system models; one on consumerism; one on the British NHS and
changes in it; one on shifting power in the Canadian System; one
on the United States; and one on planning and the health professions. Part 5 has papers on the teaching of medical sociology by
Western medical sociologists.

Stanford Research Institute. THE WORLD PHARMACEUTICAL INDUSTRY. Palo
Alto, Calif., 1969.

Susser, Merwyn W., and Watson, W. SOCIOLOGY IN MEDICINE. 2d ed.
New York: Oxford Univ. Press, 1971.

Systematic study of health and epidemiology. Has its basis in sociological concepts and illustrative field studies. Emphasis is on
the social epidemiology of disease. A first chapter compares the
patterns of illness in peasant and industrial societies using South
Africa as a case which juxtaposes the two types.

Thursz, Daniel, and Vigilante, Joseph L., eds. REACHING PEOPLE, THE
STRUCTURE OF NEIGHBORHOOD SERVICES. Social Service Delivery Systems:
An International Annual, vol. 3. Beverly Hills, Calif., and London: Sage
Publications, 1977.

This volume directs itself to two major themes: styles of delivering
social services at the neighborhood level, and the conceptual work
available to planners involved in organizing and analyzing local
service systems. The various contributors examine such issues as
the nuances of ethnicity in delivery systems, linkages between
neighborhood services and higher levels of government, and neighborhood delivery systems in Switzerland, UK, Zambia, Israel, France,
India, and Norway.

Titmuss, Richard M. THE GIFT OF RELATIONSHIP. New York: Pantheon
Books, 1971. Tables, appendixes, index.

Investigates political, economic, and philosophic questions related
to the provision of blood for transfusion. With emphasis on the
UK and the United States, utilizes an eclectic research method to
compare donor systems, statistics of distribution, and demand for
transfusions in various national settings. Inquires into such matters
as characteristics of the donor, motivation for his donation, and
the gift relationship of donor and recipient.

U.S. Department of Health, Education and Welfare. REHABILITATION OF THE DISABLED IN FIFTY ONE COUNTRIES. Washington, D.C.: Government Printing Office, 1964.

> Examines government policies and formal statements of approaches to payment and services. Provides some useful assembly of data on this large number of countries, but is uncritical in the use of official data. Includes no on-site studies of numbers and types of disabled and their treatment and outcomes.

U.S. Department of Health, Education and Welfare. Social Security Administration. HEALTH INFORMATION FOR INTERNATIONAL TRAVEL, INCLUDING UNITED STATES DESIGNATED YELLOW FEVER VACCINATION CENTERS. Supplement to MORBIDITY AND MORTALITY 23 (September 1974).

> Valuable guidance on innoculations and other travel preparations according to areas of the world.

_____. Social Security Administration. SOCIAL SECURITY PROGRAMS THROUGHOUT THE WORLD--1969. Social Security Administration, Research Report no. 31. Washington, D.C.: Government Printing Office, 1969.

> A periodically issued compendium begun by Daniel Gerig (see US Social Security Administration, 1967, in chapter 3.1). A valuable information source. Notes the relative lack of provision of social security programs in largely agricultural countries and the confusing array of partial and special coverages in most other countries including special medical benefits. However, most industrial countries have a more complete, integrated system than does the US. Summarizes social security provisions of 123 independent nations, alphabetically arranged in tabular form by country. Categorizes programs under the following headings: old age; invalidity; death; sickness and maternity; work injury; unemployment; and family allowance. Condenses existing statutory provisions to indicate main administrative regulations of reported systems.

Wade, O.L., and Beeley, Linda. "Monitoring Adverse Reactions to Drugs: Toward a Therapeutic Audit." INT'L. J. H. SERV. 4 (1974): 109-23. 37 refs.

> From the author's summary: "Information about adverse drug reactions comes from many sources, including reports in the medical literature and reports to national monitoring organizations. The World Health Organization has played an important role . . . Studies of patterns of drug use in Northern Ireland have been conducted and a working party of the World Health Organization has been set up to compare drug use in different countries. The epidemiologic study of adverse reactions to drugs, an important new field for clinical pharmacology, should be viewed as only a part of a much larger, more embracing discipline: the therapeutic audit."

Wolstenholme, Gordon E.W. "Florence Nightingale: New Lamps for Old."
PROCEEDINGS OF THE ROYAL SOCIETY OF MED. 63 (December 1970):
22-28.

> In commemorating Florence Nightingale's contributions, the author
> puts forth the notion of a world medical service: "an international
> organization of medical service . . . for the use of medical teams,
> extended by voluntary service of the kind I have suggested."

Wolstenholme, Gordon E.W., and O'Connor, Maeve, eds. HEALTH OF MAN-
KIND. Boston: Little, Brown and Co., 1968.

_____. TEAMWORK FOR WORLD HEALTH. London: J. and A. Churchill,
1971. Refs., index.

> A collection of papers from Ciba Foundation in honor of Professor
> S. Artunkal held at the Tarabya Grand Hotel, Istanbul, June 8-
> 12, 1970. Contents: "Florence Nightingale--Handmaid of Civili-
> zation"; "Response to Emergencies, National and International";
> "The New Priorities in Tropical Medicine"; "The Health Corps in
> Iran"; "The Turkish National Health Services"; "Experiments in Ex-
> panding the Rural Health Service in People's China"; "Backcloth
> to the NHS in England and Wales"; "The Family Care Team:
> Philosophy, Problems, Possibilities"; "Pediatrics and the Community";
> "Paramedical Paradoxes--Challenges and Opportunity"; "New Con-
> cepts in Medical Education"; "Philosophy of Management: The
> Place of the Professional Administrator"; "Teamwork at Ministry
> Level"; "Mental Health Care: A Growing Concern to Communities";
> "Volunteers--Their Use and Misuse"; "Teamwork for World Health:
> Personal Conclusions and Recommendations"; and closing speeches
> by S. Artunkal, E.S. Egeli, and R.V. Christie.

"Women and Health." INT'L. J. H. SERV. 5 (1975): 162-346 (entire issue).

> Important contribution to a topic of growing importance. In ad-
> dition to original articles on discrimination against women in medical
> treatment and involvement in medical work, there are several re-
> view articles of recent books on this topic and replies by some of
> the authors. The last piece in the volume (pp. 343-46) is a com-
> munication from Ruth Roemer on the International Conference on
> Women in Health held at PAHO in Washington, D.C., June 16-18,
> 1975, as part of the activities of International Women's Year.

World Health Organization (WHO). FIFTH REPORT ON THE WORLD HEALTH
SITUATION, 1969-1972. Geneva, 1975.

> Fifth in a series covering four-year periods. General survey of
> health problems, the organization and administration of health ser-
> vices, planning, personnel, and research. Also a comprehensive re-
> view by territory and country, though information on many UDCs is
> lacking. One of the most valuable information sources for CNSHS.

_____. "Organizational Study on Methods of Promoting the Development of Basic Health Services." Annex II to OFFICIAL RECORDS OF WHO, no. 206. Geneva, 1973.

Important policy statement reorienting WHO's priorities toward general, basic health services rather than disease-specific programs. Considers such factors as resistance from vested professional interest groups in the difficult task of providing coverage to all of a nation's people.

_____. ORGANIZATION, STRUCTURE AND FUNCTIONING OF HEALTH SERVICES AND MODERN METHODS OF ADMINISTRATIVE MANAGEMENT. WHO Technical Discussions, 26th World Health Assembly. Geneva, 1973.

Contains basic working document and the deliberations of the discussion groups as well as summary report concerning the worldwide problem of lack of adequately prepared health services administrators and planners.

_____. "Participation of Health Centres in Ambulatory Care." Geneva: WHO/OMC/33, February 11, 1959.

An expert committee defines the health center as "a place where the appropriate basic services are rendered." These should be linked with other services such as education and agriculture. The patterns of organization in a range of countries are considered including the polyclinic and health stations in rural areas of the USSR where staffing by feldshers plays an important part. Some countries emphasize geographic extension while others seem to highlight proximity to the hospital. There are also different emphases on cure, prevention, or integration. The trend historically seems to be from the provision of preventive care for rural areas to comprehensive health care for whole national populations through regionalized structures with health centers at the periphery of the systems.

_____. "Report of the Technical Discussions at the Twenty-Seventh World Health Assembly on 'The Role of the Health Services in Preserving or Restoring the Full Effectiveness of the Human Environment in the Promotion of Health.'" Geneva: A27/Technical Discussions, 1974.

A comprehensive overview emphasizing socioeconomic and cultural factors.

_____. "The Urban and Rural Distribution of Medical Manpower." WHO Chronicle 22 (March 1968): 100-105.

_____. URBAN HEALTH SERVICES. FIFTH REPORT OF THE EXPERT COMMITTEE ON PUBLIC HEALTH ADMINISTRATION. Technical Report Series, no. 250. Geneva, 1963.

This study was an early recognition of urban-rural imbalances in health services and the growing problem of providing service to displaced, impoverished persons (urban nomads) and residents of periurban slums (shack towns).

World Health Organization. Regional Office for Europe. HEALTH SERVICES IN EUROPE. Copenhagen: WHO, 1965.

This document deals with such problems as background and evolution of the health services in Europe, preventive services, organization of medical care, administration, personnel, and main trends in health care organization. It presents a synopsis of health services in thirty-one countries, including all countries of the EEC.

Young, Alan A., ed. "Cross Cultural Studies in Health and Illness." MEDICAL ANTHROPOLOGY 2 (Spring 1978): entire issue.

Authors in this special issue include Alan Young, Horacio Fabrega, Jr., Mark Nichter, Carl E. Taylor, and Arthur Kleinmann. One additional paper by Charles Leslie appears in a later issue of this journal. The articles in this issue were originally presented as papers at a conference titled "Rethinking the Western Health Enterprise," held in Cleveland on the sixth and seventh of March, 1978.

Chapter 4

WORKS WITH A COMMON STATED FRAMEWORK
COMPARING TWO OR MORE COUNTRIES

From the point of view of developing the CNSHS field, this is the most important chapter in this book. Unfortunately, it is also one of the shortest. Short as it is, it includes some works which might have been categorized elsewhere because they deal with a particular facet or problem in more than one system more than with the overall health systems of two or more countries. The book by Glaser on negotiating structures is an example. But such works are included here when they spell out their comparative framework and place the study, even of a facet, in the overall contexts of the health systems and political economies of the countries studied. The ideal is the study which (1) lays out a logic for comparing or contrasting two or more countries; (2) spells out a framework; and (3) employs this framework in examining available as well as specifically gathered empirical data on the health systems broadly and their political-economic, social, cultural, and epidemiologic contexts, including historical developments. Such work is extremely rare. Perhaps the works of Anderson, Fry, Roemer, and Weinerman come closest to the ideal. And among these, there are important divergences in framework and not always a clear logic for selection of countries. Clearly, much work remains to be done in this young but growing field.

Altenstetter, Christa. HEALTH POLICY MAKING AND ADMINISTRATION IN WEST GERMANY AND THE UNITED STATES. Administration and Policy Studies Series, no. 03-013. Beverly Hills, Calif.: Sage Publication, 1974.

> Although focused only on policymaking and administration, the author lays out a framework for studying these two national systems, the one with the oldest compulsory NHI in the world. In a concluding chapter the author offers revisions in the framework she suggested at the outset. These suggested revisions are based on the study as well as her discussion and implications drawn.

Anderson, Odin W. HEALTH CARE: CAN THERE BE EQUITY? THE UNITED STATES, SWEDEN AND ENGLAND. New York: John Wiley and Sons, 1972.

> Cross-national comparative analysis of three health care systems utilizing a general system approach. A model of modern health

service is constructed and its elements are discussed as indicators in each system. One of the few CNSHS which spells out (however partial or selective it may be) a framework used in examining each of several systems. The overall political-economic dimension of main concern to the author in these three generally "liberal-democratic" systems is whether distribution occurs through a maximized market (the United States approaches this more than the other two) or a minimized market. Health services framework deals with organizational characteristics, facilities, personnel, funding, utilization, and "payoff" in terms of health levels, accessibility, and family solvency. Each of these is complex and the most specific aspects of each may not be exactly comparable in the three systems; thus the author's depth of experience and understanding of each system is important in analyzing and comparing the whole picture for each country.

Separate reviews by A. Peter Ruderman, Julian Tudor Hart, and Samuel Wolfe and the author's reply are published in INT'L. J. H. SERV. 3 (1973): 521-33. One reviewer (Ruderman) says the data seem to have been assembled from an administrative perspective whereas a patient perspective would be required to get at the question of equity. In spite of the title, all these reviewers are sharply critical of Anderson's failure to recognize that Sweden and England have moved toward erasing income inequalities in care more than has the United States, and "dynamism" applied to the latter may be a euphemism for confusion.

Blanpain, Jan, et al. NATIONAL HEALTH INSURANCE AND HEALTH RESOURCES: THE EUROPEAN EXPERIENCE. Cambridge, Mass. and London: Harvard Univ. Press, 1978.

Author's annotation: "This book discusses health resources development in England and Wales and Sweden where direct government provision of health services is the dominant feature and in France, the Federal Republic of Germany and the Netherlands in which compulsory, contributory health insurance prevails. . . . Although primarily conceived to relate the European experience to the emerging national health insurance in the United States, the study also offers European policymakers and scholars a unique perspective on resource development within neighboring systems."

Christie, Ronald V. MEDICAL EDUCATION AND THE STATE. THE CHANGING PATTERN IN TEN COUNTRIES. DHEW pub. (NIH) 76-943. Bethesda, Md.: John E. Fogarty International Center for Advanced Study in the Health Sciences, 1976.

An important study of medical education and state support in ten countries which reports on several common points of concern for each country, even though it fails to examine adequately the overall medical care and political economic contexts.

Conder, Brigitte, and Sandier, Simone. "Le Système des Soins Médicaux en France et aux États Unis. [The system of medical care in France and the United States]." LE CONCOURS MÉDICAL, April 21 and 28, 1973, pp. 3001-4. In French.

> One of the few pieces in the literature directly comparing the general outlines of the medical care systems in the United States and France according to an outline of key concerns. Not extensive and detailed enough to be more than suggestive.

Elling, Ray H., and Kerr, Henry. "Selection of Contrasting National Health Systems for In-depth Study." See chapter 7.

> Suggests approach and framework for studying contrasting cases, i.e. countries with similar levels of overall resources but widely divergent health outcomes as indexed by such general measures as infant mortality.

Empkie, Timothy M. "The Organization of Tuberculosis Prevention: A Comparison of the Federal Republic of Germany and the German Democratic Republic." Required research paper, Univ. of Connecticut Medical School, Farmington, April 1976. Reproduced. Available from the Program in CNSHS, Univ. Conn. Health Center, Farmington, Ct., 06032.

> Based on original field work in both countries as well as document study. In what was a common system before World War II, and using the subnational regional system as his unit of analysis, the author examines differences in organization for tuberculosis prevention and care which have developed since the two Germanies came under different forms of political control. The record of accomplishment in the East is at least as good as in the West, even though overall resources have been shorter. One of the main organizational differences is the greater degree of melding or merger of tuberculosis services into the polyclinic, the local form of health services in the East, while in the West, follow up of patients may be more complex and difficult in the private office form of practice which predominates.

Falk, Isidore S. "Medical Care in Two Areas of Southeast Asia--Malaya and Singapore." AJPH 48 (April 1958): 448-53.

Field, Mark G. "Comparative Health Systems: Differentiation and Convergence." Unpublished final report on Research Grant HS00272 submitted to the National Center for Health Services Research, Health Resources Administration, DHEW, March 31, 1976. Bibliography, appendixes.

> Reports on a comparative study of the health systems of six industrialized nations: France, Japan, Sweden, UK, United States, and USSR. A conflict theorist would argue with the framework, but the work has the merit of clearly spelling out a guiding thought structure for the study which the author characterizes as "structural-

functional, macro-sociological; evolutionary-historical; dynamic; comparative; and relevant." The health system is seen as needing the following supports: legitimacy; knowledge and techniques; personnel; and economic resources. These are always limited and problematic, yet in all the countries studied the health systems are seen as having "grown at a faster rate than almost any other sector of society, and . . . in that process, they all have tended to become increasingly internally differentiated and complex." Thus all systems have an imbalance away from primary care. There develops then a "Kafka-like Medicine of the Absurd, where therapeutic poverty flourishes in the midst of biomedical abundance." Ten problem areas for future study are cited: (1) the evolving mandates of health systems; (2) limits (or lack of limits) of demand for health services; (3) the bureaucratic-managerial logic and the individual patient; (4) the question of such a logic at all; (5) the recycling or relicensing of physicians; (6) flexibility or rigidity in organizational medicine; (7) the patient-consumer role; (8) auxiliaries and "the greater medical profession"; (9) moral dilemmas of modern medicine; (10) the chimera of the "ideal" health system.

Foulon, Alain. "Les Services Médicaux en Suède et en France (1960-1967)." CONSOMMATION (Paris) 4 (1970): 3-31. In French.

A valuable description of the Swedish and French systems and point-for-point comparison on major aspects and trends.

Fraser, R.D. "An International Study of Health and General Systems of Financing Health Care." See chapter 3.4.

Attempts to explain infant mortality levels in eighteen developed countries by the proportion of health care financing devoted to nonpersonal health services.

Fry, John. MEDICINE IN THREE SOCIETIES--COMPARISON OF MEDICAL CARE IN THE USSR, USA AND UK. New York: Elsevier, 1970; and Aylesbury Bucks, England: MTP Publisher, 1969. Tables, figures, appendixes, index.

Describes and contrasts medical systems of USSR, United States, and UK in terms of a series of levels of care determined by required specialist services (e.g., family unit, first-contact physician, specialist services for ambulatory patient). Explores operational principles and philosophies applying to system components, levels of care, and their administration within each national context. A section is devoted to each level of care and the ways in which the three systems provide these services. Two specific problems-- maternal and child care and mental illness--are taken up to examine how these systems function at the several levels in relation to these problems. Training and organization of health workers are described. Difficulties in comparing the three systems are

recognized. Concludes with personal reflections and recommendation about action within existing medical care structures. Among
other interesting distinctions, the author differentiates between
generalist, specialoid, and specialist. The specialoid is like a
pediatrician or geriatrician, concentrating their care in a certain age range but serving too wide a range of problems to be a
specialist in the usual sense.

_____. "Medical Care in Three Societies, Common Problems and Dilemmas
in the USSR, USA and UK." INT'L. J. H. SERV. 1 (1971): 121-33.

A comparative study by a British general practitioner on the ways
in which three societies (USSR, United States, and UK) have organized medical services. The findings reveal that there are many
more similarities than differences. These differences need to be
examined to see, if they are successful in one system, whether
they might be more widely applied. There is a need, for example,
to examine the ways in which the medical assistants (feldshers) are
used in the USSR. The author points out the need to reexamine
the needs at the first-contact primary level of care, and in particular the place of the "specialoid" or generalist physician.

Glaser, William A. HEALTH INSURANCE BARGAINING: FOREIGN LESSONS
FOR AMERICANS. New York: Halsted Press, 1978.

Although focused on a particular problem--the kind of negotiating
structures and processes which arise between organized physicians
and the government and other insurance agencies under NHI systems--
this important book is something of a model for CNSHS in spelling
out clearly the logic of its design and a framework of concern,
at least in terms of major categories. These categories are: type
of political system; type of payment to physicians (see the author's
earlier book on this subject cited in chapter 3.4); parties to the
negotiations; and organization of the negotiations. The book places
the study problem in the context of the overall health system and
political context of the country. Chapter headings: Learning from
Abroad; Canada; France; Belgium; The Netherlands; FRG; Switzerland; Sweden; UK; Lessons for the USA. The author states that
the focus is on "how to organize the decision-making machinery
to produce the terms of service, fee schedules, and pay rate for
doctors under national health insurance." The medical association
and insurance carriers must reorganize for this and set up regular
negotiations. Government only negotiates terms of service where
the carrying of insurance has been nationalized. "Some countries
have standing committees with neutral chairmen, and this seems a
good model for the United States. . . ." NHI "will work badly
if America's health delivery remains so muddled."

Kent, Peter W., ed. INTERNATIONAL ASPECTS OF THE PROVISION OF
MEDICAL CARE. London: Routledge and Kegan Paul, 1976.

While this work does not employ a comprehensive stated framework
in its descriptions of different systems, the authors do have common
central concerns and there is attention to the national political
economic contexts of the described systems. Aspects of the provision of medical care in a wide variety of countries--including
Germany, the USSR and China--are examined in these essays. The
failures and successes of different systems are candidly discussed,
and the effects upon the relationships between doctors, patients,
hospitals, medical education agencies, and government agencies
are viewed from within widely differing political and social systems.

Marmor, Theodore R., and Thomas, David. "Doctors, Politics, and Pay Disputes: 'Pressure Group Politics' Revisited." See chapter 5.

Maxwell, Robert. HEALTH CARE, THE GROWING DILEMMA: NEEDS VERSUS
RESOURCES IN WESTERN EUROPE, THE U.S. AND THE U.S.S.R. See chapter
3.2.

Examines patterns of organization and strains toward higher costs
in nineteen, primarily European countries, but including information on Canada, the United States, and USSR.

Maynard, Alan. HEALTH CARE IN THE EUROPEAN COMMUNITY. See chapter
3.2.

Minkowski, A. "Health of Mother and Child: The Experiences in the People's
Republic of China, the Democratic Republic of Vietnam and Cuba." IMPACT
OF SCIENCE ON SOCIETY 23 (January-March 1973): 29-41.

A relatively rare kind of work comparing approaches to an important problem area in several socialist-oriented countries.

Roemer, Milton I. COMPARATIVE NATIONAL POLICIES ON HEALTH CARE.
New York: Marcel Dekker, 1977.

This important volume grew out of the life work of this well-known
scholar in CNSHS and more particularly his work with the AAMC
self-study course in international health (see vol. 5 of the AAMC
work cited in chapter 3.4). The vast amount of information brought
together in this book represents major aspects of health care. The
author breaks down the data according to seven components: (1)
economic support of health services, (2) health manpower resources,
(3) health care facilities, (4) patterns of delivering medical care,
(5) patterns of delivering preventive services, (6) regulation of
health care, and (7) methods of health administration and planning.
Likewise, to simplify the range of countries under discussion, the
author uses five categories of political structure and level of economic development which have the greatest influence on the health
care system of a particular country: (1) free enterprise states,

(2) welfare states, (3) underdeveloped states, (4) transitional states, and (5) socialist states. The author makes an effort to offer illustrations from more than one country of each of the five types. Additional readings are given for each chapter.

_____. "General Physician Services under Eight National Patterns." AJPH 60 (October 1970): 1893-99.

The countries studied were the same as for this author's study of medical care under social security (see previous entry). Describes aspects of organizing general practice in these countries. Just two general patterns are found--the indirect, in which the government social security agency contracts for service from relatively independent practitioners (Belgium, Canada, FRG, UK), and the direct pattern, in which general physicians services are offered through government facilities with physicians employed on salary (Ecuador, Tunisia, India, Poland). But the article gives essential qualifications. For example, in Ecuador only 5 percent of the population is so covered and these are mostly urban; the salary is usually for two or three hours of a doctor's time, the rest of which he devotes to private practice. Also, this way of classifying the UK sounds "looser" than the usual conception of a national health service (versus an NHI). But, as Roemer notes, "General physicians are in private practice, but each is paid fixed monthly amounts in accordance with the number of persons who have chosen him for care."

_____. MEDICAL CARE IN LATIN AMERICA. Washington, D.C.: Technical Publications and Documents, Department of Social Affairs, Pan American Union, 1963.

One of the earliest and classic works in CNSHS, employing a common framework concerning organization, financing, control, and sponsorship structures, as well as social class and the social security mechanisms and distribution of care. Compares the medical care systems of several Latin and South American countries.

_____. THE ORGANIZATION OF MEDICAL CARE UNDER SOCIAL SECURITY. Geneva: ILO, 1969. 155 refs., index.

Detailed study of the operation of medical care under social security in eight countries--Belgium, Canada, Ecuador, FRG, India, Poland, Tunisia, and UK. Discusses evaluation, structure, function, costs, and quality of programs. Employs a common stated framework in the description and analysis of each system. Major elements of this framework include the social setting of medical care patterns (whether industrialized or not and whether the political structure favors private enterprise and local autonomy or planned production and centralized government control); basic patterns of medical care organization (i.e., indirect purchase of service from independent professionals and organizations; or direct provision of service through government health institutions); and elements of medical care (quantity, quality, cost, and results). One of the most valuable works in the field.

_____. "Political Ideology and Health Care: Hospital Patterns in the Philippines and Cuba." INT'L. J. H. SERV. 3 (1973): 487-92.

Starting from a similar heritage of Spanish colonialism followed by U.S. influence, the Philippines and Cuba developed sharply divergent ideologies after Cuba's socialist revolution in 1959. In the Philippines today there is a pattern of hospital services based strongly on capitalist "free market" ideology; government facilities, intended to serve the majority of the population, are meager while private ones are relatively abundant and compete for a small market of paying patients. In Cuba, virtually all hospital resources have been placed in the public sector and urban-rural disparities have been greatly reduced. All hospital services are available to every resident on an equal basis. This work is a good example of contrasting case studies (see Elling and Kerr, chapter 7). However, the framework for contrasting the two systems should have been made more explicit.

_____. "Strategies for Increasing Rural Medical Manpower in Five Industrialized Countries." Paper presented at the Eighth Int'l. Scientific Meetings of the IEA, Puerto Rico, September 17-23, 1977. Available from the author, School of Public Health, University of California, Los Angeles.

In order to learn lessons relevant for the United States, health manpower policies and practices were investigated in five countries with differing systems of NHI or health service. Field visits were made to Australia, Belgium, Canada, Norway, and Poland for five to ten weeks each; semistructured interviews were conducted with key leaders of the Ministry of Health, other governmental and private health agencies, the universities and other educational institutions, hospitals, health centers, professional associations, and citizen organizations. The focus of investigation was on adjustments in manpower production and use to the demands for health service generated by the various systems of health insurance. In all five countries, deliberate strategies are employed to increase the settlement of physicians in rural areas. All strategies include financial incentives, but these alone never seem to be sufficient, so that various additional inducements are usually given. The nature of these supplementary inducements reflects the political ideology embodied in each country's health care system.

Roesch, Georges, and Sandier, Simone. "A Comparison of the Health Care System in France and the United States." Paper presented at the Int'l. Conference on Health Care Costs and Expenditures, Bethesda, Maryland, Fogarty Int'l. Center, NIH, June 2-4, 1975. Available from the Fogarty Center. 14 tables, diagrams, 30 refs.

A lengthy, very impressive paper employing available data on use, costs, facilities, personnel, and so forth in the two systems. Presents a set of categories of concern for developing and presenting the data. Discusses both systems as market-oriented, growing in size and cost and relatively uncontrolled.

Salkever, David S. "Economic Class and Differential Access to Care: Comparisons among Health Care Systems." INT'L. J. H. SERV. 5 (1975): 373-95. 16 refs., appendix.

Author's summary: "This paper presents a new technique for describing inequality of access to medical care. Access is described by the empirical relationship between need and the probability of entering the health care system for treatment. The need-entry probability relationship for one population group is compared with that for another population group to determine the extent of access differentials (differences in entry probabilities) at varying levels of need. As an illustrative application, the technique is employed to describe access differentials by economic class in six different geographic areas located in five different countries (Canada, England, Finland, Poland, United States) with differently structured health care systems. Although the findings for adults varied considerably from area to area, the access differentials among children were surprisingly consistent and unrelated to health care system structure. In particular, it appears that higher family income is associated with greater access to medical care among children at all levels of need. The paper concludes with suggestions for further applications of the proposed technique to problems of monitoring and evaluating the effectiveness of policies aimed at reducing the extent of access inequality."

Schicke, R.K. ARZT UND GESUNDHEITSVERSORGUNG IM GESELLSCHAFT-LICHEN SICHERUNGSSYSTEM. BUNDESREPUBLIK DEUTSCHLAND, ENGLAND, U.S.A. [Physician and health organization in the social security systems in Germany, England, and the United States]. Freiburg im Breisgau, FRG: Verlag Rombacht, 1971. In German.

The writer compares social security systems, health organization, and role of the physician in the United States, England, and West Germany. Society and the social position of social security are emphasized. The latter is analyzed through its structure, functioning, financing, and the role of the physician.

Seham, Max. "An American Doctor Looks at Eleven Foreign Health Systems." See chapter 3.2.

Article gives data and general observations on certain common points from eleven health systems. Not a comprehensive systematic study of these systems.

Simanis, Joseph G. NATIONAL HEALTH SYSTEMS IN EIGHT COUNTRIES. DHEW Pub. No. (SSA) 75-11924. Washington, D.C.: Government Printing Office, January, 1975. 107 p. Charts, refs.

> Done as an extension of the Office of Research and Statistics publication, Social Security Administration, on NHI proposals for the United States. Using secondary material, this book compares the health systems of Australia, Canada, FRG, France, Netherlands, New Zealand, Sweden, and UK. A standard outline is used to describe each system: (1) background; (2) organization of health care delivery; (3) coverage; (4) benefits; (5) procedures for obtaining care; (6) role of private insurance; (7) financing; (8) reimbursement procedures.

Stone, Deborah. "Professionalism and Accountability: Controlling Health Services in the United States and West Germany." Paper presented to the annual meeting of the American Political Science Association, Palmer House, Chicago, August 29-September 2, 1974. 23 notes and refs.

> This paper examines the new Professional Standards Review program in light of a similar program (Economic Monitoring) used in West Germany for over forty years. Professional Standards Review Organizations (PSROs) were created by Congress to help control the quality and costs of the health services purchased by the federal government through Social Security programs. In the first section, the PSRO program is described as government-mandated peer review by professional organizations, and this is compared and contrasted with the West German system. The second section argues that the PSROs are likely to strengthen the organization of established medicine, to increase the bargaining power of professional organizations, and to further insulate professional behavior from public scrutiny. The third section describes some of the effects of bureaucratic rigidities in peer review on the practice of medicine; these are the preservation of old technologies, the development of fixed patterns of practice, and the strengthening of the technical and interventionist biases in medical care. The final section evaluates the PSRO program as a failure of Congress to set any rules for the development and application of norms and standards. The lack of any mechanism for accountability of the PSROs to the public is emphasized. Based on the author's Ph.D. thesis work, Duke University, 1975, which spells out a framework for comparing the distribution of power as between public and professional interests in FRG and the United States.

Tait, H.P. "Health Services in India and Burma: Their Evolution and Present Status." MED. HISTORY (London) 16 (April 1972): 169-78.

> After expressing a set of key concerns with respect to health services development generally, the author outlines developments in the health field and indicates health objectives of the government of India. He summarizes the structure of India's health admini-

stration and points out that India was the first country to adopt
family planning as a national policy. Trained doctors and medical
teachers are urgently needed. Distribution of doctors is uneven
with most engaged in private practice. The Fourth Five-Year Plan
proposes further training and hospital facilities. Although there
have been improvements in education of nursing and paramedical
staff, much remains to be done. Construction of health facilities
is being undertaken in rural areas. The fields of public health,
general sanitation, nutrition, maternal and child health, school
health, and communicable disease control are discussed. In Burma,
the overriding problem is a financial one. Special programs deal
with malnutrition and communicable diseases. Burma has attempted
to unify curative, preventive, and social medicine; a system of
rural health centers staffed by health assistants is well established.
The author outlines Burma's health administration and such public
health activities as sanitation, nutrition, and maternal and child
health. There is only one doctor per 9,000 population and the
shortage of nurses is acute, but a school of paramedical science
has been established at Rangoon, and teaching programs for other
medical personnel are being expanded.

Terris, Milton. "The Three World Systems of Medical Care: Trends and Prospects." Paper presented at the 105th annual meeting of the APHA, Washington,
D.C., October 30-November 3, 1977. Available from the author through
the APHA, Washington, D.C.

There exists in the world today three basic systems of medical care:
public charity, health insurance, and national health service. The
public charity system is dominant in 115 countries with 49 percent
of the world's population; the health insurance system, 25 countries with 17 percent of the world's population; and the national
health service system, 16 countries with 34 percent of the world's
population.

The basic characteristics of each system are described with regard
to types of nations, their location, degree of industrialization, and
their economic system. In addition, the population coverage,
methods of financing, scope of services, methods of providing service, and type of administrative agency are described. The author
concludes that the most logical and rational system is the national
health service. Compares Sweden's and the UK's transitions from
health insurance to health service, and discusses the prospects for
transition of other industrial countries to a national health service.

Troupin, James L. "Medical Care and Public Health in Finland, Soviet Union,
Czechoslovakia and Yugoslavia." AJPH 59 (April 1969): 705-10.

Although not extensive enough and explicit enough as regards a
general health systems framework used in comparing systems to be
included in this section, this work does give a brief overview of
these four systems and focuses on the integration of medical care

VANDERBILT MEDICAL CENTER LIBRARY

with public health in each system. It is at least suggestive of the kind of work that is needed in comparing more than one system.

Viel, Benjamin. LA MEDICINA SOCIALIZADA Y SU APLICACIÓN EN GRAN BRETAÑA, LA UNION SOVIETICA Y CHILE [Socialized medicine and its application in Great Britain, USSR and Chile]. Santiago: Universidad de Chile, 1964. In Spanish.

> After laying out what is meant by socialized medicine and its dimensions, the author examines, primarily through available information, how and to what extent these dimensions have been achieved in the three countries.

Weinerman, E. Richard. "The Organization of Health Services in Eastern Europe: Report of a Study of Czechoslovakia, Hungary, and Poland." MED. CARE 6 (July-August 1968): 267-78.

> A preview with summary and discussion of key points in the framework with related findings reported more fully in the authors monograph (see following item).

Weinerman, E. Richard, and Weinerman, Shirley B. SOCIAL MEDICINE IN EASTERN EUROPE: THE ORGANIZATION OF HEALTH SERVICES AND THE EDUCATION OF MEDICAL PERSONNEL IN CZECHOSLOVAKIA, HUNGARY AND POLAND. Cambridge, Mass.: Harvard Univ. Press, 1969.

> Comprehensive investigation of these three countries, whose political economic similarities are influenced by traditional national differences. Discussed are organizational levels, authority linkages with government, medical schools, physician distribution, polyclinics, and access of citizens to medical care. Has the virtue of employing an explicit common framework for the description and analysis of the three systems.

Zayed, Marlene. "Contrasting Case Studies of National Health Systems in Arab Countries." Required student research paper, University of Connecticut School of Medicine. Available from Program in CNSHS, Univ. Conn. Health Center, Farmington, Ct. or on interlibrary loan from the Univ. Conn. Health Center Library, Farmington, Ct. 06032.

> A valuable student research paper comparing socioeconomic conditions, health systems, and regionalization of health services in Arab countries, particularly Syria versus Saudi Arabia, and Iraq versus Egypt. Has a wealth of information on these systems not otherwise treated in the comparative health system literature.

Chapter 5

FRAMEWORK STATEMENTS

Not all the items in this chapter explicitly and deliberately formulate an interrelated set of concepts which might guide researchers to the important aspects of total national realities to be observed and compared or contrasted in CNSHS. But all items contribute in one way or another and to one degree or another to providing this kind of much needed but as yet not well-developed guide. Most work in the field is ignorant of this need. Usually, a particular health system is described or more than one compared along lines which the author presumes to be the important or possibly the only ones. Or maybe these are simply the traditional aspects of health systems about which information is usually available--such as health status indicators (usually limited to mortality rates), health personnel-population ratios, hospital bed-population ratios, payment arrangements, and costs for health care (often as a percent of GNP). Or one finds different authors, for example, in a collection of descriptions of different systems such as HEALTH SERVICES PROSPECTS (see Douglas-Wilson and McLachlan in chapter 3.4) describing some more or less similar aspects and other very different ones. This descriptive work may be useful in theory construction insofar as it tells the theorist what other students of health systems have found important to describe. One seldom finds any deliberate discussion of why certain aspects are described or should be described.

For the most part only such deliberate attempts to provide a framework are included here. And generally these are comprehensive attempts, that is, directed toward conceiving of health systems as wholes in relation to their national socioeconomic, political, cultural, and epidemiologic contexts (though one of the key points of variation in frameworks is the amount and kind of attention paid to the political-economic context especially).

Perhaps the most inclusive review of the theoretical literature is given by Miguel. He attempts to show a historical progression toward greater inclusiveness as regards the whole health system, and, most recently, attention to the political economic context. While Miguel's work is important and valuable for its completeness, and classificatory suggestion, it does not provide an in-depth review and analysis of work in the field. Such a review and analysis remains to be done.

Perhaps the major watershed between theorists is the way they conceive of
health systems as fitting into and being determined by their surrounding societies.
The bulk of work in the field, wittingly or otherwise, adopts a set of assumptions which sees society as a generally harmonious system of functionally interrelated parts, with the health system as one of these parts directed toward maintaining the members of society in a productive, useful (healthful) role. This
can be termed the consensual or integrative view. The fundamental assumption
involved is that society is held together by common values and beliefs. Perhaps
Field's work is most clear in this view.

The contrary view focuses on disparities and associated class struggles in capitalist political economies. This view sees the health system as favoring the
elite and ambivalently helping the worker and peasant classes when it is in the
interest of the ruling class, but ignoring or primarily serving as an instrument
of social control when there might be danger of the masses developing greater
consciousness and solidarity, and taking state power into their own hands. This
can be termed the conflict or coercion perspective. Perhaps its clearest spokes-
person is Navarro (see, for example, the last chapter of his MEDICINE UNDER
CAPITALISM). In this view, society is seen as held together by force, ultimately the armed force of army and police, with values and beliefs peddled
through the media and "acceptable" political organization as an ideology supportive of the ruling class. The worker-peasant class, insofar as it develops
consciousness and moves toward revolutionary struggle, includes different medical
and public health priorities, values, and beliefs. The contrast in the two perspectives can be seen in the emphases of the health systems of the PRC and the
United States.

Perhaps the sharpest focus on picking out the different assumptions involved in
the conflict and consensual perspectives is given in chapter 5 of Dahrendorf's
CLASS AND CLASS CONFLICT IN INDUSTRIAL SOCIETY. As theory develops
further in CNSHS, it seems likely to follow one or the other of these lines.
No integration is available, nor does it seem likely that one can be developed.

Abel-Smith, Brian. "Health Priorities in Developing Countries: The Economist's
Contribution." INT'L. J. H. SERV. 2 (1972): 5-12.

> Though many new techniques have been developed to assist countries
> in allocating their resources, there are special difficulties in using
> these techniques in health services. The key problem is finding an
> acceptable measure of health output. The author argues that health
> should not be measured in crude economic terms and points out why
> no alternative measure has yet been evolved.

Agency for International Development. Office of Development Program Review
and Evaluation. "Project Evaluation Guidelines." 3d ed. M.O. 1026.1
Supplement I. Washington, D.C., August 1974.

> While directed toward health demonstration and other development
> projects, rather than overall health systems, this statement is useful

for laying out many of the variables of concern to an external
administrative center of interest. Thus this statement provides
data for framework development rather than a framework per se.

Aiken, Michael, and Hage, Jerald. "Organizational Interdependence and Intra-
Organizational Structure." ASR 33 (1968): 912-30.

One of the best empirical-research-based conceptual statements of
factors affecting the development of joint programs between agencies and the effect of joint programs on internal agency structure
and function. One of the major factors in a competitive market-
type political economy is the actual or promised receipt of greater
support for both agencies establishing a joint program. Important
in its implications for coordination among health agencies. Reprinted in Brinkerhoff and Kunz (see below).

Alford, Robert R. HEALTH CARE POLITICS: INTEREST GROUP AND IDEO-
LOGICAL BARRIERS TO REFORM. Chicago: Univ. of Chicago Press, 1975.

Carries further the analysis first laid out in his article "The Political Economy of Health Care" (see below). While very valuable
for identifying health-related organized interest groups, particularly
in the United States, this work does not elaborate sufficiently
the political economy as a whole and its control as related to the
class structure and government. For this, one must consult Krause,
Navarro, Waitzkin, and others.

_____. "The Political Economy of Health Care: Dynamics without Change."
POLITICS AND SOCIETY 2 (Winter 1972): 127-64.

Analysis of US health reforms in the context of the struggle between
interest groups. The health system resists change. The problem is
seen in terms of the domination of the private sector and the inability of the political system to effect changes. Although major
interest groups such as corporate rationalizers are identified, the
work fails to articulate these with the class and power structure
of the United States and does not connect government actions to
the interests of the ruling class. Some combination of this perspective with that of Navarro should be developed in which the
role of government health legislation and programs would be seen
more clearly as protecting or enhancing the position of the ruling
class vis a vis the health sector. The book by Krause, POWER
AND ILLNESS, cited below, may come closest to providing this
combination.

American Public Health Association. FAMILY PLANNING, MATERNAL & CHILD
HEALTH, AND NUTRITION: GUIDELINES FOR DEIDS PLANNING-I. Washington, D.C., August 1973.

Under contract from AID the APHA undertook to establish and

evaluate health services development projects in several countries. This DEIDS project sought to establish guidelines for individual projects. While suggestive of commonly recognized considerations, it is not especially creative. Nor does the bland approach to political economic differences (almost as if they could be ignored) recommend this work.

Andersen, Ronald. "Cross-National Comparisons of Health Services Systems." In CROSS-NATIONAL SOCIOMEDICAL RESEARCH: CONCEPTS, METHODS, PRACTICE, edited by Manfred Pflanz and Elisabeth Schach, pp. 25-35. Stuttgart, Germany: Thieme, 1976.

Framework for study of health systems particularly valuable in identifying health services-population links and sociopsychological variables. The broad categories (and subparts) of concern are (1) societal characteristics (wealth-technology, political norms, physical environment), (2) health service system (organization, resources), (3) individual characteristics (predisposing factors, enabling factors, need), (4) health services utilization (type, site, purpose, time interval), (5) satisfaction (of consumers, providers, third-party payers, public, government), and (6) health level (mortality, morbidity, disability). Some figures are provided to clarify suspected interrelations. Personal and sociopsychological characteristics are elaborated in figure 2.

Anderson, Odin. "Towards a Framework for Analysing Health Services Systems." SOCIAL AND ECONOMIC ADMINISTRATION 1 (January 1967): 16-21.

Outlines the framework which served for the author's study of the health systems of Sweden, UK, and United States (see chapter 4).

Badgley, Robin F., et al. "International Studies of Health Manpower: A Sociologic Perspective." In ASILOMAR CONFERENCE ON INTERNATIONAL STUDIES OF MEDICAL CARE, edited by John H. Mabry, pp. 235-52. Special issue of MED. CARE 9 (May-June 1971). 45 notes and refs.

With concern for the supply of health manpower in the face of a worldwide rising demand for adequate health care, the report of this workshop group first takes up general considerations and definitions. It is noted that units are not comparable since the division of labor between physicians and other workers differs along with organizational relationships (e.g., general community physicians in the United States can usually practice in hospitals, while such work is reserved to specialists in the UK). A second part critiques traditional approaches to health manpower planning, such as designation of some health personnel-population ratio as a policy goal, demographic projection added to the last approach, estimation of health services needs, estimation of supply and demand, analysis of health services functions, and target setting. The third section of the report offers a sociologic perspective focusing on the system of organization of health manpower in different countries. "Each system develops distinctive patterns for the recruitment of new members which regulate the behavior of individuals." In the final section, a set of topics are suggested for future research: health occupational group membership, group organization, occupational roles, socialization and recruitment, incentives and career mobility, social controls (e.g., on the extent of private practice allowed to government physicians), professions and bureaucracy, sociopolitical implications of health manpower recommendations.

Battistella, Roger M. "Rationalization of Health Services: Political and Social Assumptions." INT'L. J. H. SERV. 2 (1972): 331-48.

The application of managerial and organizational principles characteristic of large-scale business and industry (i.e., quantification of decision-making, consolidation of production, money rewards for cost savings, and economies of scale) is increasingly seen as the key to controlling health care costs. Because of the tendency toward convergence in the problems governments face in the financing and delivery of health care, it is suggested that developments in the United States may be relevant to other countries in similarly advanced stages of economic growth. Accepts the assumptions of convergence theory, that is, that all industrial countries' health systems share certain problems. This view has been critiqued by Navarro and others on grounds that political economic transformations can and do make real differences in whether the primary emphasis of health services is on high technology and special care for the few or on adequate general and preventive care for the many.

Beck, R.G. "Economic Class and Access to Physician Services under Public Medical Care Insurance." INT'L. J. H. SERV. 3 (1973): 341-55.

Examines the effects of public medical care insurance on access to physician services. Access is measured as the inverse of the proportion of families of a given economic class who have not used physician services in a given year. Data are presented for the period 1963-68 for a large sample of families in the Province of Saskatchewan in Canada. The evidence suggests that low-income classes have less contact with physicians than high-income classes. This disparity in accessibility is reduced, but not removed, as experience with Medicare increases. Concludes that public medical care insurance does increase relative accessibility to physicians for the low-income classes.

Belmar, Roberto, and Sidel, Victor W. "An International Perspective on Strikes and Strike Threats by Physicians: The Case of Chile." INT'L. J. H. SERV. 5 (1975): 53-61. 51 refs.

Author's summary: "The program for health services developed by
the government of Dr. Salvador Allende Gossens in Chile is outlined, as well as its early effects. A review of this development
is necessary to an understanding of the systematic opposition of
the organized medical profession to this program in particular, and
to the broad socialist goals of the government in general. Three
periods of activity by the medical profession are traced, beginning
in September 1970 and culminating in September 1973 with the
military coup and overthrow of the democratically elected government of Chile and the murder of its president, a physician. While
the medical profession was opposed to the government program for
community participation in health care and to changes in the models
for delivery of care, and feared a changed status for the physician,
clearly there were broader political links between the organized
medical profession and the political opponents of the government
which sought its overthrow."

This report clearly links the medical profession of the presocialist
period to the ruling class, and shows a connection between the
medical profession's resistance to the Allende government and US
intervention, including the CIA and economic sanctions. The
medical profession was linked to the ruling class more through land
holdings, other economic interests, and political economic ideology,
than through specific or general philosophic concerns with regard
to the changes in the health system under Allende.

Benjamin, B. SOCIAL AND ECONOMIC FACTORS AFFECTING MORTALITY.
The Hague: Mouton, 1965.

Similar to work of Thomas McKeown in challenging the contribution
of health services to longer life. Instead, nutrition, sanitation,
and improved living conditions are seen as primary. Whatever the
contribution of health services, it seems clear that in UDCs greater
benefits are to be derived from preventive health programs than
from modern curative care.

Bonnet, Phillip D., and Ruderman, A. Peter. "Health Care Systems and Fi-
nancing." In HEALTH PLANNING: QUALITATIVE ASPECTS AND QUANTI-
TATIVE TECHNIQUES, edited by W.A. Reinke, pp. 208-18. Baltimore: Johns
Hopkins Univ. Press, 1972.

Each country has its particular political, cultural, and historical
tradition. Decision making may be centralized, resulting in a
formal, easily recognized system, or diffused, and less formal.
Neither the centralized nor the decentralized system guarantees
great effectiveness or economy, although the centralized is generally assumed to provide a more equitable system of health care
where resources are scarce. Sponsorship may be public or private,
but comprehensive care is rarely provided. Discusses advantages
and disadvantages of various types of financial sponsorship of health
care systems. Lists additional readings.

Boulding, Kenneth E. THE IMAGE: KNOWLEDGE IN LIFE AND SOCIETY.
Ann Arbor: Univ. of Michigan Press, 1956.

> Considers the dynamics of behavior in terms of individual and
> shared world images. Examines the processes of organization, em-
> phasizing communication and feedback of information and know-
> ledge for organized growth. One of the best attempts at a uni-
> fied theory for the social sciences. An image is defined as the
> way any social unit (person, group, organization, nation, etc.)
> presents itself to the world of significant others and receives im-
> pressions (knowledge information) from the world.

Brenner, M. Harvey. "Health Costs and Benefits of Economic Policy." INT'L.
J. H. SERV. 7 (1977): 581-623. 133 refs.

> From the author's abstract: "The purpose of this study is to trans-
> late research findings on pathological effects of unemployment and
> other forms of economic distress into a form that would be useful
> for national economic policy decisions. . . . Overall, it is evi-
> dent that significant relationships exist between economic policy
> and measures of national well-being. This study indicates that
> actions which influence national economic activity--especially the
> unemployment rate--have a substantial bearing on physical health,
> mental health, and criminal aggression. To the extent, therefore,
> that economic policy has acted to influence economic activity, it
> has always been related to the nation's social health. It would
> appear that on a day-to-day basis, nearly all political and deli-
> berate economic policy decisions which affect the national, re-
> gional, and local economic situations also are associated with many
> aspects of the nation's well-being. Indeed, significant ameliora-
> tion of many of our basic social problems may depend, in part,
> on national economic policy considerations."

_____. MENTAL ILLNESS AND THE ECONOMY. Cambridge, Mass.: Harvard
Univ. Press, 1973.

> Shows that mental hospital admissions in the United States rise as
> the business cycle declines and vice versa. Discusses this phe-
> nomenon in terms of the tensions of a capitalist economy and so-
> ciety in times of recession and depression. Conflicts with Eyer
> (see below, this chapter) who sees a time lag between business-
> cycle trends and illness occurrence. Although both Brenner and
> Eyer see a relationship between economics and illness, they differ
> on data presentation and interpretation. Also see Stark, this chapter.

Breslow, Lester. "Research in a Strategy for Health Improvement." INT'L. J.
H. SERV. 3 (1973): 7-16.

> Author's summary: "A strategy for health improvement should in-
> clude personal health care, environmental control measures, and
> means of influencing health-related behavior. All three of these

ways of improving health are applicable in the present state of knowledge to most major health problems, including trauma from automobile accidents, dental caries, myocardial infarction, lung cancer, and infant deaths. Research as an integral part of this strategy should be directed toward both what to do and how to do it. The problems of dental caries and lung cancer are examined in some detail to indicate the role of research in a strategy for health improvement."

An important contribution by an outstanding figure in public health, but one which runs the risk of making health primarily a personal matter leading possibly to a new version of "victim blaming." See Crawford, this chapter.

Brinkerhoff, Merlin B., and Kunz, Phillip R., eds. COMPLEX ORGANIZA-TIONS AND THEIR ENVIRONMENTS. Dubuque, Iowa: Brown, 1972. Bibliography, no index.

The most valuable collection of sociological work with implications for the interdependencies of health institutions with elements of their environments, such as other institutions, occupational groups, governmental and other control agencies, sources of support, and the class and power structure of their society (though this last aspect is not as well or fully developed as in the work of Navarro, cited below). The general model of organizations implied if not explicitly developed in these articles is the open systems view: "Open-systems theory suggests that the organization, which is the object of analysis, is only a part of a larger system, and is in continual interaction with other parts of the system because it is dependent upon them for resources as input and for recipients of the output" (xiii).

Bryant, John H. "Principles of Justice as a Basis for Conceptualizing a Health Care System." INT'L. J. H. SERV. 7 (1977): 707-19. 9 refs.

Author is concerned with the causes of the worldwide maldistribution of health care. Explores briefly the question of entitlement to health care, focusing on the appropriateness of expressing that entitlement in terms of social justice. Formulates some principles of justice as related to health care, drawing on the thinking of John Rawls and Nicholas Rescher. In short, a survival or "adequate" minimum is to be provided to the least fortunate (not like the socialist alternative which is to strive for equality). These principles are then used as a basis for planning a theoretical health care system in an LDC. This theoretical health care system is intended to reflect a just distribution of health care under conditions of varying limitations of resources, including those in which resources are not adequate to provide care for all of the people. Discusses some of the technical, social, and political implications of such a system.

Critical commentaries on this article are given in the same issue
by George Silver, Michael Stewart, and Sander Kelman. Kelman
critiques the metaphysical perspective Bryant offers and ties the
problems of health and health services to real political economic
structures from a Marxian perspective.

Brzeski, Andrzej. "Social Engineering and Realpolitik in Communist Reorgani-
zation." In ESSAYS IN SOCIALISM AND PLANNING IN HONOR OF CARL
LANDAUER, edited by Gregory Grossman, pp. 148-83. Englewood Cliffs,
N.J.: Prentice-Hall, 1970. 70 refs.

Important for conceptualizing the political economic context of
health systems. Opening with a quote from Lenin as his motto--
"Politics cannot but have priority over economics. To argue differently is to forget the ABC of Marxism"--the author offers numerous examples and illustrations of economic reorganizations drawn
mostly from USSR and Poland, with some contrasting examples from
Yugoslavia, which he maintains, show that political struggles within
a sometimes divided collective leadership form the base for change
or resistance to change rather than some rational solution to economic efficiency or direction. "The new communist realpolitik is
that of checks and balances among 'collective leaders.' The organizational complement of this delicate political equilibrium is
a progressive fragmentation of authority (including economic decision making), fostered as a safeguard against a takeover a la
Stalin, Bierut, or Rakosi. In this new environment, ministries can
challenge the planning commissions, central boards and trusts can
defy ministries, and so on down the hierarchical line." Officials
are seen as building constituencies in relation to organizations and
sectors of the economy based on shared personal experiences and
other "nonrational" or "nonplanned" identities and interests. But
these constituencies and loyalties are seen as unconnected with
relatively enduring interest issues as is true for pluralist, interest
group politics in Western countries--labor, farmers, industry, and
so forth. Instead loyalties are fast shifting. Thus he recommends
a restudy of Machiavelli and "Kremlinology." In any case, according to this author, some of the organizational phenomena are
seen to be occuring--such as striving for survival and growth, competition and coalition and cooptation in interorganizational relations--
and there is a general trend toward decentralization and reform of
the economy in terms of markets versus a centralized "commercial
economy." Does not deal with the class issue.

Cartwright, Anne. PATIENTS AND THEIR DOCTORS. London: Routledge and
Kegan Paul, 1967.

A thorough sociological consideration of physician-patient relations
in the UK. Generally, a patient's satisfaction is seen as a function of the degree to which his or her hopes and expectations of
relief and reassurance are met and the degree to which his or her
problem was handled expeditiously and with personal attention and

compassion. As care passes more and more into large impersonal, bureaucratic settings, a curious contradiction develops. The technical and knowledge base may be improved in the institutional setting, but patient satisfaction may decline. Thus this study indicates a substantial degree of approval of individual providers such as personal physicians and a large residue of dissatisfaction with doctors in general and particularly with institutions such as hospitals, outpatient departments, and emergency rooms.

Cassel, John. "Psychosocial Processes and 'Stress': Theoretical Formulation." INT'L. J. H. SERV. 4 (1974): 471-82. 51 refs.

Author's summary: "Despite widespread belief that psychosocial processes may be important in disease etiology, attempts to document the role of such factors in epidemiologic studies have led to conflicting and often confusing results. It is the thesis of this paper that this is largely a result of inadequacies in our theoretical framework. The point of view is presented that this stems from an uncritical subscription to and often erroneous interpretation of stress theory, a failure to recognize that psychosocial processes are unlikely to be directly pathogenic (in the way that, for example, a microorganism is) and unlikely to be unidimensional. An alternative point of view with data from animal and human studies is presented, and the implications for research strategy and the delivery of health care are discussed."

A most significant statement from one of the foremost social epidemiologists. Implies that health prevention and service efforts must be directed toward high risk groups exposed to pathogenic social conditions, not just those exposed to infectious agents, though these will often turn out to be the same groups, since the stressful social conditions prepare the groundwork for various disease agents to have their effect.

Chance, Norman. "China: Socialist Transformation and the Dialectical Process." Paper presented at the symposium "China: The Socialist Transformation" at annual meeting of the American Anthropological Assn., Toronto, December 2, 1972. 11 refs. Available from the author, Dept. of Anthropology, Univ. of Conn., Storrs, Conn. 06268

An important paper clarifying the way in which ideological struggle was used to change social reality and human consciousness in the PRC during the Cultural Revolution.

Cleaver, Harry. "Malaria and the Political Economy of Public Health." INT'L. J. H. SERV. 7 (1977): 557-79. 52 refs.

Malaria has been making a dramatic resurgence in the 1970s. Government response has been inadequate despite appeals by public health officials and the availability of adequate resources. This article seeks an understanding of this decontrol in the history of the political economy of public health and in an analysis of the current international economic crisis. The current world crisis is another period of social conflict--one in which various sectors of business and various governments are trying to restore the conditions of growth and accumulation which were ruptured in the late 1960s by an international cycle of social instability. Allowing malaria to spread, like allowing drought and flood to turn into famine, thus appears as a de facto repressive use of "nature" to reestablish social control. These circumstances raise hard questions regarding the most effective means of reversing these trends.

Cole, S., and Lejeune, R. "Illness and the Legitimation of Failure." ASR 37 (1972): 347-56.

A study of welfare mothers which builds a case for the interpretation that reported illness is used to legitimate failure. Comment: This is a version of "blaming the victim." Fails to ask: Whose failure or the failure of what: A system with high unemployment and welfare support which splits families? or the individual who chooses not to run like Sammy in such a system?

Conover, Patrick W. "Social Class and Chronic Illness." INT'L. J. H. SERV. 3 (1973): 357-68.

This paper traces a three-stage history of theorization on the causal relationship between social class and chronic illness, focusing on the contributions of Kadushin and Mechanic. Five areas of agreement between Kadushin and Mechanic are presented as a basis for further analysis: (1) the importance of data from the National Health Survey; (2) the necessity for studying chronic disease problems within comparable age categories; (3) the more severe measure of chronic diseases, as shown by activity limitation or work loss, are clearly class related, with the greatest magnitude of change between the lowest income category and the next highest category; (4) no reliable data oppose the above evidence; (5) it is more likely that persons will accurately report more severe episodes of chronic illness than less severe episodes. Two central research questions are then addressed: What is the true shape of the relationship between socioeconomic status and chronic disease? What are the most reasonable of the possible causes of this relationship? New material from the National Health Survey is analyzed to answer these questions. Certain relationships are noted: There is a strong relationship between income and measures of chronic disease for both whites and nonwhites. With a threefold division of the income category, there are large differences between income levels. These relationships hold over a wide range of specific chronic diseases. The author concludes that Kadushin's hypothesis of overreaction to illness by the lower classes is of little significance. More study is needed of the downwardly mobile effects of chronic illness. The effects of poor health and low socioeconomic status are presumed to be circular.

Framework Statements

Cox, Caroline, and Mead, Adrianne, eds. A SOCIOLOGY OF MEDICAL PRACTICE. London: Collier-MacMillan, 1975.

> A work with important conceptual material on the meaning and perception of illness and doctor-patient relations in different (primarily US and UK) systems. An article by Cassee examines nurse-patient communication in Dutch hospitals. There is little on the health system level, though a valuable piece by Derek Gill traces out the embeddedness of the NHS in the UK political economic context by examining its roots in sociopolitical history. About half the book is made up of previously published classic pieces by Renee Fox, Eliot Freidson, Erving Goffman, Julian Hart, Anselm Strauss and Barney Glaser, Arnold Rose, and Irving Zola. In addition, there are several pieces with general concepts but an empirical base in the British experience. There are also articles by Nancy Milio, "Values, Social Class and Community Health Services"; Ernest Becker, "Socialization, Command of Performance and Mental Illness"; Fred Davis, "Professional Socialization as Subjective Experience: The Process of Doctrinal Conversion among Student Nurses." The article by Michael J. Bloor and Gordon W. Horobin, "Conflict and Conflict Resolution in Doctor/Patient Interactions," seems particularly potent in its critique of the Parsonian view. Instead of doctor-patient harmony, they see inherent conflict with the patient in a "double-bind."

Crawford, Robert. "You Are Dangerous to Your Health: The Ideology and Politics of Victim Blaming." INT'L. J. H. SERV. 7 (1977): 663-80. 52 refs.

> Describes the emergence of an ideology which blames the individual for her or his illness and proposes that, instead of relying on costly and inefficient medical services, the individual should take more responsibility for her or his health. At-risk behavior is seen as the problem; changing lifestyle, through education and/or economic sanctions, is seen as the solution. The emergence of the ideology is explained by the contradictions arising from the threat of high medical costs, popular expectations of medicine along with political pressures for protection or extension of entitlements, and the politicization of environmental and occupational health issues. These contradictions produce a crisis which is at once economic, political, and ideological, and which requires responses to destabilizing conditions in each of these spheres. These ideological responses, on the one hand, serve to reorder expectations and to justify the demand for access to medical services, while attempting to divert attention from the social causation of disease in the commercial and industrial sectors.

> While this analysis applies especially to the United States, it also has relevance to many other countries such as Canada which have taken up the ideology found in Marc Lalonde's book (cited below, this chapter).

Culyer, A.J. "The Nature of the Commodity 'Health Care' and Its Efficient Allocation." OXFORD ECONOMIC PAPERS 23 (July 1971): 189-211.

Dahrendorf, Ralph. CLASS AND CLASS CONFLICT IN INDUSTRIAL SOCIETY. Stanford, Calif.: Stanford Univ. Press, 1959.

An analysis of the social structure as capable of producing the elements of its own supersession and change. Class conflicts are seen as forces and products of structural change. Class is conceived as an analytic category within a theoretical framework. This is an exposition and critique of the Marxian conception of class and an expanded conflict theory at the societal level. Chapter 5 is especially good in contrasting point for point the assumptions and emphases of integrative theory and conflict theory.

Dingwall, Robert, et al., eds. HEALTH CARE AND HEALTH KNOWLEDGE. New York: Prodist, 1977.

The social context of medicine has changed greatly in recent years. Health care, now a substantial element of most countries' GNP, is one of the biggest single industries in any advanced country. As health care has become more industrialized, its workers have tended to adopt industrial modes of organization. This volume brings together some key papers from the 1976 British Sociological Association Conference which examined recent social changes and their implications for health care and medical sociology. It includes the feminist critique of medicine that has aroused investigation of the social processes of health care institutions and the encounters experienced by women in medical settings. Contents: Introduction; "Images of Pregnancy in Ante-Natal Literature"; "Old Age as a Social Problem"; "Therapeutic Optimism and the Treatment of the Insane"; "The Reproduction of Medical Knowledge"; "Social Control Rituals in Medicine"; "Everyday and Medical Knowledge in Categorizing Patients"; "Magical Elements in Orthodox Medicine: Diabetes as a Medical Thought System"; "When Was Your Last Period? Temporal Aspects of Gynaecological Diagnosis"; "Policy and Practice in Paramedical Organizations: The Case of the Family Planning Agencies."

Donabedian, Avedis. ASPECTS OF MEDICAL CARE ADMINISTRATION: SPECIFYING REQUIREMENTS FOR HEALTH CARE. Cambridge, Mass.: Harvard Univ. Press, 1973.

The major work by this well known student of the social system of medical care. Important in suggesting dimensions for CNSHS, particularly those related to quality of the patient care process.

_____. "Models for Organizing the Delivery of Personal Health Services and Criteria for Evaluating Them." MILBANK MEM. FUND Q. 50, pt. 2 (October 1972): 103-54.

Theoretical piece on evaluation criteria for the problem of measuring health, access, costs, consumer participation, assessment.
Aspects of this model include degree of organization, relationship
of physician and consumer, access, financing, process of health
care. The particular emphasis here as regards quality assessment
is on process (patient flow and logic of care) rather than structure
(training levels of personnel, number of beds, etc.) or mortality
levels (outcomes).

Eckstein, Harry. THE ENGLISH HEALTH SERVICE: ITS ORIGIN, STRUCTURE
AND ACHIEVEMENTS. Cambridge, Mass.: Harvard Univ. Press, 1959.

On political theory in relation to development of a health system.

Elling, Ray H. "Case Studies of Contrasting Approaches to Organizing for
Health: An Introduction to a Framework." SOC. SCI. MED. 8 (1974): 263-70.

Identifies some suggested major dimensions of a cross-national
framework for studying health systems. These interacting elements
are (1) health status as the primary objective; (2) health services
delivery, with emphasis on the elements of regionalization; (3)
planning structure and approach; and (4) the political and socioeconomic context as the underlying determining set of forces.
Selected subparts of each of these four major components of any
system are identified, interrelations discussed, and a flow diagram
presented.

_____. "Occupational Group Striving in Public Health." In ADMINISTERING
HEALTH SYSTEMS, edited by M. Arnold, L.V. Blankenship, and J. Hess, pp.
70-86. New York: Aldine/Atherton, 1971.

Discussion of the field of public health in the United States, levels
of authority in the profession, and the strategies of occupational
group establishment in terms of interest group theory. This framework may be limited to competitive capitalist societies. By way
of contrast see "Levelling the Chinese Physician" by Record, below,
this chapter.

Elling, Ray H., and Halebsky, Sandor. "Organizational Differentiation and
Support: A Conceptual Framework." ADMINISTRATIVE SCIENCE Q. 6 (1961):
185-209.

Examination of organizational sponsorship and its relation to environmental support. Empirical study of 136 short-term general
hospitals, and their community support in the form of financial
donations, admissions, volunteers, and worker participation (nursing
turnover). Local governmental hospitals were found to receive
lower support than private religious or voluntary hospitals. This
was interpreted in terms of hospital differentiation and social class
links in US society.

Ellwood, Paul M., Jr. "Models for Organizing Health Services and Implications of Legislative Proposals." MILBANK MEM. FUND Q. 50, pt. 2 (1972): 73-101.

> The U.S. notion of HMO (health maintenance organization) is laid out--a renamed version of the prepaid group practice of Kaiser-Permanente origin. Of some general interest, since this general form of local health service is found under the names "health center" or "polyclinic" in many countries.

Emery, F.E., and Trist, E.L. "The Causal Texture of Organizational Environments." HUMAN RELATIONS 18 (February 1965): 21-32.

> Study of organizational change in the context of environmental change, in order to arrive at determinants of organizational form. Develops a typology of causality in organizational environments, with varying degrees of uncertainty and control. Rather abstract and possibly irrelevant, but suggestive.

Evan, William M. "The Organization-Set: Toward a Theory of Interorganizational Relations." In APPROACHES TO ORGANIZATIONAL DESIGN, edited by J.D. Thompson, pp. 173-191. Pittsburgh: Univ. of Pittsburgh Press, 1966.

> Develops the concept of organization-set as the interorganizational environment. Theoretical discussion of interorganizational relations as intersocial system relations. Takes its cues from Merton's concept of role-set applied to persons. Reprinted in Brinkerhoff and Kunz (see above, this chapter).

Eyer, Joseph. "Does Unemployment Cause the Death Rate Peak in Each Business Cycle? A Multifactor Model of Death Rate Chance." INT'L. J. H. SERV. 7 (1977): 625-62. 139 refs.

> Author's abstract: "Natural time series and prospective studies are combined to determine the contribution of many causal factors to the business cycle variation of the death rate. The variation of housing and nutrition together accounts for roughly a tenth of the death rate fluctuation. Drug consumption accounts for about one-sixth, with 11 percent of the total variation due to alcohol and 6 percent due to cigarette smoking. Social relationship changes, both as sources of stress and as means of relief, account for the greatest part (72 percent) of the business cycle variation of the death rate."

Fabrega, Horacio, Jr. "The Function of Medical Care Systems: A Logical Analysis." PERSPECTIVES IN BIOLOGY AND MED. 20 (Autumn 1976): 108-19. 16 refs.

> Conceives of Western, "scientific" medical care systems (MCSs) as more geared to biomedical disease and as having more control over such disease. This orientation "is made possible by a distinctive

cultural perspective--the Western--a scientific perspective." In this perspective the individual is seen impersonally and as distinct from a body which itself is conceived as made up of interconnected structures and functions. Among nonliterates a "social-behavioral" view of disease presupposes a "folk perspective in which the individual is seen holistically, morally, and as almost continuous with his social and nonmaterial world." While this perspective affords relatively little control of disease, it also affords little currency to the idea of disease as a biological form, and it is hard to apply standards of disease control linked to the scientific perspective. Instead, preservation of the social and sometimes social-spiritual nexus is critical. "A conclusion that follows would appear to be that, since there is no universally valid or veridical view of what disease is or what its causes are, there is no universally valid or veridical way of evaluating MCS. What obtain, instead, are culturally specific perspectives associated with cultural constructions of disease, each of which predicates a different type of MCS. The important issue then becomes the degree of control a cultural group achieves over what it defines as disease, so that what is being controlled becomes critical in the evaluation of the efficacy of a group's MCS." A penetrating, provocative statement but one ignoring the origins of the medical cultural hegemony which is seen to vary between societies. Krause and others would derive the medical cultural hegemony from the political economic structure and character and power of the ruling class as well as the state of medical technology.

Fee, Elizabeth. "Women and Health Care: A Comparison of Theories." INT'L. J. H. SERV. 5 (1975): 397-415.

Author's summary: "There are three distinct approaches to the analysis of women's position in society, and thus of women's relation to the health care system. Liberal feminists seek equal opportunity 'within the system,' demand equal opportunity and employment for women in health care, and are critical of the patronizing attitudes of physicians. Radical feminists reject the system as one based on the oppression of women and seek to build alternative structures to better fill their needs. They see the division between man and woman as the primary contradiction in society and patriarchy as its fundamental institution. They have initiated self-help groups and women's clinics to extend the base of health care controlled by women in their own interests. Marxist-feminists see the particular oppression of women as generated by contradictions within the development of capitalism. Women's unpaid labor at home and underpaid labor in the work force both serve the interests of the owners of capital. The health care system serves these same interests; it maintains and perpetuates the social class structure while becoming increasingly alienated from the health needs of the majority of the population."

Reasoning from this important statement, one would expect both an ideology and actual arrangements more supportive and engaging of the human potential of women in a Marxist-oriented political structure such as the "democratic centralist" regime in China (as described in Mao's collected works--see especially the passages "On Ultra-Democracy"; "On the Disregard of Organizational Discipline"; "On Absolute Equalitarianism"; "On Individualism"; and "Combat Liberalism").

Feldstein, Martin S., et al. RESEARCH ALLOCATION MODEL FOR PUBLIC HEALTH PLANNING, A CASE STUDY OF TUBERCULOSIS CONTROL. Geneva: WHO, 1973. Supplement to BUL. OF THE WORLD HEALTH ORGANIZATION 48 (1973).

Mathematical modeling and economic theory applied to control of tuberculosis in an UDC.

Field, Mark G. "The Concept of the 'Health System' at the Macrosociological Level." SOC. SCI. MED. 7 (1973): 763-85.

A restatement of the convergence theory suggesting that growth of medical knowledge and technology have had such a fundamental influence in shaping health care delivery systems that nations with very different political ideologies and economic arrangements have surprisingly similar forms of medical care and face many common problems. The difficulties with this view are that although a general structural-functional framework is offered suggesting that the health system fulfills a maintenance and social control function on behalf of the society, (1) "the society" is seen as an integrated entity rather than one held together by force (state power) on behalf of an elite ruling class in capitalist societies (with modifications in this for working- and peasant-class control in democratic socialist societies) and (2) no criteria are given for what should be considered convergent or divergent. Thus a system which has rural polyclinics but has trouble filling all positions may be seen as sharing the problem of urban-rural imbalance with another system lacking almost any form of modern rural care when in fact it does not share the problem in the same way or degree.

_____. "A Conceptual Approach to the Comparative Examination of Health Systems." Geneva: WHO/RECS/BHS, 1969. Reproduced.

From the stance of integrative, consensual theory, examines health and medical care systems as functional elements in their overall societies.

_____. "The Health System and the Social System." In HEALTH, MEDICINE, SOCIETY, PROCEEDINGS OF THE INTERNATIONAL CONFERENCE ON THE SOCIOLOGY OF MEDICINE, WARSAW (JABLONNA), AUGUST 20-25, 1973, edited by Magdalena Sokołowska et al., pp. 315-29. Dordrecht, Netherlands, and Boston: D. Reidel; Warsaw: PWN--Polish Scientific Publishers, 1976.

A summary of this author's previous theoretical work. The conference version of the paper included a very helpful precis and a valuable fifty-nine-item bibliography which unfortunately were omitted from this publication. The health system function of maintaining social actors for society's benefit occurs more or less successfully, according to a number of structural problems now developing which are seen to show convergence between different modern industrial societies. These problems include rising cost and complexity of medical technology, depersonalization of care, gaps in general care at the periphery of systems, and the relative position of health systems vis à vis other sectors of society. A typology of health systems is offered: (1) pluralistic (e.g., US); (2) insurance (e.g., France or FRG); (3) national health service (e.g., UK); (4) socialized medicine (e.g., USSR). There are several figures indicating the "inputs" to health systems and their "metabolism." A valuable statement from this point of view.

_____. "Stability and Changes in the Medical System." In STABILITY AND SOCIAL CHANGE, edited by Bernard Barber and Alex Inkeles, pp. 64-83. Boston: Little, Brown and Co., 1971.

Foster, George M. "Medical Anthropology and International Health Planning." MED. ANTHROPOLOGY NEWSLETTER 7 (May 1976): 12-18.

Recounts some stages of US-aided involvement in health services development in other countries and the anthropological conceptions involved. Lays out a more adequate set of anthropological conceptions, stressing structural arrangements or conditions rather than cultural values regarding health. Fascinating to see the conceptual development reflected in this statement as compared to the item by this same author cited below.

_____. PROBLEMS OF INTERCULTURAL HEALTH PROGRAMS. New York: Social Science Research Council, 1958. Booklet.

Valuable early consideration of cultural variations in understandings of health problems and appropriate measures as a way of explaining the difficulties in acceptance of modern or so-called Western medical practices by Indian and other indigenous populations. But gives some recognition to structural factors, thereby challenging a purely diffusionist model. For example, it is reported that resistance to use of the hospital in Peru quickly broke down as soon as experience with deliveries and "coming out alive" became known. Does not give adequate attention to political economic structures in determining medical structure and culture.

Frankenberg, Ronald. "Functionalism and After? Theory and Developments in Social Science Applied to the Health Field." INT'L. J. H. SERV. 4 (1974): 411-27. 35 refs.

The author argues that empirical work in the health field, while useful, suffers from the inadequacy of attempts to apply sociologic theory to medicine. This inadequacy arises out of the social position of sociologic theory to medicine, specifically the social position of sociologists, their elitist view of administration, and their desire to influence doctors. To correct this situation, sociologists must identify with patients and accept class conflict and contradiction. The author suggests that in this respect Mao Tse-tung might be seen as a successful medical sociologist. A parallel is drawn with problems of realism and naturalism in art. The article successfully counters the main consensual, integrative, or structural-functional theorists of medical sociology and health systems by presenting a Marxian conflict view.

Fraser, R.D. "Health, Health Services, National Prosperity and General Systems of Providing Health Care." Ph.D. dissertation, Univ. of London, 1965.

Broad conceptual work employing data available through Able-Smith's study of financing of health services in a number of countries. A later analysis and "boil down" of this work is found under chapter 7 in this author's article titled "Health and General Systems of Financing Health Care."

Freidson, Eliot. "Applications of Organizational Theory: Models of Organization and Service for Health Care." In HEALTH, MEDICINE, SOCIETY, edited by Magdalena Sokołowska et al., pp. 349-61. Dordrecht, Netherlands, and Boston: D. Reidel; Warsaw: PWN--Polish Scientific Publishers, 1976.

The problem of health systems today "has shifted from the medical-technical discoveries needed to allow the control of health problems to the means of organizing health manpower to assure that known medical techniques are made available to all the people who need them" (p. 349). Sees, historically, a shift in medical systems from a free market model to a professional or craft model: "In essence, I suggest that a model which includes within it an untraditionally active role for the patient, or consumer, is both appropriate for the typical health problems in advanced industrial societies and for discouraging the characteristic pathologies of professional and bureaucratic systems." Does not give details or consider the difficult problems of class and differential power.

_____. PROFESSIONAL DOMINANCE, THE SOCIAL STRUCTURE OF MEDICAL CARE. Chicago: Aldine, 1970.

Sociological analysis of the medical care system and the role of professionals, especially physicians, as dominating the problematic relations with those being served. Discusses the organization of health care and delivery. Particularly relevant to the United States but has more general import for problems of organization, especially relations between occupational groups in the health field. Does not clearly link the politics of occupational groups striving to the class and power structures of the society along the lines of Navarro's analysis (see Navarro, "An Explanation of the Composition, Nature, and Functions of the Present Health Sector of the United States," below, this section).

Gallagher, Eugene B., ed. DOCTOR-PATIENT RELATIONSHIP IN THE CHANGING HEALTH SCENE. Papers and Proceedings from International Conference held April 26-28, 1976 in Bethesda, Md. DHEW Pub. No. (NIH) 78-183. Bethesda, Md.: John E. Fogarty Int. Center for Advanced Study in the H. Sciences, 1978.

A valuable collection produced by an international gathering, primarily of medical sociologists. Most of the presentations and discussions focus on the doctor-patient relationship in France, FRG, UK, and United States. Some system level papers are included, among them a provocative paper by Howard Waitzkin (see below, this chapter).

Georgopoulos, Basil S. ORGANIZATION RESEARCH ON HEALTH INSTITUTIONS. Ann Arbor, Mich.: Institute for Social Research, 1972.

An extremely valuable pulling together of the research literature, mainly on hospitals, in the United States.

Gish, O. "Social Security and Medicine in the USSR: A Marxist Critique." In ANNUAL REVIEW OF SOCIOLOGY, vol. 3, edited by Alex Inkeles et al., pp. 144-56. Palo Alto, Calif.: Annual Reviews, 1977.

An important book critiquing the Soviet health system from a Marxian perspective.

Gitter, A. George, and Mostofsky, David I. "Toward a Social Indicator of Health." SOC. SCI MED. 6 (April 1972): 205-9.

Glaser, William A. "From National Findings to Cross-National Generalizations." In TRANSACTIONS OF THE FIFTH WORLD CONGRESS OF SOCIOLOGY, vol. 4, pp. 465-71. Montreal: Int'l. Sociological Assn., New York: Columbia Univ., Bureau of Applied Social Research, 1962.

_____. SOCIAL SETTINGS AND MEDICAL ORGANIZATION. New York: Atherton Press, 1970. Appendix, index.

Draws on data from some hundred hospitals in sixteen countries. Examines effects of social setting on medical care organization. Specifically investigates cross-system variation among hospitals within a framework of comparative organizational sociology. Provides systematic comparisons of conditions existing in regions in Europe, Middle East, the Soviet bloc, United States, and UK. Offers generalizations on medical care and hospital organization relevant to sociologic and organizational theory.

Goss, Mary, et al. "Professional Organization and Control." Paper presented at the annual meeting of the ASA, New York City, 1973. Available from the author.

> The control of decision making in medicine is a crucial issue because the definition of illness at the societal level may be used as a means of social control. Sociologists have not carried out extensive studies in different nations of the loci of control of decision making in medicine, of extramedical responsibilities assumed by physicians, and the implications in different social orders. With growing bureaucratization of medicine and increased regulation of medical activities, sociologists will be called upon more and more to address these issues.

Greenhill, Stanley. "What Does the Public Want of Health Services? The Need for Some Health Indices." CANADIAN J. OF PUB. H. 63 (March-April 1972): 108-12.

Grzegorzewski, Edward. "Studies in Comparative Public Health: References to People's Health in the National Constitutions." Unpublished English version of a paper published in Spanish in BOLETIN DE LA OFICINA SANITARIA PANAMERICANA 67 (1969): 134-41.

> Calls for comparative studies of patterns of organizing for public health as a basis for teaching of public health administration. Recommends examining such patterns in relation to national cultural histories, legal and political concepts, psychological traits, education, and "socio-economic realities" and trends. The present paper is offered as an exercise of this sort, limited to whether or not health is mentioned in national constitutions. Of 142 countries studied, 122 had constitutions and 75 of these mentioned health (some 17 of the 20 countries in Africa which mentioned health did so by including "The Universal Declaration of Human Rights" which includes reference to medical care and is quoted in the paper). Socialist countries, French-speaking countries of Africa (as compared with English-speaking ones), and countries with constitutions adopted since 1940 all were more likely to have a mention of health. There is no necessary connection between a constitutional recognition of health and adequacy of health care, however, as illustrated the Scandinavian countries which have very adequate health care systems but do not mention health in their constitutions.

Haber, Lawrence D. "Some Parameters for Social Policy in Disability: Cross-National Comparison." MILBANK MEM. FUND Q./H. AND SOCIETY 51 (Summer 1973): 319-40.

Hart, Julian Tudor. "The Inverse Care Law." LANCET 1 (February 27, 1971): 405-12.

A fundamental critique of the NHS from the point of view of a practicing physician who adopts a Marxian perspective. Points out that even with the NHS, in a capitalist political economic structure which leaves an elitist ruling class in charge, the least care and least adequate care still goes to those with the greatest needs.

Harvey, David. "Ideology and Population Theory." See chapter 2.

Helt, Eric H. "Economic Determinism: A Model of the Political Economy of Medical Care." INT'L. J. H. SERV. 3 (1973): 475-85. 18 refs.

Helt argues that the medical care system under capitalism promotes not the health of the people, but instead, economic, political, and cultural inequality in favor of the health profession and the other economic elite of such a society. When stresses within the medical system threaten the institutional conditions that sustain this inequality, they are reestablished through state-sanctioned collective action. A clear, penetrating statement.

Holst, Erik, and Wagner, Marsden. "Primary Health Care is the Cornerstone." In HEALTH CARE IN SCANDINAVIA, 1976, edited by Donald E. Askey, pp. 30-39. Bethesda, Md.: NIH, John E. Fogarty Center for Advanced Study in Med. Science.

Describes the important role of primary health care in the various Scandinavian health systems. The primary focus is on Denmark, but there are comparisons with other systems. Attempts to apply the Scandinavian experience to the problems of the United States, especially with respect to the recruitment of general practitioners and administrative and motivational arrangements for keeping them actively serving where most needed. Denmark appears to have found ways of solving this problem.

Hyman, Herbert H., et al. METHODS TO INDUCE CHANGE AT THE LOCAL LEVEL, A SURVEY OF EXPERT OPINION. Geneva: UNRISD, 1965.

Jahn, Erwin. "Integriertes System der medizinischen Versorgung--Ein Modell" [Integrated system of medical care--a model]. Duesseldorf, Germany: Wirtschafts--und Sozialwissenschaftliches Institut des Deutschen Gerwerkschaftsbundes [Business and Social Science Institute of the German Labor Union], April, 1974. In German. Available from the institute.

Develops a conception of a medical services system in relation to different units--subregions and regions--highlighting two special components--the medical technology center and the central information System. The technology center is conceived as a primarily diagnostic unit built near the regional or district hospital, perhaps connected with the hospital by passageways. The information system is a computerized limited access component. The author envisions group practice as the basic form of practice within this system. Although it sounds rather idealistic and does not give serious attention to payment systems and socioeconomic variables, this is a thought-provoking statement. Has seventeen pages. Makes reference to other studies by this institute on the FRG's health insurance system.

Jeffers, J.R., et al. "On the Demand versus Need for Medical Services and the Concept of 'Shortage.'" AJPH 61 (1971): 46-63.

Kane, Cheikh Hamido, and Mandl, Pierre Emeric. "Vers une remise en cause des politiques de santé publique on Afrique de l'Ouest et du Centre?" [Toward a questioning of the politics of public health in West and Central Africa?]. In POLITIQUES ET PLANIFICATIONS DE LA SANTÉ DANS LES PAYS EN VOIE DE DEVELOPPEMENT [Politics and planning of health in developing countries]. Special issue of REVUE TIERS-MONDE 14, no. 53 (January-March 1973).

A particularly valuable and potent critique of colonial leftovers and misguided development efforts and their impact on health, particularly of mothers, infants, and children. Notes the concentration of modern services in urban areas; the financial impossibility of covering the whole (mainly rural) population with such service; the real gaps--such as inadequate water supplies, nutrition, sanitation, protection of women; and the reasons why efforts to raise production often ends up harming the health of women and children. Draws these conclusions after examining 2,000 pages of studies in eight African countries; working papers and revisions for a UNICEF conference on "Infancy, Youth Women and Plans of Development," held in Lomé, Togo in May 1972; and his own analysis of institutional inadequacies.

Kaprio, Leo A. "The Future of Health and Social Services (Europe)." Paper prepared for the Int'l. Conference on Med. Sociology, Warsaw (Jablonna) August 20-25, 1973.

A seemingly rambling statement by the regional director for Europe of WHO, but actually one full of important insights. The concern for health and social services is first set in the world picture of resources, population, and consumption of goods and services. "The 'rich' part of the world will have to limit its use of resources while at the same time aiding development in the 'poor' countries; development not aimed at economic growth alone but balanced social well-being." In Europe, there is increasing concern for social well-being as compared with an earlier concern solely for economic growth. It is more and more clearly realized that health levels are determined by education, employment, distribution of income, and other socioeconomic conditions; yet health services are not designed to deal with such matters. In turn, effective health preventive work can contribute to improved socioeconomic conditions, and good care arrangements can provide some of a people's feeling of security. With regard to social services per se, a person's disease even if medically well-treated can turn into a social and personal disaster without social support. And if social needs are met in the community, the person does not need to "misuse" or "escape" into the medical care system at great cost to society. He sees increasing need for improved joint health and social services administrative arrangements and predicts improvements on a subnational regionalized basis but notes current variety and trends, including the separation of social and health services in UK under the reorganization of the NHS.

Kasl, S., and Cobb, S. "Health Behavior, Illness Behavior and Sick Role Behavior." ARCHIVES OF ENVIRONMENTAL H. 12 (February 1966): 245-66.

Good discussion of some distinctions important to consider in conceptualizing the interface between health services and users.

Kelman, Sander. "The Social Nature of the Definition Problem in Health." INT'L. J. H. SERV. 5 (1975): 625-45.

Kelman argues that through the adoption of the appropriate theoretical approach and the derivation of suitable analytical categories, the problem of defining health can be seen as operational, nontrivial, and highly problematic to the determination of health care policy. Attempts to isolate the social basis of the definition of health. Notions of health are traced paradigmatically, then a historical materialist approach is employed to develop the social basis of an operational, contemporary definition of health. This statement is of major significance for understanding the thrust of health systems in relation to their supporting political economic structures.

King, Maurice. "Personal Health Care: the Quest for a Human Right." In HUMAN RIGHTS IN HEALTH, edited by K. Elliot and J. Knight, pp. 227-43. Amsterdam: Elsevier, 1974. 5 refs.

Delivered at the CIBA Symposium on Human Rights in Health Care, London, July 1973. A discussion follows the paper. A health care package is defined as an integrated set of components promoting the application of a particular group of "interventions"--a convenient name for such medical procedures as administering a polio vaccine or penicillin, or even transplanting a kidney--for the improvement of health care under specific socioeconomic conditions. Such interventions, which constitute health care, can be simple or complex, expensive or cheap, but many are closely clustered or associated, so that if one is available, another can be provided at little extra cost. Hierarchical scales of interventions can be constructed for clinical pathology, surgery, radiology, and so forth in terms of what health units in developing countries are capable of doing. The well-designed health care package is one that augments scarce technical, administrative, and educational skills.

Priority needs for developing countries are delivery of outpatient rather than inpatient care, maternal and child care, simple surgical and laboratory services, such as blood transfusion. The contents of such packages by their nature define basic rights in personal health care and establish a basis for judging quality as well as quantity of services provided. Comment: The managerial technological base of this "package" conception allows no clear room, and certainly no determining role for matters of human meaning in varying political-economic and cultural contexts.

Klarman, Herbert. THE ECONOMICS OF HEALTH. New York: Columbia Univ. Press, 1965.

A general coverage of health economics showing the "irrationalities" of the field such as an imperfect market due to professional monopoly practices and imperfect knowledge and fear on the parts of clients. Along with a number of works by others, notably Roemer, this study suggests that use of services has more to do with availability of beds than with morbidity levels. Also considers difficulties in defining and measuring "health" outcomes and "quality" medical inputs.

Kleczkowski, Bogdan M. "The Spectrum of Activity of the Modern Health Care (an Attempt to Systematize the Concepts)." SANTÉ PUBLIQUE; REVUE INTERNATIONALE (Bucharest) 10 (1968): 255–65.

Kleinman, Arthur M. "Explanatory Models in Health Care Relationships." In HEALTH OF THE FAMILY, pp. 159–72. Washington, D.C.: National Council for Int'l. H., 1975.

A cultural linguistic approach to understanding traditional and modern approaches to illness. Focused more at the user-provider interface than toward the health care system's organization.

Kohn, Robert, and White, Kerr, eds. HEALTH CARE, AN INTERNATIONAL STUDY: REPORT OF THE WHO INTERNATIONAL COLLABORATIVE STUDY OF MEDICAL UTILIZATION. Foreword by Robert F. Bridgman. London, New York, and Toronto: Oxford Univ. Press, 1976. 588 p.

Reports the most ambitious CNSHS ever undertaken. Lists thirty authors and two consultants besides the two editors.

Krause, Elliott A. "Health Planning as a Managerial Ideology." INT'L. J. H. SERV. 3 (1973): 445–63. 58 refs.

Author's summary: "This paper examines health planning as a form of technocratic ideology in use both by proponents inside government and by outside interest groups in the health field. Ideology and the nature of technocratic power are defined. Health planning is analyzed as occupation, process, and ideology. The ideology in use is analyzed for the following American programs: Hill-Burton, Comprehensive Mental Health Planning, OEO Neighborhood Health Centers, Regional Medical Program, Comprehensive Health Planning. It is concluded that health planning cannot operate in the present sociopolitical context except as an ideology to justify the status quo in health services."

_____. POWER AND ILLNESS, THE POLITICAL SOCIOLOGY OF HEALTH AND MEDICAL CARE. New York, Oxford, Amsterdam: Elsevier, 1977.

A book with major conceptual implications oriented primarily to the US "health" system, drawing on both liberal and Marxian sociological studies. Employs the idea of "cultural hegemony" drawn from the Italian Communist, Antonio Gramsci (LETTERS FROM PRISON) to understand the thrust of a health system as determined by a political economic structure and the power of the ruling class.

Kunitz, Stephen J., and Levy, Jerrold E. "Changing Ideas of Alcohol Use among Navaho Indians." Q.J. OF STUDIES ON ALCOHOL 35 (March 1974): 243.

Author's abstract: "Current definitions propose that alcoholism is a disease marked by deviant and maladaptive behavior. This concept is based on experience with non-Indians, and may therefore not be appropriately applied to Indians. The common pattern among Navahos is to drink publicly and in groups; the drinker who drinks alone and does not share his liquor is considered deviant by the Navahos; the group Navaho drinkers are labeled deviant by Anglos. Style of drinking reflects social organization and determines the incidence of associated illnesses: the highly visible Navaho drinkers have lower death rates from liver cirrhosis than do the more covert Hopi drinkers while the incidence of delirium tremens is similar among them and much higher than among Anglos or Blacks."

A piece with important theoretical implications which are not fully drawn out. Tends to support the framework offered by Krause in his POWER AND ILLNESS. The dominant US society, particularly the capitalist ruling class, benefits from the exploitation of mineral and other resources on Indian lands. Much earlier work by Graves and recent work by Levy and Kunits--SOUTHWEST J. OF ANTHOLOGY 27 (Summer 1971): 97-128--give this as the background against which to view a range of social pathologies including homicide, suicide, and "inappropriate" use of alcohol among American Indians with different forms of social organization and different levels of acculturation to US society. The way such "pathologies" are defined allows different degrees of social control, as we see from the present article.

Lalonde, Marc. A NEW PERSPECTIVE ON THE HEALTH OF CANADIANS, A WORKING DOCUMENT. Ottawa, Ontario: Information Canada, 1975. Also in French in the same vol.

Conceives of health systems in four parts: human biology, environment, life styles, and health services and sees most money and attention as having gone to the last. Has received wide notice and attention in official health circles. May be a sophisticated new way of "blaming the victim" by placing major weight on personal health behavior.

Last, J.M. "The Iceberg--Completing the Clinical Picture in General Practice." LANCET 2 (July 6, 1963): 28-31.

Points out the considerable unrecognized disease in the population beyond that brought to clinical recognition among those seeking treatment. This statement subsequently became a foil for, on the one hand, socially liberal health planners who urged epidemiologic studies to uncover the vast unmet need and design service systems to meet it, and, on the other hand, conservatives, those Alford might term "corporate rationalizers" and "professional monopolists" who use this rationale for restricting medical services because one could never hope to fill the bottomless pit of medical need. From the perspective of Illich, concerned with the medicalization of too much of modern society, this statement of Last's might appear suspect, though it can be taken as a call for prevention, rather than more and more treatment.

Lehman, Edward W. COORDINATING HEALTH CARE, EXPLORATIONS IN INTERORGANIZATIONAL RELATIONS. Foreword by Amitai Etzioni. Sage Library of Social Research, vol. 17. Beverly Hills, Calif., and London: Sage Publications, 1975.

Excellent coverage of the literature. Offers a paradigm for the study of literal interorganizational bonds in a complex multicontrol structure and multisupport channel health system and recommends (as regards the United States) increased corporatism, centralization, and government intervention but with a continuing mix of pluralism involving local initiative and insight without always a "snug" fit with the corporate superstructure.

Litman, Theodor J., and Robins, Leonard. "Comparative Analysis of Health Care Systems--A Socio-Political Approach." SOC. SCI MED. 5 (1971): 573-81. 54 refs.

Cites Osler Peterson (see below, this chapter) as having observed that the traditions, organization, and institutions of each nation provide a particular legacy which not only constrains innovations but encourages differing if not contradictory health services systems to develop. This view sharply qualifies, if it does not directly oppose, the "convergence theory" (see Field, Mechanic, this chapter) in which all systems, or all modern systems, are seen as sharing overall structural properties and problems. The authors identify a number of comparative works which proceed from rather shallow unstated biases (for example, that by Helmut Schoeck, commissioned by the AMA--see chapter 3.2--or the frank antisocialist bias which pervades Lynch and Raphael's MEDICINE AND THE STATE--see chapter 3.2). Is also critical of the general focus of past work on (1) discrete parts of systems rather than overall systems of health and medical care in relation to their sociopolitical contexts; (2) organizational, financial, and operational arrangements to the exclusion of theoretical and ideological bases; (3) uncritical assumption of transferability of approaches from one system to others; (4) use of a "rational policy setting" as opposed to a "bureaucratic politics" model of health policy (as in the work of Eckstein on the NHS or Badgley and Wolfe on the doctor's strike in Saskatchewan).

Offers some headings (but does not elaborate, specify indexes, or discuss interrelationships) of an analytic sociopolitical framework which essentially lays out organized interest groups to be considered in comparing different systems. Major headings are sociopolitical forces which have led to present arrangements, the present policy-making structure for health service (informal and formal, i.e., the effective structure), major sociopolitical forces inhibiting change. Does not seem to offer a clear view of the class-related role of government, but is generally very valuable.

Mabry, John H. "International Studies of Health Care." In his ASILOMAR CONFERENCE ON INTERNATIONAL STUDIES OF MEDICAL CARE, pp. 193-202. Special issue of MED. CARE 9 (May-June 1971). Appendix, 64 notes.

An introductory statement by the editor of this conference report based in part on questionnaire replies of conference participants. Notes that there were six workshops: (1) epidemiologic studies and medical care systems; (2) perceptions and responses to symptoms; (3) planning of health services; (4) health manpower; (5) utilization; (6) and comparative health systems. The papers are briefly introduced and some key concepts and methods mentioned. "All the papers agree that cross-national research is essential to lend credence to tests of hypotheses which result from studies in nations with different health care systems and varying influences upon the use of health services" (p. 199). Appendix lists research questions under the following headings: health problems and status; use of services; outcomes of illness episodes and health behavior events; personal, family, and group characteristics; environmental influences (demography, economy, etc.). While stimulating with regard to theoretical considerations, this article and the volume do not generate and contrast different comprehensive theories of health systems in relation to their national contexts. The paper by Weinerman (see below, this chapter) perhaps goes furthest in this direction.

McKeown, Thomas. "A Background of Health Care Planning." In INTERNATIONAL ASPECTS OF THE PROVISION OF MEDICAL CARE, edited by Peter Kent, pp. 1-12. Stocksfield, Engl., London, and Boston: Oriel Press, 1976.

Considers merits of and challenges to the NHS in the UK. The most
tangible achievement was to make medical care available to all
and remove the burden of direct payment. The system has not
victimized doctors or public, and it has not stifled initiative.
Outlines limitations of administrative and organizational structure,
what evidence there is that any kind of medical care system affects
health levels (the author's forté), and the changing character of
health problems. A major section, "Issues in Health Planning,"
has the following subsections: emphasis on the main influences on
health; evaluation of medical procedures (assessment of quality is
uncommon in the UK); hospital services (considers the prospect of
separating technological and psychological needs, as in the care
of the dying); medical practice (there are vast differences between
countries, especially in the relation between general and special
care; for the future all doctors will be pediatricians, general
physicians, or geriatricians); relation of doctors to other health
workers (the relations will remain dynamic because of changing
technology, demands, and rationalization).

_____. "A Conceptual Background for Research and Development in Medicine."
INT'L. J. H. SERV. 3 (1973): 17-28.

From the author's summary: "This paper attempts to establish a
background against which the balance between basic and applied
research and the mechanisms needed for effective research and development can be considered. . . . The author concludes that
conceptualization of the medical task has hitherto been inadequate
and has led to deficiencies in the approach to both medical science
and medical services. . . . Against this background the paper
considers briefly the mechanism of research and development. It
suggests that at the highest level, all problems of medical research
and development should be examined together."

_____. MEDICINE IN MODERN SOCIETY. New York: Hafner, 1966. Index.

Reviews complexities of modern medical care through discussion of
historical trends in improvement of health. Explores influence of
factors other than modern medical achievements. Considers organization of contemporary medical practice, the concept of a balanced hospital community, local public health services, and the
role of the teaching center. Concludes with examination of financing and administration of medical services.

_____. THE ROLE OF MEDICINE, DREAM, MIRAGE OR NEMESIS? London:
Nuffield Provincial Hospitals Trust, 1976.

An important work by a noted sceptic concerning the efficacy of
medical care. His position is not as radical as that of Illich
(MEDICAL NEMESIS) but he does give full recognition to circumstances and way of life as major determinants of health levels.

Marmor, Theodore R., and Thomas, David. "Doctors, Politics and Pay Disputes: 'Pressure Group Politics' Revisited." BRITISH J. OF POLITICAL SCIENCE 2 (October 1972): 421-42.

One of the most potent theoretical contributions in the CNSHS field. Challenges Eckstein's explanation in his book, PRESSURE GROUP POLITICS, of the success of the British Medical Association in not only obtaining a large increase for physicians in the 1965-66 crisis but, more important, as argued here, in holding the line on method of payment. Eckstein thought the political culture important, specifically, the intimate style of bargaining between the BMA and the Ministry of Health, but these authors show that physicians' groups have also got their way in Sweden and the United States as well as where styles are very different. Marmor and Thomas hypothesize that "as producers of a crucial service in industrial countries, and a service for which governments can seldom provide short-run substitutes, physicians have the overwhelming political resources to influence decisions regarding payment methods quite apart from the form of bargaining their organizations employ." Thus it is the political economic attributes of physicians which are important, rather than political style or culture. The article also makes a methodological contribution by showing that a case study cannot be used to support Eckstein's hypothesis on intimate bargaining structures, because the bargaining structure does not vary in the single nation or case. However, these authors' work suffers from a similar limitation, since they examine three countries which perhaps do not differ emough in their organizations and distributions of authority. A case like that of China (see Record, this chapter) suggests that there are limits to bargaining power, since other groups can be created to fill medical needs. Has valuable details on decisions in the three countries.

_____. "The Politics of Paying Physicians: The Determinants of Government Payment Methods in England, Sweden, and the United States." INT'L. J. H. SERV. 1 (1971): 71-78. 13 refs.

Author's summary: "This paper most generally seeks to account for why governments pay doctors as they do. It evaluates the hypothesis that, among western industrial countries, widely known physician preferences on method of pay determine subsequent policy, whatever the bargaining arrangements and distinctive national political setting. Two bodies of data are used: primary studies of payment method decisions in Sweden, England, and the United States, and secondary information on methods of payment employed throughout the world compiled by Glaser. The data proved consistent with the hypothesis. The explanation offered stresses the structural imbalance between the political resources (and willingness to use them) of physicians and governments on questions of payment method. This account has policy implications quite different from those stressing the impact of bargaining forms and settings in payment method decisions."

Marshall, T.H. "Some Observations on Professions and Professionalism." In ESSAYS ON MODERNIZATION OF UNDERDEVELOPED SOCIETIES, edited by A.R. Desai, pp. 310-23. New York: Humanities Press, 1972.

Traces the idea of "profession" back to the Greek image of "the good life" and the Roman conception of artes liberales. In the nineteenth century the concept combined an idea of noncommercialism with autonomy and other privileges associated with a quasi-monopolistic position. That conception is being challenged because (1) the privileges are too great or unnecessary and can be easily abused and (2) the elitist flavor of the idea leads to distinctions between occupational groups which cannot be sustained by any generally recognized criteria. Marshall draws on work of Rueschemeyer to identify three essential elements of a profession: (1) service (direct personal relations between professional and client); (2) application of a systematic (Marshall says "scientifically acquired") body of knowledge; and (3) dealing with problems of central value to society. Medicine is examined as a cardinal example, but there are problems such as growing bureaucratization and impersonalization; the fact that much medical service is not based on scientifically established knowledge; the fact that hauling away the garbage is as central a value as almost anything in medicine, yet service in this area is not well-rewarded or given high prestige in most societies.

A valuable statement of the more traditional conception in social science. Does not take into account two other positions: (1) "profession" simply as an ideology to aid one group in its struggles for ascendency over others, and (2) "profession" as an ideology of the capitalist ruling class serving to keep work groups separated and antagonistic so they do not combine to assume state power.

Matthews, William H. "Developing the Concept of Outer Limits in the Context of Meeting Basic Human Needs." Paper prepared for the 1975 Dag Hammarskjold Project referred to in appendix to WHAT NOW? THE 1975 DAG HAMMAR-SKJOLD REPORT, special issue of DEVELOPMENT DIALOGUE (Summer 1975) Uppsala, Sweden.

Maynard, Alan. "Avarice, Inefficiency, and Inequality: An International Health Care Tale." INT'L. J. H. SERV. 7 (1977): 179-90.

Provides data on disparities in regional distributions of physicians in England, Ireland, France, and FRG. This appears to be a serious ubiquitous problem, almost regardless of differing health system structures, finances, and so forth. Considers the relative lack of evidence regarding the cost-effectiveness of a variety of popular surgical and other therapies in a variety of countries. "The basic economic motivation of self-interest and avarice has led this profession [physicians] to produce health care outcomes which are inequitable and inefficient." Argues that both markets and bureaucracies should be carefully monitored. Unfortunately, the author uses personalistic and moral arguments instead of grappling with the political economic changes which might be necessary to institute "pecuniary and nonpecuniary incentives" which would bring physicians "to behave in a manner which leads to more equitable and efficient health care outcomes."

Mechanic, David. "The Comparative Study of Health Care Delivery Systems." In ANNUAL REV. OF SOCIOLOGY, edited by Alex Inkeles, vol. 1, pp. 43-65. Palo Alto, Calif.: Annual Reviews, 1975. 97 refs.

Although it fails to take into account the health system conceptual work of Elling, Litman, De Miguel, and others, this is an important statement which integrates a good deal of research literature (much of it on social psychological aspects of health care utilization in the United States and studies of US prepaid group practices) in presenting a broad framework for comparative study of national health systems. The primary concern of this framework is with distribution and quality of care, rather than health status of a population. Mechanic appropriately sees the economic organization and ideology of a society as determinative background against which the level and character of medical technology work to affect professional organization (particularly medical dominance à la Freidson which he finds increasingly universal), organization and distribution of health services, and access to medical care which in turn affect quality. Suggests as do Field and others that the growth of medical knowledge, changing technology, and increased specialization are leading to convergence in modern medical systems. Yet he is ambivalent on this score, for he cites work of Rosemary Stevens and others that much of medical specialization can be best understood in terms of a professional interest group self-regulated system such as that in the United States. And although it is possible to point to widespread common problems--increasing demands for modern care along with rising costs, a desire to reduce inequalities between rich and poor, linking of service systems to defined population groups, search for more efficient and effective primary care patterns, and so forth--still, he notes remarkable differences in approach in socialist and capitalist countries. Also, he admits that no criteria for convergence have been offered.

_____. "Ideology, Medical Technology, and Health Care Organization in Modern Nations." AJPH 65 (March 1975): 241-47. 26 refs.

Following a variety of convergence theories, identifies a number of problems with the South African health system which are said to be found in other systems. But the gross inequities of this racist, fascist brand of capitalist medicine break through to give the lie to this sanitizing brand of theory.

_____. "Patient Behavior and the Organization of Medical Care." In ETHICS OF HEALTH CARE, edited by L.R. Tancredi, pp. 67-85. Washington, D.C.: Institute of Med., National Academy of Science, 1974.

Author's summary: "In theory, the organization of delivery systems has an implicit logic. Such systems, as one moves from the points of first contact to secondary and tertiary facilities, are organized to deal with more complex and specialized problems, and it is assumed that the sequence of referral reflects increasing severity or the life-threatening nature of the illness, the complexity of the clinical picture, and the need for more specialized care. In large part such factors are predictive of the flow of work, but a great deal of the variance remains unexplained by such objective variables. However, if one examines each of the components of the delivery system as a minisocial system, it is evident that the flow of patients and decision making in respect to them in part result from sociocultural and psychosocial factors unrelated to the severity of the conditions treated or the objective needs of the patients. These include the wishes and manipulations of patients to receive certain kinds of treatments irrespective of their objective value, the incentives and nonmedical needs that influence how physicians work, the actual resources available, and the pressures on varying components of the system. In addition, the fact that many hospitals and clinics are multipurpose institutions involving patient care, education, and research require that they construct their populations not only on the basis of patient care needs but in terms of existing requirements for varied goals of the institution."

Miguel, Jesus M. De. "A Framework for the Study of National Health Systems." In COMPARATIVE HEALTH SYSTEMS, edited by Ray H. Elling. Supplemental issue of INQUIRY 12 (June 1975): 10-24.

Presents a classification scheme for literature on international health comparisons; defines health systems as interrelationships directed toward the maintenance and improvement of health status of a certain human population. One of the most valuable framework statements in that it covers nearly all health systems theory literature available to date of writing and offers a position of its own. Sees health system framework development as becoming increasingly inclusive of socioeconomic, political, and cultural concerns.

Miller, S.M. "The Political Economy of Social Problems: From the Sixties to the Seventies." SOCIAL PROBLEMS 24 (1976): 131-41.

A penetrating examination of the changing political economic climate, mainly in the United States, in the 1960s and 1970s. "Social problems should be viewed in the broad context of political economy rather than in personalistic or even labeling perspectives. . . . The misinterpretation of the sixties and the economic difficulties of the seventies are producing an approach to social problems that restricts public expenditures to deal with them and advocates punitive action against those who have succumbed to them." Although focused on US experience and oriented toward all kinds of social problems, this statement clearly orients the theorist concerned with CNSHS to the dynamics within the political economies of nations as the essential background against which to view health systems.

Mills, C. Wright. THE SOCIOLOGICAL IMAGINATION. New York: Grove Press, 1959.

> A seminal statement of meaning-oriented sociology as distinct from neopositivistic, "hard" science which often ends up with carefully gathered data isolated from a larger sociopolitical context and difficult to understand or attribute social as distinct from statistical significance.

Milne, R.S. "Decision-Making in Developing Countries." J. OF COMPARA-TIVE ADMINISTRATION 3 (February 1972): 387-404.

Moore, Wilbert E. "The Utility of Utopias." In ORDER AND CHANGE, ESSAYS IN COMPARATIVE SOCIOLOGY, chap. 17, pp. 292-304. New York: John Wiley and Son, 1967. 16 refs.

> A beautifully written, conceptually clear statement of a place for sociologically derived conceptions of society as a way of working toward improving the condition of human life. Moore notes that ideas of fate, religion or God, and evolution as determining the human condition have been replaced by more mundane calls for change such as Marxism. Chance as an explanation is dismissed as too risky and ignorant. He concludes, "My only plea is for indulgence toward our brethren who think that man is worth saving and his lot in life worth improving. A little activism of this ambitious kind will do us no harm."

Morris, J.N. "Tomorrow's Community Physician." LANCET 2 (October 18, 1969): 811-16.

> A very important statement which links improved community-level care, personal preventive care, and personal treatment.

Morris, Robert. "Basic Factors in Planning for the Coordination of Health Services." AJPH 53, pt. 1 (February 1963): 248-59; pt. 2 (March 1963): 462-72.

> Factors related to coordination: simultaneous crisis in agencies to be coordinated; substantial informal contact between trustees of agencies to be coordinated; cooperation; a planning structure committed to interagency leadership of high status capable of bridging antagonistic boards; expert studies suggesting gains from cooperation; discriminating use of incentives (money alone will not do it, but it helps). Although based on US experience, appears valuable generally.

Murray, D. Stark. "Who Has the Best Health Service?" See chapter 3.4.

> Suggestive of key questions to be asked in comparing different systems.

National Center for Health Services Research. "Policy Research Series, Controlling the Cost of Health Care." DHEW Pub. no. (HRA) 77-3182. Washington, D.C., May 1977. Pamphlet. 50 refs.

> Primarily oriented toward US concerns but may have general applicability. The Policy Research Series published by NCHSR describes findings from the research program that have major significance for policy issues of the moment. These papers are prepared by members of the staff of NCHSR or by independent investigators. The publication series is specifically intended to inform those in the public and private sectors who must consider, design, and implement policies affecting the delivery of health services.

> This report summarizes some of the research findings that relate to the rising costs of health services. In particular, the report describes what is known about the effectiveness of various strategies intended to reduce costs of such services, considering supply incentives and disincentives, including hospital and ambulatory care; provider behavior (changes in treatment patterns, effects of insurance, changes in physician productivity and workload; payment of physicians, hospital reimbursement and cost control); consumer behavior. Some references reflect experience in other countries, specifically Glaser's work on modes of paying physicians in other countries, and Enterline and Evans's work on the effects of various aspects of NHI in Canada. While this is a very valuable summary of the lessons to be learned on cost containment from the research literature, the report suffers at a basic conceptual level from focusing on a whole set of factors as if they could be considered one after the other, in isolation (forward budgeting for hospitals, deductibles, etc.), when a whole system is operating. There is no consideration of more encompassing strategies like regionalization.

Navarro, Vicente. "An Explanation of the Composition, Nature and Functions of the Present Health Sector of the United States." INT'L. J. H. SERV. 5 (1975): 65-94. 76 refs.

> It is postulated that the present economic structure of the United States determines and maintains a social class structure, both outside and within the health sector, and that the different degrees of ownership, control, and influence that these classes have on the means of production, reproduction, and legitimization in the United States explain the composition, nature, and functions of the health sector. It is further postulated that the value system is not the cause (as usually stated in much sociological, economic, and medical care literature), but a symptom, of these class controls and influences. A penetrating analysis from the conflict perspective. For a comparison of this perspective with the integrative or consensual view, see Dahrendorf (cited above, this chapter), especially chapter 5.

> This article is based on a presentation at the annual conference of the New York Academy of Medicine, April 25-26, 1974. A modified version of the article appeared in the BUL. N.Y. ACAD. MED. 51 (January 1975): 199-234.

_____. "Health and Health Services in People's China and Cuba." INT'L. J. H. SERV. 2 (August 1972): 327-29.

Although numerous publications on rural health care in developing countries are available, accounts of the experience of socialist countries, such as the PRC and Cuba, are underrepresented. Experiences in China and Cuba put to question the widely held beliefs that due to lack of resources, developing nations cannot provide comprehensive care to all their people. Socialist countries' experiences indicate that failure to deliver care to the majority of people is simply a matter of poorly distributed resources. Both China and Cuba demonstrate in health services their commitment to minimizing inequalities between social classes, between cities and rural areas, and between regions. Redistribution of resources must be accompanied by development of new resources. In this sense socialist countries are defining the people as their resource and are deploying them to create health services for rural and urban population. Massive popular participation in the health sector is required rather than the training of a few to care for the majority.

_____. MEDICINE UNDER CAPITALISM. New York: Prodist; London: Croom Helm, 1976. Refs. each chapter.

A most important collection of writings presenting health systems in relation to their political economies while employing a Marxian or conflict perspective. Although most of the chapters focus on the United States, the fundamental theoretical conceptions are widely applicable. Two chapters are particularly powerful in drawing out the articulations between the health system and the class and power structure of a society. One comes to understand the underdevelopment of health in Latin America, the repression of Allende's Chile through US and Chilean capitalist ruling class forces, the maldistribution of health and health services in the United States, the exploitation of workers and inadequate occupational health protection, and the place of women in health occupations and institutions as particular health system aspects of a worldwide capitalist political economy. The key question revolves around who controls state power. In capitalist countries and in the worldwide capitalist system (see Wallerstein; also Chase-Dunn; and Rubinson, cited in chapter 2), state power is in the hands of an elite ruling class. As regards health and medical care, the state intervenes in this kind of society in such a way as to protect or enhance the interests of the ruling class. Thus, governments which encourage more women to enter medicine as physicians (instead of nurses and charwomen) are seen as intending to take the real steam out of the women's movement. As Navarro observes, "class loyalties are far stronger than sex loyalties. For example, in terms of socioeconomic behavior, the female physician is far closer to and supportive of the male physician than she is to the cleaning women in the hospital. . . . Indeed, to limit the con-

cern of women's liberation, black liberation or any other liberation movement to the fight for the advancement of those belong-
ing to the upper and upper-middle classes leads merely to a change
in the sex or racial composition of those at the top, leaving conditions for those at the bottom unchanged. . . . As Mother Jones,
that great trade union leader among the Appalachian miners said,
'It is to break with the control that the few have over our lives,
that we need the work and the struggle of all of us.' And it is
in terms of this understanding that the struggle for women's liberation
also implies the struggle for the liberation of us all" (p. 178).
The last chapter offers a useful distinction and discussion of state-
market capitalism (US), state capitalism (USSR), and democratic
socialism (PRC).

_____. "Redefining the Health Problem and Implications for Planning Personal
Health Services." H. REPORTS (Health Services and Mental Health Administration) 86 (August 1971): 711-24. 29 refs., figures.

Describes the current work and functioning of health services systems
in Western industrial societies, including gaps such as that suggested
in the iceberg conception of recognized and unrecognized need
(see Last, this chapter). Defines desirable arrangements, including
a new type of community physician, new division of labor in a
health team, regionalization of health services, and revised preparation of personnel. Considers a range of models which have
been proposed by others. Although not as penetrating and critical
in relation to the political economic context as some of his later
writings, this piece is very valuable in laying out the pieces and
parts of a health system and their relations to one another. This
paper was distributed as part of the WHO/EURO Working Group on
Health Planning in National Development meeting held in Stockholm,
June 19-22, 1972.

Neuhauser, Duncan, and Jonsson, Egon. "Managerial Responses to New Health
Care Technology: Coronary Artery Bypass Surgery." In THE MANAGEMENT
OF HEALTH CARE, edited by William J. Abernathy et al., pp. 205-13. Cam-
bridge, Mass.: Ballinger, 1974. 19 refs.

Although focused on Sweden and the United States and on a particular kind of investment in high medical technology, this piece
is of general theoretical interest for linking medical investment,
expense, and possible waste of human life to organizational form.
Allegedly, there had been some 100,000 coronary artery bypass
operations in the United States while only 100 had been done in
Sweden. The authors believe organizational differences are the
reasons why such operations are much more frequent in the United
States. One of the major organizational differences is that Swedish
surgeons are salaried while US doctors are paid a fee for service.
"For a surgeon, to do 250 such operations a year at $2,000 a
piece means a gross income of half a million dollars a year. . . .

Salaried doctors and hospitals on fixed budgets are provided fewer incentives." The authors note that US hospitals can usually pass the cost on to third-party payers while in Sweden the County Councils have been gathering more and more of total health care costs into a single pot which they control for their region or district; thus there is a tighter control on financing and hospital officials would have to justify increased technological investments before local elected officials who fear to raise taxes.

Ordonez-Plaja, Antonio. "Teamwork at Ministry Level." In CIBA FOUNDA-TION SYMPOSIUM ON TEAMWORK FOR WORLD HEALTH, edited by Gordon Wolstenholme and Maeve O'Connor, pp. 167-76. London: J. and A. Churchill, 1971.

Discusses the concept of teamwork versus "the strongman" notion, especially in the Latin American context.

Paige, Jeffrey M. AGRARIAN REVOLUTION: SOCIAL MOVEMENTS AND EXPORT AGRICULTURE IN THE UNDERDEVELOPED WORLD. New York: Free Press, 1975.

A book which makes important contributions both to theory of political order and change and to methods for cross-national research. The extension of world capitalist market forces into agrarian economies has produced disruptions, and these represent one of the greatest sources of potential change in the world political economy. Yet there has been a great diversity of responses--from passive resistance, if any, to episodic, short-lived uprisings, to militant communist revolutions. Classifies agrarian economies into sharecropping, migratory labor estate, commercial hacienda, plantation, and small free-holding systems. These types of organization reflect variations in and combinations of type of labor (constant vs. periodic); capital investment (high vs. low); and world market for the crop (strong vs. weak). These cause or are associated with variations in the kind of land tenure, the flexibility of the rural upper classes, and potential solidarity of the peasant class. Elites in sharecropping and migrant labor situations have little flexibility and cannot give in to demands of workers who have little hope in upward mobility and little vested interest in the system and organize relatively easily against the upper classes. In these situations revolution is more likely. In other situations, there may be outbursts which produce little change, or mild protest with accomodation. An important methodological innovation is the assembly of data on export sectors within nations (e.g., coffee and sugar within Brazil) rather than nations as a whole. Gives data on 135 sectors in seventy nations and uses regression analysis.

Pan American Health Organization (PAHO). FINANCING OF THE HEALTH SECTOR: TECHNICAL DISCUSSIONS. Scientific Publications no. 208. Washington, D.C., 1970.

Important for conceptualizing sources and amounts of support for health systems in different countries.

Parsons, Talcott, and Fox, Renee. "Illness, Therapy and the Modern Urban American Family." J. OF SOCIAL ISSUES 8 (1952): 31-44.

A fundamental piece from the structural-functional perspective, oriented primarily toward the middle-class US family. Generalizes to the changing function of medical systems in modern industrialized societies. With increasing secularization and modernization (adoption of individual success striving, scientific values, appreciation of technology, etc.), medicine has stepped in to deal with problems that were once under the authority of the family, religion, or the legal system. In medical institutions, particularly hospitals and long-term care facilities, the ill, aged, retarded, or those with problems which might otherwise disrupt the normal course of affairs are isolated and the society insulated from confronting them. Comment: from a conflict perspective, there are several problems with this, particularly, medicine is seen as functioning on behalf of "the society" as if the society were a value-integrated rather than a coercively integrated entity.

Patton, Michael Quinn. "An Analysis of the Effects of Environmental and Technological Contingencies on Organizational Dynamics in Colonial Africa: A Theory of Upwardly Revolving Compliance Succession." Paper presented to the Cross-National Organizational Research Section, ASA meetings, Montreal, August 24-28, 1974. Available from the author through the ASA, Washington, D.C.

A study of Tanganyika under German and later British rule with a section on postcolonial Tanzania. The focus is on agricultural development policy and the kind of compliance strategies employed by governing powers and organizations. Increasing structural differentiation, specialization, and national integration carried shifts in views of "the African." The first view was that he did not understand economic rationality, thus coercive and repressive compliance strategies were employed. Then a view developed that Africans may be motivated by economic gain, carrying with it a remunerative compliance strategy. At present, the emphasis remains on economic goals, remunerative compliance and calculative involvement. "However, ideological goals and high moral commitment represent a pattern which has become increasingly important in rural areas as the government has initiated a Tanzanian version of rural communes called 'ujaama' villages." Has an impressive coverage of organizational and historical literature.

Paul, Benjamin D., ed. HEALTH, CULTURE AND COMMUNITY. New York: Russell Sage Foundation, 1955.

One of the earliest works in medical anthropology examining failures in health services developments in a wide range of countries--

mostly UDCs--for reasons which the several authors see as mis-
matching of traditional and modern thinking about disease and
medical care. This kind of conception has since been revised by
a better understanding of how the ruling class of a country may
develop (to use Gramsci's term) a cultural hegemony defining what
is to be believed and valued. In short, culture is seen as a product of power. See also Elliott Krause, POWER AND ILLNESS
(cited above, this chapter).

Payne, Anthony M.M. "Innovation out of Unity." MILBANK MEM. FUND Q.
4 (October 1965): 397-408.

Advocates the unifying of approaches to health issues through health,
social, and political science innovation. Disease must be classified
by agent and circumstances, implying a marriage between medical
and behavioral sciences. General health or, negatively, disability,
is seen as worthy of major epidemiologic attention, rather than or
in addition to disease-specific studies. Impressive array of data
is presented from many parts of the world, showing that nearly all
diseases have higher incidence in poverty groups.

Peterson, Osler. "What is Value for Money in Medical Care? Experiences in
England and Wales, Sweden and the U.S.A." LANCET 1 (April 8, 1967):
771-76.

Compares health status, expenditures, resources, and utilization of
medical care services in these three affluent countries. In the context of noting that traditions, overall organization, and particular
institutional arrangements leave a legacy in each country which
constrains innovation and has created differing if not contradictory
programs of health service, discusses the essential difficulty in defining common meanings and weights for seemingly similar elements
in different systems. Throws the feasibility of CNSHS in question
on any but an in-depth case study basis. The picture of difference
offered here seems to challenge the popular conception that modern
health systems are converging in their structural arrangements and
the challenges they face (see Field, Mechanic, this chapter).
Neither the convergence idea, nor the (seemingly) unpredictable
variance view, takes account of what others see as fundamental
variations determined by real differences in underlying political
economic orders (see Krause, Navarro, Waitzkin this chapter).

Popov, M., et al. "Theoretical and Analytical Model of Society's Health Needs
and Scientific Guidance of Health Activity." SANTÉ PUBLIQUE; REVUE IN-
TERNATIONALE (Bucharest) 14 (1971): 15-26.

Powles, John. "On the Limitations of Modern Medicine." SCIENCE, MED.,
AND MAN 1 (1973): 1-30.

A thorough, scholarly work which suggests that much of the efficacy

of modern technologically based medicine may be due to the pla-
cebo effect because our modern scientific culture leads us to have
faith in such things in the same way that traditional medicine systems may be effective because of the supporting belief systems of
those cultures.

Purola, Tapani. "A Systems Approach to Health and Health Policy." MED.
CARE 10 (September-October 1972): 373-79.

Attempts to analyze medical and sociologic concepts of illness,
morbidity, medical care, and health policy, as well as their relationship as integrated components of the same macro system."

Raikes, P.L., and Meynen, W.L. "Dependency, Differentiation and the Dif-
fussion of Innovation: A Critique of Extension Theory and Practice." Paper
presented to the East African Universities Social Science Council Conference,
Nairobi, Kenya, 1972. Available from the authors.

An important paper clearly bringing the political economy and
power bases thereof into the understanding of changing cultural
orientations. A statement from the conflict or dependency theory
perspective.

Read, Margaret. CULTURE, HEALTH, AND DISEASE: SOCIAL AND CULTURAL
INFLUENCES ON HEALTH PROGRAMMES IN DEVELOPING COUNTRIES. See
chapter 3.3.

A book on the cultural background of medical care, especially of
traditional approaches in rural areas of UDCs.

Record, Jane Cassells. "Leveling the Chinese Physician: Permanent Revolution
and the Medical Profession in the People's Republic of China." Paper presented at the ASA meetings, Montreal, August 1974. Available from the author, Kaiser Research Foundation, Portland, Oregon.

Examines the many and apparently somewhat successful ways (at
least during the Cultural Revolution) in which medicine has been
destratified, demystified, deprofessionalized, and made more generally available in China. Clearly associates the stratification
system of medicine with the stratification system of society. A
classless society will have a destratified medical system.

Reinke, W.A. "International Comparative Aspects of Health Delivery Systems."
In GLOBAL SYSTEMS DYNAMICS, edited by E.O. Attinger, pp. 306-20. New
York: John Wiley & Sons, 1979. 17 refs.

From the Global Systems Dynamics International Symposium, Char-
lottesville, Virginia, 1969. Outlines a conceptual framework for
comparing health delivery systems in various countries. Health
services draw upon resources in response to certain health problems

to produce improved health status, but higher health status is dependent on more than per capita expenditure. Within this framework, health problems, resources, and expenditures are broken down
for an analysis of their interrelationship. Such models are useful
in planning health services. This one was applied in the development of a national health plan in Chile, pre-Allende. A project
directed by the Department of International Health, Johns Hopkins
University, is using this model in a functional study of health
workers in two provinces in India and three in Turkey, to discover
how much activity can be shifted onto workers with the lowest
level of skill commensurate with adequate care. The objective of
these studies is to be able, eventually, to predict the impact of
certain system interventions on the magnitude of problems, distribution of functions, and requirements for training health workers.
Offers a strictly "managerial" perspective.

Renaud, Marc. "On the Structural Constraints to State Intervention in Health."
INT'L. J. H. SERV. 5 (1975): 559-71. 24 refs.

Author's summary: "This paper explores the general structural constraints which are imposed upon all states in capitalist societies in
their problem-solving endeavor relative to health. The general
argument is that capitalist industrial growth both creates specific
health needs and institutionalizes solutions to these needs that are
compatible with capital accumulation. The key mechanism in this
institutionalization is the engineering model of modern scientific
medicine, which transforms health needs into commodities for a
specific economic market. When the state intervenes to cope with
some health-related problems, it is bound to act so as to further
commodify health needs, and without ameliorating the health status
of the population."

Roemer, Milton I. "National Systems of Personal Health Service in Comparative
Perspective." 1969. Unpublished. Available through WHO, Geneva.

A conceptual statement by a major student of health systems worldwide. Key distinctions are between more and less organized systems
in sociopolitical-economic contexts supportive of these systems.

_____. "Primary Care and Physician Extenders in Affluent Countries." INT'L.
J. H. SERV. 7 (1977): 545-55. 44 refs.

Author's abstract: "The worldwide growth of specialization in
medicine has led to a perceived shortage of primary care. A
major response in the United States has been the training of physician extenders (both physician assistants and nurse practitioners).
Other industrialized countries have rejected this approach, in favor
of strengthening general medical practice through continuing education, provision of ancillary personnel, use of health centers,
and by other methods. Developing countries use doctor-substitutes

as a reasonable adjustment to their lack of economic resources. All countries use ancillary personnel for selected procedures, such as midwifery, which involve only limited judgment and decision making. The American strategy on use of doctor-substitutes for primary care, however, follows from willingness to train greater numbers of primary care physicians and to require them to serve in places of need. This results in an inequitable concentration of doctor-substitutes on service to the poor in both urban and rural areas."

_____. "Social Insurance as Leverage for Changing Health Care Systems: International Experience." BUL. N.Y. ACAD. MED. 48 (January 1972): 93-107. 29 refs.

International experience shows that the growth of health insurance has had some impact on the patterns of health services. Where the political ideology is more collectivized and where the economic level is somewhat lower, the degree of influence is greater. In some countries, these changes have provided the structural basis for development of national health services. Social insurance provides leverage for health system innovations in disease prevention, medical teamwork, regionalization, and general quality control. Social insurance for medical care has led to the establishment of health centers with innovative staffing patterns.

Roemer, Milton I., and Axelrod, Solomon J. "A National Health Service and Social Security." AJPH 67 (May 1977): 462-65.

A most penetrating and valuable statement offering a typology of medical care systems in the world according to form of organization (individual vs. regionalized salaried system) and basis of financing (social security or insurance vs. general tax revenues). These noted and long-term students of medical care organization see risks of cutbacks and deterioration of services financed through general tax revenues for special groups in a capitalist system (e.g., medicaid for the poor and the Indian Health Service in the US) and see these same risks in other capitalist countries where a national health service system is adopted without first going through a national health insurance type of system. In such instances, the public service undergoes cutbacks as the ruling class decides that "economies" must be instituted and the deprived groups begin to seek care through the private system which may be expensive for them and not proper for their needs but may not have long lines or other drawbacks. This brief statement does not take up issues such as overmedicalization, an issue raised by Illich, nor considers whether "practical politics" in an inequitable system can be a kind of retrogressive reform.

Ronaghy, Hossain A., and Solter, S. "The Auxiliary Health Worker in Iran." LANCET 2 (August 25, 1973): 427-29.

An article reporting the failure of an attempt to adopt the Chinese barefoot doctor idea in Iran with important conceptual implications concerning the "fit" between political and health systems.

Saunders, Lyle. CULTURAL DIFFERENCES AND MEDICAL CARE. New York: Russell Sage Foundation, 1954.

An important early work drawing out the difficulties of "giving," "providing," "taking" modern medical care to peoples of other cultural orientations. Most of the examples are drawn from Spanish-speaking groups in Colorado and the southwest of the United States.

Schulz, Rockwell, and Bjorkman, James. "Strategies for Implementing Changes in National Health Policies." Paper presented at the 105th annual meeting of the APHA, Washington, D.C., October 30-November 3, 1977. Available from the authors through APHA, Washington, D.C.

This study examines literature on change, innovation and implementation in order to explain the relative success or failure of national policies for changing the health care delivery system. Although change may be either unintended or purposeful, a national policy implies at least some intent. If a policy is centrally coordinated and directed, changes may be abrupt, massive, and comprehensive; if not, changes in policy will be incremental, experimental, and diverse. A model of change must include at least four components: (1) characteristics of the target group, (2) characteristics of the change-agents, (3) the proposed changes per se, and (4) environmental characteristics. Drawing on evidence from the United Kingdom, the United States, and Libya, the authors develop a model to help policy makers implement change. They recommend that policy makers systematically consider all four components of the model when devising strategies for implementing proposed changes.

Scrimshaw, Nevin S. "Myths and Realities in International Health Planning." AJPH 64 (August 1974): 792-98. 14 refs.

The following myths are considered:

Knowledge of the agent of a disease is sufficient to understand its causation and to design programs for its prevention.

The first need of populations in unfavorable circumstances is medical care.

Modern medical care is the priority need of all societies and has been responsible for the marked drop in mortality rates and the population explosion of recent decades.

Population growth is such a major threat to the world that family planning should have absolute priority over other expenditures for health in developing countries.

The poorer a person and the greater his need, the more
time he will have available to wait in clinics, bring
children to health centers, make repeated visits, or at-
tend lectures and demonstrations.

Each of these is refuted or seriously qualified in discussion ranging
over a wide field of experience in different countries. The focus
is to some extent on health-nutrition programs in which the author
has gained a well-deserved reputation.

Segovia, Jorge. "La salud como sistema social" [Health as a social system].
MEDICINA ADMINISTRATIVA 3 (1969): 89-108. In Spanish.

An important statement departing from the Parsonian conception of
a social system in that it brings in the sociopolitical dimension.
Discusses the struggle of occupational groups and complex organizations over limited support in a sociopolitical system.

Seipp, Conrad, et al. "Coordination, Planning and Society: Cases in Coordination: Six Studies of State Mental Retardation Planning." Pittsburgh: University
of Pittsburgh, Graduate School of Public Health, 1968. Reproduced; available
from the school.

Discusses the relationships of power bases, sources of leadership,
societal values, and conceptions of health planning in varying
agencies.

Sherif, M. "The Formation of Group Standards or Norms." In AN OUTLINE
OF SOCIAL PSYCHOLOGY, pp. 156-82. New York: Harper and Brothers,
1948.

Organized group interaction gives rise to norms which shape and
regulate attitudes and behaviors of members. Experiments with
autokinetic effect applied to groups shows common frames of reference arising. In short, the social definition of reality occurs
in relation to power position in the group within some broad limits
established by the reality itself.

Sidel, Victor W. "Quality for Whom? Effects of Professional Responsibility
for Quality of Health Care on Equity." BUL. N.Y. ACAD. MED. 52 (January 1976): 164-76. Refs.

Within a market-oriented capitalist system, concern with measuring
and improving quality can have a damaging effect on quantity and
availability of care. A careful scholarly statement.

Sokołowska, Magdalena, et al., eds. HEALTH, MEDICINE, SOCIETY. Warsaw:
PWN--Polish Scientific Publishers; Dordrecht, Netherlands, and Boston: D.
Reidel, 1976.

Valuable collection of papers in medical sociology first presented
at the International Conference on the Sociology of Medicine,

Jablonna (Warsaw), 1973. Although oriented primarily toward therapist-patient relationships and conceptions of illness and care, the volume includes papers with both conceptual and methodological value for CNSHS.

Somers, Anne R. "The Rationalization of Health Services: A Universal Priority." See chapter 3.2.

On the concept of rationalization of health services and its relation to regionalization in Denmark, Sweden, and UK.

Stark, Evan. "The Epidemic as a Social Event." INT'L. J. H. SERV. 7 (1977): 681-705.

Using a broad historical sweep, the author presents disease as both a product of society and as a social force affecting, even reordering, the usual forms of production and control. Agrees with Foucault's analysis to the extent that structural conditions bring about a medical cultural hegemony called "the objective clinical gaze." But finds the links between ideology, disease, and social structure in the evolving capitalist political economy, rather than in the clinic structure. "As the rural population moved cityward, it naturally brought its own medicine. But the proletarianization of the farmer both in the city and in the country left him a dependent, passive in the eyes of the urban professions, and a fitting object for 'the clinical gaze'." The author presents an outline of a Marxian epidemiology:

> What alternative does Marxist epidemiology offer? If health and sickness are social processes, they can also be identified with real historical expressions of freedom and their negation. In this context alone, the positive dimension of social breakdowns such as riots and epidemics makes sense. Health may actually improve during strikes, rebellions, and riots, even if measured by conventional means. Reich, Mitchell, Laing, Marcuse, and Fanon each argue convincingly that prevailing modes of personality, family, and social life are 'sick' and that health, starting from social needs and capacities, may include such 'illness behaviors' as angry outbursts, biological passivity, regression, and so forth. This is a long way from health as 'harmony with nature'!

> We have argued that disease is not simply implanted by capitalism but that, conversely, insofar as it is a social process, it also shapes politics, economics, and thought. More than this, the logic of capitalist development and of the disease process must be traced, in part, to the dynamic contradictions that arise from their interaction. So, capital takes social forms to manage 19th-century crises in health and safety; but 'social capital,' by in-

corporating the disease process more directly into centralized economic mechanisms, creates the diseases of
chronic stress. As disease and disorder broke out of
the factory and working-class neighborhood and circulated
'wildly' in 19th-century cities, they were politically
reconstituted as epidemics and riots. But this very process gradually helped dissolve the distinction between
factory and community.

Today, the disease process reflects the vertical extension of work in time as well as its expansion through
social space. 'Stress' as a major factor predisposing the
physical/psychic system toward breakdown signifies the
homogenization and integration of the disease and the
processes used to extend and protect profit taking.
Ironically, just as the causes of disease coincide almost
exactly with the factors responsible for economic growth
in capitalist society, the epidemic, as a visible community of disease, seems to disappear behind a clinical
medicine- and hospital-based technology developed to
comprehend the most outrageous symptoms of progress,
to individuate collective mortality, and to time-grade
death according to the relative value placed on different classes of victims as labor. Clinical medicine
situates collective alienation biologically by reshaping
the disease process into patterns that appear unique in
time, social space, and intensity. The distribution of
symptoms along an apparently arbitrary time-space con-
tinuum makes illness seem 'individual' and conceals its
epidemic nature. The patient's complaint that he feels
like just another statistic reflects both his particular
alienation in the urban clinic and his sense that he is
being urged to experience the meaning of his existence
retrospectively, as a function of his prior determination
as abstract labor.

Starkweather, David B. "Health Facility Mergers: Some Conceptualizations."
MED. CARE 9 (1971): 468-78. Adapted from a paper presented to the Con-
ference on Interorganizational Relationships in Health, sponsored by Johns Hopkins
Univ. and National Center for Health Services Research and Development, New
York City, January 1970.

Discusses health facility mergers, using several different classification schemes. There are two general classification types. The
first defines health service integrations as static arrangements,
identifying seven "dimensions": (1) organizational pattern, (2)
legal bonds, (3) nature of combined services, (4) stages and forms
of production, (5) geography of population served, (6) facility location, and (7) organizational impact. The second classification
presents health facility combinations as a process, emphasizing the
dynamic state of health organizations and the important dimension

of time. Seventy-two reported variables are grouped into five
stages of the merging process. These conceptualizations attempt
to bring together the worlds of theory and practice, contributing
to further research and policy development concerning the rationalization of health care delivery systems.

Starobinski, J. "Gazing at Death: Review of Michel Foucault's 'The Birth of
the Clinic: An Archeology of Medical Perception.'" N.Y. REV. OF BOOKS
22 (January 22, 1976): 18, 20-22.

A stimulating, provocative, phenomenological approach to understanding modes and styles in medical conceptions and approaches.

Stevens, Rosemary. AMERICAN MEDICINE AND THE PUBLIC INTEREST. New
Haven, Conn.: Yale Univ. Press, 1971.

Based on comparative studies of medical specialization which differ
remarkably in the United Kingdom and the United States, this work
suggests the complexity of health and medical organizational issues,
the lack of clear universal, rational principles for such organization, and the extent to which organizational features are embedded
in unique historical forces that have come to shape the evolution
of each system of care. A valuable contribution which tends to
counter the convergence school of thought, but may do so without
adequate recognition of underlying general political economic forces.

Strauss, Anselm, et al. "The Hospital and its Negotiated Order." In THE
HOSPITAL IN MODERN SOCIETY, edited by Eliot Freidson, pp. 147-69. New
York: Free Press, 1963.

Development of a model for the study of psychiatric hospitals in
the context of social change. The key factor is the interaction
between professionals and nonprofessionals resulting in the "negotiated order" of formal organizations. This conception offers a
striking alternative to the conception of organizations according to
Weber's ideal typical elements of bureaucracy.

Susser, Merwyn. CAUSAL THINKING IN THE HEALTH SCIENCES. London
and New York: Oxford Univ. Press, 1973.

Although directed more toward problems of social epidemiology,
this book is valuable for considering the role of models in CNSHS.
After considering the evolution and historical development of key
concepts in epidemiology--environment, agent, host, and immunity--
the author offers an ecological model for schistosomiasis to illustrate
the several functions of models: (1) prediction, (2) representation,
(3) organization (putting a complex of related factors into coherent
forms), and (4) mediation. The ecological model is said to mediate
"between the traditional epidemiological formulation of agent, host,
and environment and the multivariate formulations that quantify the
relationships among the many variables of the ecological system."

There is also an analytic or explanatory function of models in which alternatives are posed among the possible relations between variables. The limits of models in relation to "the continuing unfolding of interacting events" as determined by significant social and political contexts are also discussed. A valuable contribution.

_____. "Ethical Components in the Definition of Health." INT'L. J. H. SERV. 4 (1974): 539-48. 23 refs.

The author maintains that definitions of health contain ethical components that rest on value systems, and that these definitions have certain consequences. The following examples illustrate changes through time and with social circumstance: (1) the relation of organized obstetrics to family planning and abortion, (2) the relation of psychiatry to the law, and (3) the historical evolution of the responsibilities of public health.

Tannenbaum, Arnold S., et al. HIERARCHY IN ORGANIZATIONS, AN INTERNATIONAL COMPARISON. Foreword by Daniel Katz. San Francisco: Jossey-Bass, 1974.

Through a survey research approach to samples of workers in "linked chains of authority" in comparable types of factories in socialist factories (kibbutzim plants in Yugoslavia) and capitalist factories (Austria, Italy, US), these researchers examine feelings of efficacy, power, and reported levels of participation in decision making. As Katz notes, "The findings do indicate the significance of common ownership; the socialist factories do show the flatter control curves." There are also significant differences among the capitalist factories, those in north Italy showing the highest centralization of power and authority. The book is remarkable for its frank and clear discussion of the ideologies of management in these countries (chapter 2), particularly for laying out the Marxist-Leninist view offered officially in Yugoslavia (pp. 27-32).

Terreberry, Shirley. "The Evolution of Organizational Environments." ADMINISTRATIVE SCIENCE Q. 12 (1968): 590-613.

Provides a conceptual framework for the study of organizational environments which are seen as evolving along three lines--increasing turbulence, less organizational autonomy, and the increasing importance of other formal organizations as components of the environment. Administrators as well as organizational researchers must be aware of the dynamics of the environment, external pressures as well as internal aspects.

Terris, Milton. "The Three World Systems of Medical Care: Trends and Prospects." See chapter 4.

An important paper presented at the 1977 APHA meetings examining and locating the three major patterns of health care organization in the world--public charity, health insurance, and national health service.

Tomasson, Richard F. "The Mortality of Swedish and U.S. White Males: A Comparison of Experience, 1969-1971." AJPH 66 (1976): 968-74.

An important empirical piece with theoretical and practical implications. The life expectancy of males in the United States is lower than that of males in most of the MDCs and in some of the LDCs. US females, by contrast, do much better in international ranking. Life expectancy at birth in 1969-71 was 67.9 for US white males compared with 71.9 for Swedish males. Greater US white male mortality is found at all ages from birth through ages 75-79. At the oldest ages there is a reversal of the differential with US white males having lower mortality than their Swedish counterparts. The greatest relative differentials between the two male populations is found at ages under 1, ages 20-24, and ages 50-59. At ages under 1 the greatest US white male mortality is accounted for mainly by higher death rates from infectious diseases, at ages 20-24 by higher rates from the external causes of death (specifically accidents and homicide), and at ages 50-59 from most of the major organic causes of death. The author examines seven aspects of life in the United States and Sweden which probably contribute to the remarkably lower death rates from nearly all causes in Sweden (suicide, tuberculosis, and stomach cancer show higher rates in Sweden). These are the better health services system; lower proportion of births to women under 20 and over 35 (specific to the much lower infant mortality rate in Sweden); less disparity between classes and higher living level for "lower" classes in Sweden; a more integrated social structure; active preventive efforts, for example, to lower smoking, accidents, and alcoholism in Sweden; lower consumption of cigarettes and alcohol; and more favorable diet and exercise in Sweden.

Ueber, Mary Susan. "Health Policy Making in Africa and the Middle East: You Have to Play to Win." Paper presented at the 105th annual meeting of the APHA, Washington, D.C., October 30-November 3, 1977. Available from the author through the APHA, Washington, D.C.

Health professionals have not been consistently successful in playing, or being willing to play, the political game that policymaking requires. This paper seeks to analyze this ecology of health policymaking and resource allocation at the national policy level in selected African and Middle Eastern nations. Based on coalition and decision-making theories in political science, the work identifies crucial actors, goals, and perceptions, and the relative acceptability of various health care delivery alternatives to each actor. This overall goal addresses two gaps in current health policy and planning: (1) the lack of a cross-national theoretical

framework for research in and analysis of policymaking at the
national level, and (2) the lack of a tool to design practical strategies for achieving technically optimal health programs through
use of, rather than opposition to, the political process. Presents
a model to be used in further research and teaching.

Ugalde, Antonio. "A Decision Model for the Study of Public Bureaucracies."
POLICY SCIENCE 4 (1973): 75-84.

Work done by the author, a political sociologist, while serving as
a consultant to WHO, Division of Research in Epidemiology and
Communications Sciences, Behavioural Science Unit. Introduces
the concept "series of decisions," defined as the total number of
decisions made in the attainment of a goal. Decisions are ana-
lytically divided into two types--programming and implementation.
Programming decisions are made during the process of converting
policy goals into programs; implementation decisions are made
during the implementation of the programs. The distinction is important because different actors and institutions are involved in
the two phases. The author hypothesizes that the relation between
the time of programming decisions and the time of implementation
of decisions tends to be zero the less effective and the less numerous the organizations participating in the programming phase.
A list of factors which could be useful in the process of testing
and modifying the hypothesis is presented. The division of health
environment of the health ministry of Colombia is used to exemplify
this concept. The concept is especially useful for understanding
the multiplicity of external and internal contingencies and interest
groups faced by a health ministry such as that in Colombia where
the tenure of ministers of health has averaged something less than
a year.

_____. "Health Decision Making in Developing Nations: A Comparative
Analysis of Colombia and Iran." SOC. SCI. AND MED. 12: 1A (January
1978): 1-8.

Follows the methods outlined for the previous item on Colombia,
this time applied in comparative fashion to Iran. Notes that in
both countries, efforts to coordinate divided interests and institutional segments of the health sector by creating a super agency--
A National Health Council--did not succeed.

United Nations. Public Administration Division. "Some Aspects of Administration
of Projects within the Context of Development Planning." New York: UN
Document ST/ECLA/Conf. 30/L.13, 1968.

Avoids the problem of project versus overall approach by saying,
"The main difference between the two is generally one of emphasis;
they do not constitute different approaches to development." Goes
on to offer many valuable considerations in relation to each of the
following phases of any sort of project, large or small, health or

other: (1) conception; (2) formulation; (3) analysis and evaluation; (4) approval; (5) implementation; (6) reporting and feedback; (7) transition to normal administration; (8) evaluation of results. Notes that "the foremost question relates to the organizational arrangement for implementing a project." Considers various aspects of new, old, and contract organizations, including the need for a project manager who is "dynamic, development-oriented, and able to get things done quickly and effectively." Seems to skirt the issues of social power and the power base (or what Howard Freeman has called "the social competence") of the organization selected to implement a project. Nevertheless, this is a valuable work, especially for cross-national study of health projects, either those developed internally or with international assistance.

Von Bertalanffy, L. "The Theory of Open Systems in Physics and Biology." SCIENCES 3 (February 1950): 23-29.

The first statement of the open systems model later applied in the study of complex human organizations instead of the relatively self-contained Weberian conception of bureaucracy. Valuable in that it focuses attention on causal forces in health organizations and health systems.

Waitzkin, Howard. "How Capitalism Cares for Our Coronaries: A Preliminary Exercise in Political Economy." In THE DOCTOR-PATIENT RELATIONSHIP IN THE CHANGING HEALTH SCENE: AN INTERNATIONAL PERSPECTIVE, edited by Eugene B. Gallagher, pp. 317-32. DHEW Pub. No. (NIH) 78-183. Bethesda, Md.: John E. Fogarty Int'l. Center, 1978.

Cites a British study which randomly assigned coronary patients to home care or to intensive in-hospital treatment in coronary care units (CCUs) and which showed no significant difference; if anything, the home situation was more favorable (H.G. Mather et al. BRIT. MED. J. 2 (1971): 334-37). Notes the vast proliferation of CCUs and their adoption as the treatment of choice in spite of lack of evidence as to their effectiveness, and much evidence as to their high capital cost and operating cost. Interprets this phenomenon in a Marxian framework of surplus capital having to work and finding the developing field of high medical technology a lucrative outlet in spite of contrary demands for holding down costs, and in spite of more pressing needs of the people for primary and preventive care (see Mahler, chapter 3.4). Waitzkin concludes, "We see that the apparent irrationalities of the health system are not irrational for a capitalist system in crisis. This framework also raises the question whether we can correct the irrationalities of the health system without fundamentally changing our capitalist economic system."

Waitzkin, Howard, and Waterman, Barbara. "Social Theory and Medicine." INT'L. J. H. SERV. 6 (1976): 9-23. 24 refs.

Authors' summary: "Three sociologists--Talcott Parsons, Eliot Freidson, and David Mechanic--have explained medical phenomena within a broader theoretical framework. Although all three have made significant contributions, their conclusions remain incomplete on the theoretical level and seldom have been helpful for workers concerned with ongoing problems of health care. Our purpose here is to summarize some of the strengths and weaknesses of each theoretical position. Parsons has elucidated the sick role as a deviant role in society, the function of physicians as agents of social control, and the normative patterns governing the doctor-patient relationship. The principal problems in Parsons' analysis center on an uncritical acceptance of physicians' social control functions, his inattention to the ways in which physicians' behavior may inhibit change in society, and overoptimism about the medical profession's ability to regulate itself and to prevent the exploitation of patients. . . . Freidson has formulated a wide range critique of the medical profession and professional dominance. On the other hand, Freidson's work neglects the full political implications of bringing professional autonomy under control. Mechanic's conceptual approach emphasizes the social psychologic factors, rather than the institutional conditions, which are involved in the genesis of illness behavior. Mechanic also overlooks the ways in which illness behavior, by permitting a controllable form of deviance, fosters institutional stability. In conclusion, we present a brief overview of a theoretical framework whose general orientation is that of Marxian analysis. Several themes recur in this framework: illness as a source of exploitation, the sick role as a conservative mechanism fostering social stability, stratification in medicine, and the imperialism of large medical institutions and health-related industries."

Weinerman, E. Richard. "Research on Comparative Health Service Systems." In ASILOMAR CONFERENCE ON INTERNATIONAL STUDIES OF MEDICAL CARE, edited by John H. Mabry. Special issue of MED. CARE 9 (May-June 1971): 272-90.

Valuable conceptual overview of the field. Focuses primarily on personal health services but defines "health service" as "all of the activities of a society which are designed to protect or restore health, whether directed to the individual, the community, or the environment" (p. 272). Health services are seen as determined by needs which create expectations, from which demands are made. When these demands are met, the outcomes determine additional needs. This cycle is related to a wide set of societal characteristics--social, cultural, political, economic, intellectual, technical, clinical, functional, genetic, biological, and environmental. Gives four important answers to the question, "Why cross-national research on comparative health service systems?" Provides an outline of a typology for the study of personal health service systems. Discusses a classified annotated bibliography of sixty-four items. Points out nine areas of needed future research. A cardinal piece in the field. Does not make sharp distinctions between types of political economies or suggest hypotheses, but notes structure may be a more powerful determinant than culture.

Weisbrod, Burton A. "Research in Health Economics: A Survey." INT'L. J. H. SERV. 5 (1975): 643-61. 107 refs.

This paper surveys the types of issues with which health economists have been concerned. Includes a valuable table showing remarkable variations in prices for the same seven drugs by the same manufacturer in the United States, Australia, Brazil, Canada, Ireland, Italy, New Zealand, Sweden, and the UK. The analgesic Doloxene by Lilly, for example, cost $7.86 in Italy but $1.66 in Ireland for 65 mg. in January 1970. Most drugs in the table cost more in the United States. This article provides a useful examination of conceptual apparatus in health economics.

Weiss, Joseph W., and Williamson, John B. "The Convergence Theory Reconsidered: Political and Economic Determinants of Social Welfare Effort: A Cross-National Analysis." Paper presented to the 72nd annual meetings of the ASA, Chicago, September 5-9, 1977. Available from the authors through the ASA, Washington, D.C.

Using national level aggregate data from thirty-nine countries, evidence is presented indicating that socialist parties and labor unions have a substantial impact on a nation's social welfare effort. This is contrary to what would be expected on the basis of most interpretations of convergence theory (that political factors are unimportant in shaping the common welfare state toward which all industrial nations are converging. One effect is on the development of a social welfare bureaucracy. The authors propose a refinement in the specification of the convergence theory with respect to political factors. An important conceptual contribution of likely relevance not only to cross-national studies of social welfare effort but to CNSHS as well.

Wennberg, J., and Gittelsohn, A. "Small Area Variations in Health Care Delivery." SCIENCE 182 (1973): 1102-8.

Cross-national as well as within country or even within region variations in rates of hospitalization, length of stay, rates of surgical procedures, and so forth, suggest that there is no clear rational basis for these variations in relation to the likely rates of morbidity in the populations in question. Availability of hospital resources is the best single predictor of gross rates of services, but it is difficult to demonstrate "unnecessary use."

White, Kerr L. "International Comparisons of Medical Care." SCIENTIFIC AMERICAN 233 (August 1975): 17-25.

On need to take the whole health care resource picture as well
as financial and behavioral patterns into account to predict use of
a specific kind of service. Has a number of other theoretical implications. For example, "where the apparent unmet need for physicians is highest, the total of hospital nights is also highest."
And, perhaps of greatest significance, looking at the social and
political characteristics of the countries, in terms of "health as a
societal value," "collectivism versus individualism," and "distri-
butional responsibility" (centralization-decentralization of health
care resource allocation), the study found all of these attributes
tending to vary together, with the highest levels for all attributes
in the European countries, Canada intermediate, and the lowest
levels in Argentina and the United States. In Saskatchewan and
Liverpool there appears to be a greater balance of levels of need,
resources, and use. Liverpool, particularly, with a lower supply
of physicians than Buenos Aires, Baltimore, or Vermont, has higher
physician use and less unmet need, suggesting greater efficiency
and effectiveness. Patterns between similar places within a country are similar while there are great variations between similar
places in different countries (the number of places for this analysis
was small).

Wise, Harold, et al. "The Family Health Worker." AJPH 58 (October 1968):
1828-38.

Describes an attempt in the South Bronx, an impoverished area in
New York City, to integrate medical and social service skills in
a team approach--with physician, public health nurse, and family
health worker. Describes training, duties, and problems of the
family health worker, who attempts to coordinate services and resources for poor patients. Presents a way of integrating preventive
and curative health services. The health team, assigned to a
certain area, attempts to develop and pursue a complete health
plan (preventive, ameliorative, curative, and rehabilitative) for
each member of each household.

Whyte, Martin King. "Bureaucracy and Modernization in China: The Maoist
Critique." AST 382 (April 1973): 149-63.

An important article analyzing the theoretical contribution of Mao
Tse-Tung to institutional and societal development in an egalitarian
direction.

World Health Organization (WHO). "Organizational Study on Methods of Promoting the Development of Basic Health Services." OFFICIAL RECORDS v.
206, Annex 11, pp. 103-15. Geneva, 1973.

A seminal statement which has influenced WHO policy for some
years in its efforts to strengthen health services. Clearly conceives
of health systems as embedded in their socioeconomic, political,

cultural, and epidemiologic contexts and calls for improved knowledge as to this relationship. Such improved knowledge would
imply CNSHS. In the absence of much work in this field, the
statement asserts that the relationship between political structures
and health systems is not so tight that there is no room to improve
services in important ways without altering the political structure.
This may not be true, if any important change is at issue (e.g.,
see Alford on the US situation, cited above, this chapter).

World Health Organization. Eastern Mediterranean Regional Office (WHO/
EMRO). "Integration of Mass Campaigns into the National Basic Health Ser-
vices." WHO/EM/RC17/Technical Discussion no. 2. Alexandria, Va.: WHO,
August 18, 1967. Unpublished document.

Integration of mass health campaigns into basic health services
demands reconsideration of priorities. Demographic and epidemiological variables need to be examined during planning, since health
care has an impact on these. In countries of WHO's Eastern Mediterranean Region the population is predominantly rural with a high
proportion under fifteen years of age. The services developed over
the past twenty years are mostly in urban areas. Integration of
health services to produce basic services requires creative reorganization; old structures must be coordinated with new orientations.
This is often difficult and demands a high level of cooperation
among interest groups that have been accustomed to fighting among
themselves for scarce financial resources. Organizational, technical, administrative, and training aspects of this progress are outlined.

Yoffee, William M. "New International Standards for Medical Care and Sickness under Social Security Programs." SOCIAL SECURITY BUL. (Washington,
D.C.) 32 (October 1969): 21-28.

Zola, Irving Kenneth. "Medicine as an Instrument of Social Control." Paper
presented at the Medical Sociology Conference of the British Sociological Association, Weston-Super-Mare, U.K., November 5-7, 1971. Available from
the author, Department of Sociology, Brandeis University, Waltham, Mass. 17
refs.

A powerful statement of the medicalization of all manner of problems (along lines similar to Ivan Illich's MEDICAL NEMISIS) and the
interpretation of such problems in moral terms. In short, good
people don't get sick, for even though the sick person is no longer
condemned, his disease is. The distinction between illness and
crime based upon the person's responsibility is disappearing. Further, those who do not properly use medical services and facilities
(break appointments, etc.) are also condemned in moral terms and
by efforts to bring them into line. Considers the potential and
consequences of this greater medical control and concludes by
quoting C.S. Lewis from over a quarter century ago: "Man's power

over Nature is really the power of some men over other men, with
Nature as their instrument." The paper has the serious weakness
of not considering the social control function of medicine under
differing political economic structures. Presumably, to the extent
that a society is truly democratic-socialist, this function will differ
remarkably from what it is in a fascist dictatorship or a state capitalist or state-market capitalist society.

Zubkoff, Michael, and Roskin, Ira E. HOSPITAL COST CONTAINMENT,
SELECTED NOTES FUTURE POLICY. New York: Prodist, 1977.

This collection of original papers provides analyses and perspectives
critical to an understanding of the design, implementation, and
consequences, often unplanned, of alternative hospital cost containment strategies. The volume draws upon recent US federal and
local experiences in assessing future options of significance for
policymakers, administrators, health service planners, and researchers. One chapter gives an international overview. The
work lacks any adequate consideration of the question of what
unit is appropriate to contain costs. Many feel that this unit
must be a subnational regional system and not an individual hospital.

Chapter 6

REGIONALIZATION OF HEALTH SERVICE SYSTEMS

In many respects this chapter can be seen as an elaboration of the last chapter on theory of health systems. It is also very practically oriented toward how best to organize health service systems. If one asks, "What should be the most encompassing yet smallest unit of organization within a national health service?" the answer, for reasons of effectiveness as well as efficiency, cannot be the doctor-patient relationship for there is much more to health and medical care. Nor can it be each town, for the provision of a relatively complete health system for every town or community, assuming this was desirable, would be beyond the means of any known country. Nor can it be a single monolithic system covering a whole nation (except perhaps in certain small, single-island countries). Something intermediate like the regional system of care seems to be the only answer.

There is much more to the idea of a regional system than geographic definition incorporating, usually, between 500,000 and 3 million people. A regional system must deal with service arrangements, payment, authority relations, involvement, and other elements. It is an idea rich in historical background and experience in many countries. Yet few if any places in the world have achieved complete regionalization of health services. Thus it is proper to think of regionalization not only as a concept of structure and function but as a process of social change toward a more ideal arrangement of the health services. While there are several reports in the literature on the experience of particular countries, there is a remarkable lack of comparative or contrasting studies of regionalization. Papers by Empkie and by Zayed, cited in chapter 4, are an exception, as well as those by Shannon and Dever, below.

Arbona, Guillermo, et al. "The International Experience." In THE REGION-ALIZATION OF PERSONAL HEALTH SERVICES, edited by Ernest W. Saward, pp. 123-33. New York: Prodist, 1976.

> Although reflecting primarily on his experience with regionalization
> in Puerto Rico, the author provides a broader overview of world
> literature and experiences on the subject. Valuable, but more
> selective than comprehensive.

Regionalization of Health Service Systems

Arbona, Guillermo, and Curt, J.N. "A Progress Report on Regionalization of Comprehensive Health Services in Puerto Rico." Working paper for the Expert Committee on Organization of Local and Intermediate Health Administrations. Geneva: WHO/Community Health Services, October 26–November 2, 1971. Reproduced. Available through WHO, 1211 Geneva 27 Switzerland.

> Updates the conception and experience described in the paper by Seipp published in LANCET (see below, this chapter). The authors disappointment over a private entrepreneurial system of medical care cutting into the coordinative ability of the public system is evident. In short, multiple authorities and streams of finance make regionalization difficult.

Arbona, Guillermo, and Ramirez de Arellano, Annette B. REGIONALIZATION OF HEALTH SERVICES: THE PUERTO RICAN EXPERIENCE. Preliminary version distributed in paperback book form at the 8th meeting of the IEA in San Juan, September 18-24, 1977.

> Arbona was minister of health in Puerto Rico. Ramirez de Arellano is responsible for much of the fine scholarship and writing. Provides a rich view of the historical background as well as a detailed statement of gains and pitfalls in the important Puerto Rican experience with regionalization. The widespread poverty and lack of medical resources in the hundred years prior to World War II make up an important part of the background. Contents: Preface; (1) Introduction: The Components of Regionalization; (2) Historical Antecedents to Regionalization in Puerto Rico; (3) The Bayamon Project; (4) The Extension of Regionalization; (5) Politics and Regionalization; (6) Regionalization Twenty Years Later; (7) Epilogue: Lessons from the Puerto Rican Experience; Appendix A Selected Data on Puerto Rico; Appendix B Chronology of Major Events in the Regionalization of Health Services in Puerto Rico; Sources Consulted.

> The Puerto Rican effort at regionalization cannot be considered a success. Political economic changes and changes in financing health care led to greater use of private doctors and hospitals and an undercutting of the regionalization scheme. Also, social workers successfully lobbied for their own social welfare structure. But many important lessons have been gleaned from this important experience, including the fact that the structure has been fairly durable although the process of regionalization has deteriorated.

Backett, E. Maurice. "Local and Intermediate Health Service Administration in Britain, A Personal Note on Problems and Progress." Working paper for the Expert Committee on Organization of Local and Intermediate Health Administrations. Geneva: WHO/Community Health Services, October 26-November 2, 1971. Reproduced. Available through WHO, 1211 Geneva 27 Switzerland.

> Anticipates the major reorganization of the UK's NHS which took effect in April 1974. Over the years since its enactment in 1946

and its beginning "on the appointed day" in 1948 as a tripartite system of general practitioners, hospitals, and local public health authorities, it became clearer that the principles of regionalization as identified in the Dawson report (see Consultative Council, below) should be applied to a whole unified health service and not just to a system of hospitals. Thus, instead of the complexity and relative lack of coordination of care under three different authorities, the reorganization put the whole system under single regional authorities in each geographic region. While this paper does not fully lay out the reorganization of the NHS, it does point up the less than desirable degree of coordination under the tripartite system.

Berfenstam, Ragnar. "Regionalization of Health Services: Learning from the Swedish Experience." In HEALTH CARE RESEARCH: A SYMPOSIUM, edited by Donald E. Larsen and Edgar J. Love, pp. 106-14. Calgary, Alberta: Univ. of Calgary, 1974.

Brief, clear description of the seven health regions in Sweden, each containing up to six counties (or parts of counties) with regional populations ranging from 600,000 to 1.6 million. In this system the counties are the primary units (though regional hospitals serve as back-up, highly specialized units for several counties). Counties contain between 2 and 400,000 persons. Within these units are district hospitals serving between 75,000 and 100,000 people and below the district hospital is the district health center serving between 30 and 400,000 persons. Problems include imperfect coordination of services and flow of patients between the levels and somewhat greater expense than might be expected perhaps due in significant part to overconcentration on in-hospital care rather than ambulatory and preventive care.

Berfenstam, Ragnar, and Elling, Ray H. "Regional Planning in Sweden: A Social and Medical Problem." In HEALTH: A MAJOR ISSUE, edited by Donald E. Askey, Special issue of SCANDINAVIAN REV. 63 (September 1975): 40-52. Republished as HEALTH SYSTEMS OF SCANDINAVIA. Bethesda, Md.: John E. Fogarty Center for Int'l. H., NIH, 1976.

Discusses the strengths and weaknesses of the Swedish health care system in relation to nine ideals of regionalization: (1) defined geographic regions; (2) graded hierarchy of services; (3) integrated authority structure in each; (4) coordinated two-way flows between levels; (5) thrust of the system toward primary and preventive care at the periphery; (6) closed-ended financing; (7) continuing education to facilitate updating and flexibility; (8) authentic citizen involvement; (9) local service units focused on the goal of developing and pursuing a complete preventive and therapeutic health plan for each member of each household. A tenth ideal often seen as essential to full regionalization was not explicitly identified; that is, that health services tasks should be performed by the person with the least formal preparation adequate for the tasks.

Bodenheimer, Thomas S. "Regional Medical Programs: No Road to Regionalization." MED. CARE REV. 26 (December 1969): 1125-66.

One of the best analyses of programs which failed to regionalize health services in the United States. Identified the following reasons for the failure of the Regional Medical Programs legislation: competing or conflicting institutional interests (hospitals, nursing homes, etc.), splits in public-private authority and sponsorship, varied streams of financing, competing or conflicting occupational group interests, locality interests, and competing planning legislation and structures (Comprehensive Health Planning designed to work through state health departments). The Regional Medical Programs legislation was designed to build health services regions around medical schools and their hospitals. The study does not give adequate attention to the theory of regionalization nor to the underlying social class and power structure conflicts in the political economy. Review of the US literature related to regionalization is especially valuable.

Boudreau, Thomas J. "The Regionalization of Health Services: Implementation and Research." In HEALTH CARE RESEARCH: A SYMPOSIUM, edited by Donald E. Larsen and Edgar J. Love, pp. 99-105. Calgary, Alberta: Univ. of Calgary, 1974.

Quotes the Castonguay Commission Report (Montreal, 1968) definition: regionalization of health services is the integrated organization of a health care system possessing multiple coordinated functions and serving a delimited geographical territory." The author clearly identifies regionalization as a process of social change and notes that most research on the subject has laid out the economic reasons for establishing regions. But there has been very little research on the process of regionalization.

Boukal, J. "Regionální systém sítě sdravotnecký́ch zařizerí v ČSSR a v zahraničí [Regional systems of the network of health institutions in Czechoslovakia and abroad]. CESKOSLOVENSKE ZDRAVOTNICTVI [Czechoslovakia's health] 17 (1969): 220-32. In Czech.

Bridgman, Robert F., and Roemer, Milton I. HOSPITAL LEGISLATION AND HOSPITAL SYSTEMS. Public Health Papers, no. 50. Geneva: WHO, 1972.

Although not devoted exclusively to regionalization, this is clearly the interest these authors have in describing and to some extent evaluating hospital legislation and systems in countries of the world. Most attention is given to industrialized or so-called developed countries.

Clark, Henry T., Jr. "The Challenge of the Regional Medical Programs Legislation." J. MED. ED. 41 (1966): 344-61.

Although targeted toward the opportunities for regionalization under the just-adopted US legislation indicated in the title, this work is important more generally and conceptually for the understanding it presents of the role of university medical centers (schools and hospitals) not only in providing back-up specialty care for a region, but in providing in-service education and on-the-job training throughout the region and in providing planning guidance through evaluative research. Draws on the works of Grant, "Health Centers etc." and Seipp, "Puerto Rico etc." (see below, this chapter). The article suffers somewhat from a lack of consideration of non-medical perspectives. The study also does not adequately consider the role of user participation particularly minority and working class users of health service, in building a fully regionalized service designed to reach all members of the population.

Cohen, Joshua. "Regionalization of Personal and Community Health Services." Working paper for the Expert Committee on Organization of Local and Intermediate Health Administrations. Geneva: WHO/Community Health Services, October 26–November 2, 1971. Available through WHO, 1211 Geneva 27 Switzerland.

One of the best conceptual statements of regionalization. Discusses, among other important points, the need to provide mass preventive measures out of district or regional public-health units, while personal, preventive care should be linked with the coordination of personal therapeutic care at the periphery of the regional system (point of patient's first entry). Is also clear about regional systems making sense only within a national system which sets overall priorities and standards and plays a role in allocating and redistributing resources.

Consultative Council on Medical and Allied Health Services. INTERIM REPORT ON THE FUTURE PROVISION OF MEDICAL AND ALLIED SERVICES. London: HMSO, 1920. [The Dawson Report].

Known as the Dawson Report, this work is of seminal importance for the theory and practice of health services regionalization. Has continuing as well as historical interest. Elements of regionalization were practiced prior to this statement; for example, in Sweden, the system of decentralized decision making, organization and financing of services through elected county councils had been practiced since the mid-1800s. But the Dawson Report was the first relatively complete written statement of regionalizing a health system. Sir Dawson of Penn, personal physician to King George V, served as chairman of the Consultative Council. Drawing on experience as a surgeon at the Western Front in World War I, he emphasized in the report a defined geographic area (the sector of a military front); a graded hierarchy of services (the front had triage in the trenches, first aid station, base hospital and regional hospital); and heavy emphasis on in-service training and upgrading

VANDERBILT MEDICAL CENTER LIBRARY

of public understanding of health problems. Concise and otherwise well written, the report has had an important influence on many health systems and health systems theorists and planners.

Da Cunha, José Correia. REGIONALIZAÇÃO DO TERRITÓRIO METROPOLITANO [Regionalization of the metropolitan (Portugal proper) territory]. Estudos de Planeamento Economico, no. 5. Lisbon: Secretatiado Technico da Presidencia do Conselho, n.d. [study conducted in 1966]. In Portugese.

An exercise in prerevolutionary Portugal to define economic regions, including hospital and military regions. The concept of subnational regions is considered. Briefly considers the identification of regions in a number of other European countries: UK, Holland, Finland, Norway, Sweden, Austria, FRG, Italy, and Spain. The history of regions in Portugal is reviewed with the aid of a series of interesting historical maps. The work proposes four regions for the future--one dominated by Lisbon, a northern, a central, and a southern one. In the appendix are a series of interesting maps showing current regions for electric service, hospitals, psychiatric service, and so forth. These all differ in important respects from each other. Useful study for confronting the problems of regional definition where a capitalist conception of economics prevails and no integral political organization has been established at the subnational regional level.

Daniels, Robert S., et al. "An Example of Sub-Regional Health Planning." INQUIRY 7 (December 1970): 25-33.

Not specifically directed toward the problem of regionalization, but is important in offering an understanding of the problems and possibilities of citizen involvement in health planning along with institutional and professional representatives in an urban area which is divided along social class and ethnic lines--South Chicago. Regional plans can not take hold or even properly evolve without the kind of organization and process described here. The article also gives the highlights of the by-laws adopted by this citizen-professional planning body.

Dixon, C.W. "Regional Medical Planning in New Zealand." NEW ZEALAND MED. J. 69 (1969): 371-74.

Dyck, Robert G. "The Regional Approach to Health in the Republic of Slovenia." In TOPIAS AND UTOPIAS IN HEALTH, edited by Stanley R. Ingman and Anthony E. Thomas, pp. 357-72. The Hague: Mouton; Chicago: Aldine, 1975.

Describes the relatively advanced concept and experience with regionalization of personal health services, health insurance (unified for workers and farmers) and environmental health in this Northwestern Republic of Yugoslavia. With some 1.5 million population, this republic is about the appropriate size for a region. In important ways it is the effective regional unit, for example, in the negotiation of "social agreements" laying out the general financing and mode of operation of hospitals, "health homes" (preventive and ambulatory care centers), and other institutions. Since 1950, health conditions have improved, personnel and services increased, and overall experience with regionalization has been favorable, though costs have also risen from 3.4 to 6.0 percent of GNP. Still there have been moves to effect efficiencies. Hospitals declined in number from thirty-two to twenty-four and health homes from 170 to 19 by 1972 with better staffing and a more complete range of services in each. The principles of Andrija Stampar (one of the founders of WHO) are listed and briefly discussed.

Elling, Ray H. "The Local Health Center and the Regional Board." In NATIONAL HEALTH CARE: ISSUES AND PROBLEMS IN SOCIALIZED MEDICINE, edited by Elling, pp. 245-62. New York: Atherton, 1973.

Anticipating (in 1971, when first published) some form of NHI in the United States, the author projects a somewhat idealistic conception of local health centers serving defined geographic areas backed up by a regionalized system controlled by a citizen board composed of at-large and local-health-center elected members. Draws an analogy with functioning combined school district boards to suggest the feasibility of such a form in the United States, since school boards also allocate scarce resources to tasks which "professionals" (teachers) usually wish to define for themselves.

_____. "Medical Systems as Changing Social Systems." In THEORETICAL FOUNDATIONS FOR THE COMPARATIVE STUDY OF HEALTH SYSTEMS, edited by Charles Leslie, Special issue of SOC. SCI. MED. 12, no. 2B (April 1978): 107-15.

The special issue of this journal was based on a conference of this title supported by the National Science Foundation and the Werner-Gren Foundation. Medical systems are seen as dependent components of their political economic contexts. A set of ten ideals are identified for achieving a fully regionalized health service as a system offering equity of access and adequate services for all along with user control. The most supportive national political economic context for this kind of health service system is seen as democratic centralism directed toward achieving a socialist economy. With regard to how inequitable systems might move, or be moved, toward the ideal, some phases of human liberation are identified as found in the work of Frantz Fanon, especially THE WRETCHED OF THE EARTH (New York: Grove Press, 1963).

_____. "Regionalization of Health Services: Sociological Blocks to Realization of an Ideal." In TOPIAS AND UTOPIAS IN HEALTH, edited by Stanley R. Ingman and Anthony E. Thomas, pp. 175-204. The Hague: Mouton; Chicago: Aldine, 1975. Bibliography.

Drawing on much of the published literature on regionalization and selected WHO reports, nine ideals of regionalization are identified (see Berfenstam and Elling, cited above, for list) and discussed briefly. Asking why these interwoven ideals have rarely if ever been fully realized, a number of conditions reflecting varied organized interests and ideological orientations are identified and discussed. Nations are categorized as wealthy or poor, with corresponding medical institutional environments termed "overstaffed" or "a vacuum." Nations are further classified according to the way political authority is organized: centralized-decentralized; or fractionated (divided)-concerted (cohesive). Hypothesizes that the ideal of regionalization will be most fully achieved in the decentralized concerted form without too many already established competing hospitals and other institutions. The cases of the PRC and Yugoslavia are cited as illustrations.

Empkie, Timothy M. "The Organization of Tuberculosis Prevention: A Comparison of the Federal Republic of Germany and the German Democratic Republic." See chapter 4.

Engel, Arthur. PERSPECTIVES IN HEALTH PLANNING. London: Athlone Press, 1968. Refs., tables, figures, appendixes, index.

Presents compilation of lecture series delivered by author upon his retirement as director-general of Swedish National Board of Health. Discusses role of national health planning in modern society. Stresses necessity for accurate vital statistics and asymptomatic disease screening as public health methods. Concludes with description of function, growth, and transition of Swedish regionalized hospital and health system to exemplify effective operation with minimal organizational requirements.

_____. PLANNING AND SPONTANEITY IN THE DEVELOPMENT OF THE SWEDISH HEALTH SYSTEM. The Annual Michael M. Davis Memorial Lecture. Chicago: Center for Health Administration Studies, Graduate School of Business, Univ. of Chicago, 1968.

The Swedish system of health services regions and other levels proceeding to the districts and health centers is built upon a hundred-year-old system of local county government control and financing of hospitals. Actually, county governments still pay some 75 percent of all health care costs (and a higher percent of hospital costs). The regions combine more than one county but can impose very little, since the real determinations are made at county level. This allows also for local initiative and variation even though there are also regional and national standards. See also American College of Hospital Administrators, chapter 3, section on Sweden in Ray H. Elling, CROSS-NATIONAL STUDY OF HEALTH SYSTEMS BY COUNTRY AND WORLD REGIONS, INCLUDING SPECIAL PROBLEMS. Detroit: Gale Research Co., 1980.

Ferrer, Reinaldo. "Regionalization in Puerto Rico--Problems and Progress."
AJPH 50 (1960): 1258-63.

Quotes John Grant on the fundamental character of regionalization
which assumes that "the education of the health care professions,
and the development of health care services form an inseparable
whole together with scientific research." To achieve this, Grant
said, "requires the re-examination and re-orientation of existing,
conventional policy in terms of an organization for the distribution
of health care services on a completely coordinated basis; and for
the inservice education and training of the technical personnel
within the health profession to undertake rendering such services
efficiently." The article identifies many of the obstacles in achieving
such a system, primarily in terms of divergences in orientation
and interest within the health professions in Puerto Rico. The article does not deal adequately with difficulties in Puerto Rico's
political economic system and colonialist ties to the United States.

Friedman, John, and Alonso, William, eds. REGIONAL POLICY: READINGS
IN THEORY AND APPLICATIONS. Cambridge: MIT Press, 1975.

A new version of the same editors' REGIONAL DEVELOPMENT
AND PLANNING published in 1964. This present volume shows
that regional planning has become a discipline in its own right
two decades after Walter Isard founded the International Regional
Science Association. Provides a thorough review and examination
of past and current work. Part 1 examines the concept of socioeconomic space and its utility for understanding the process of development. Part 2 deals with the role of cities in national development. A shortcoming of the book is its lack of any discussion
of foreign dependency and unbalanced power relationships as these
affect regional and national development plans of UDCs. There is
no special focus on health or health care systems.

Glasgow, John, et al. REGIONALIZATION OF HEALTH SERVICES: POLICY
IMPLICATIONS OF A NATIONAL EXPERIMENT. Boise, Idaho: Health Policy
Analysis and Accountability Network, 1977. 41 refs., 7-item bibliography.

An article-length monograph (20 p.) attempting to pull out "lessons
learned" from several US partial attempts at regionalization, though
the focus here is on the Regional Medical Programs legislation and
does not dwell on the Hill-Burton Hospital Construction Act or the
Comprehensive Health Planning and does not mention legislation in
the mental health field directed toward "catchment areas" and so
forth. The thrust of the analysis and recommendations is on clear
administrative and planning structures for regional systems. A
valuable contribution.

Godlund, S. "Population, Regional Hospitals, Transport Facilities and Regions."
Lund Studies in Human Geography, Series B in HUMAN GEOGRAPHY 21.
Lund, Sweden: Royal Univ. of Lund, 1961.

Presents a method for locating regional hospitals under the assumption that the average travel time and cost for the population to be served should be minimized and no one should have to travel more than four hours, thereby cutting down on overnight stays. Includes the drawing of "isochrone" lines on a map at one-hour travel time separation from each other in relation to a proposed regional hospital center. Then a population density map is superimposed to allow calculation of average travel time. By this method, Sweden adopted seven centers (actually two in Stockholm counted here as one): Stockholm, Upsala, Lund-Malmoe, Gothenburg, Umei, Linkoeping, and Karlstad.

Grant, John B. "Health Centers and Regionalization." AJPH 43 (January 1953): 9-13.

This work builds upon the Dawson Report (see Consultative Council on Medical and Allied Health Services, above) and experience in prerevolutionary China. Makes a distinct contribution to the theory and practice of regionalization.

_____. "Medical Regionalization and Education." J. MED. ED. 30 (1955): 73-80.

Gross, P.F. "Urban Health Disorders, Spatial Analysis, and the Economics of Health Facility Location." INT'L. J. H. SERV. 2 (1972): 63-84.

An analysis of a number of contemporary bed-planning methodologies, either in use or under development, reveals a number of limitations. In particular, the linkage between the optimal size of health facilities and the optimal size of their service areas has often been ignored; in addition, the determinants of utilization of services have often been ignored. An alternative approach to the size-location problem is proposed. Working from health-economics-medical-sociology concepts, a behavioral model of health services utilization is proposed on the demand side. The interface to the supply side is through a model of the consumer's perception of the total costs facing him in hospital care.

Haraldson, Sixten. "Health Services among Scattered Populations." ACTA SOCIO-MEDICA SCANDINAVICA 6, supplement (1972): 50-56.

"H[ealth] I[nsurance] P[rogram of Greater New York] Completes First Major Reorganization in 25 Years." GROUP H. AND WELFARE NEWS 12 (January 1972): whole issue.

Discusses and analyses the problems of regionalizing a health insurance and services program which covers only a part of a metropolitan population (subscribes through labor unions and other groups) and faces competing interests in teaching hospitals which raise the costs of care in these settings. Describes reorganization measures intended to deal with these problems. This article was reviewed in MED. CARE REV. 29 (March 1972): 251-54.

Hechter, Michael. "The Persistence of Regionalism in the British Isles, 1885-1966." AJS 79 (September 1973): 319-42.

Although not focused on health, this article provides some of the sociocultural and political economic context for understanding such regional disparities in health resources as those observed by Julian Tudor Hart, "The Inverse Care Law." See chapter 5.

Heller, P.S. "The Strategy of Health-Sector Planning in the People's Republic of China." Univ. of Michigan Discussion Paper, no. 24. Ann Arbor, 1972. Reproduced.

Identifies the emphasis on decentralization and self sufficiency at the local level which is so supportive of a relatively complete degree of regionalization in the PRC.

Infante, A.D. "Regionalización Como Estructura Docente" [Regional confinement of the teaching structure]. REVISTA MEDICA DE CHILE (Santiago) 96 (May 1968): 348-59. In Spanish. 12 refs.

The division of Chile into health regions closely follows the structure of the NHS in the UK. The hospitals of Santiago are assigned to broad health zones into which the country has been divided. East Hospital is the area base and, as such, acts as the regional hospital for other smaller hospitals located in the same zone. The geography of the country presented certain problems to this concept of regionalization, which, at the time of the publication of the paper, were referred back for further study. The endemic lack of medical personnel and their inability to meet the demands upon their services were reasons for the establishment of the Postgraduate School of the Faculty of Medicine of the University of Chile. Patients go to the regional hospital seeking services the zone hospital cannot provide, and doctors from zone hospitals go to regional hospitals to seek advice or supplementary training. Specialists from the regional hospitals give consultations at zone hospitals, thus providing feedback to the faculty through field experiences. The NHS although a national structure, allows zone units to operate with a degree of autonomy to meet regional needs. The paper suggests that the chronic shortage of professional staff could be met by using people in rural areas as auxiliary health workers. The extent of their training should be proportional to the difficulty of obtaining the services of a physician.

Isard, Walter, and Reiner, Thomas A., "Regional Science." In INTERNATIONAL ENCYCLOPEDIA OF THE SOCIAL SCIENCES, edited by David Sills, vol. 13, pp. 382-90. New York: Macmillan, 1968.

Valuable general consideration of regional theory and planning; not specific to health.

Klarman, Herbert E. "Some Technical Problems in Area Wide Planning for Hospital Care." J. OF CHRONIC DISEASES 17 (1964): 735-47.

Kulinski, Antoni R., and Petrella, Riccardo, eds. GROWTH POLES AND RE-GIONAL POLICIES, A SEMINAR. The Hague: Mouton, 1972.

Not directed toward health services, but important in considering regional political economic arrangements in development which have important implications for health. For a critical review of this and other theories of development, see Brookfield, cited in chapter 2. Rather than "spreading" their developmental influences throughout a region, growth poles (urban centers, usually) extract from and exploit their hinterlands. This view makes good sense in the health field when one considers the almost worldwide problem of concentration of modern facilities, personnel, and services in urban areas, as well as the problem of the "brain-drain."

Lavoipierre, Guy J. "Economic Development and Health, The Lake Volta Schistosomiasis Epidemic." FEATURES, no. 21, October 1972, pp. 1-4. Geneva: WHO.

Good discussion of the interweaving of socioeconomic, political, cultural, and epidemiologic conditions of a region in Ghana.

Lawson, Ian R. "Some Determinants in the Management of Long-Stay Care--The Substance of an Address to the Conference on Continuing Care." Sponsored by the Connecticut Regional Medical Program, the Yale New Haven Health Center, and the Connecticut Hospital Assn. New Haven, Conn.: CRMP, December 2, 1969. Reproduced. Available from the author, vice-president for medical affairs, Danbury Hospital, Danbury, Conn.

At the time of writing, the author was assistant professor of clinical medicine, University of Connecticut and had served as consultant physician in the Scottish North-Eastern Regional Geriatric Service. The paper is not highly systematic but nevertheless succeeds in adumbrating the key elements of a comprehensive regionalized system of care for the elderly. Using his own experience, Lawson contrasts the US system of treating patients with the Scottish system. He finds the US system is partial (many pieces such as organized home care and day or weekend care are usually missing), imbalanced (far too much of elder care is concentrated in human warehousing in nursing homes, and necessary social support services are not adequately covered under Medicare), and uncoordinated (no hospital-based problem assessment unit is linked in a responsible way into a full range of other services and the patient care coordinating responsibility shifts with each new service). He presents a very sensitive view of elements needed in a properly regionalized system.

Leavell, Hugh, R. "Regionalization of Health Services, An Examination of the Regionalization Concept and of WHO's Possible Role in Relation to this Concept." Geneva: WHO/Organization of Health Services, 1969. Reproduced. Available through WHO, 1211 Geneva 27 Switzerland.

> This consultant's report reviews and digests a great amount of material on the subject. Although one of the best overviews, it is limited in its coverage of non-Western experience and is not particularly forceful and clear as to what WHO should do about regionalization.

Long, M.F., and Feldstein, Paul. "Economics of Hospital Systems: Peak Loads and Regional Coordination." AMERICAN ECONOMIC REV. 57 (May 1967): 119-29.

McNerney, Walter, and Reidel, Donald C. REGIONALIZATION AND RURAL HEALTH CARE. Ann Arbor: Univ. of Michigan, 1962.

> A sound empirical study of some limited attempts at regionalizing hospitals in a rural region of Michigan. Esentially no movement was achieved in such vital areas as exchange of staff and patients. Some movement was achieved in sharing continuing education resources and experiences.

Maynard, Alan. "Avarice, Inefficiency, and Inequality: An International Health Care Tale." See chapter 5.

> The author considers the lack of evidence for the cost-effectiveness of many popular surgical and other treatments and calls for changes in health system organization.

Meade, James. "A Mathematical Model for Deriving Hospital Service Areas." INT'L. J. H. SERV. 4 (1974): 353-64.

> Author's summary: "The basic premise explored in this paper is that patient flow in rural areas is based on the proximity to medical care. The hospital is defined as the center of care and hospital catchment areas are defined by patient movements. A methodology is described to analyze patient flow among an assemblage of hospitals. Finally, a model which mathematically replicates patient movement is introduced to act as an aid in the hospital planning process." The study is based on Idaho data.

Ministry of Health for Western Australia. "Regionalization of Hospital Services." Perth, Australia; August 19, 1975. Available through the ministry.

> An interesting document with maps and data on beds and use attempting to delineate three rationally defined hospital service regions for the vast land area of western Australia. Does not provide much discussion, particularly of such interesting aspects as the flying doctor service.

Myrdal, Jan, and Kessle, Gunn. THE REVOLUTION CONTINUED. New York: Random House, Pantheon Books, 1972.

> See especially the chapter entitled "The Health Insurance Reform." The whole work is important for understanding the impact of the Cultural Revolution in the PRC. A particularly potent statement, because Myrdal was able to study the same village both before and after the Cultural Revolution. The chapter on health indicates what Mao's theme, "In health, place the emphasis on the countryside," has meant. The realization of the collective value of health at the local brigade and commune levels brought with it extensive and authentic citizen involvement in health policy and action including payments toward an insurance for barefoot doctor and other services. Thus, although a regional back-up system of commune and central hospitals is in place in most areas, the thrust of the system is properly toward the periphery to anticipate and deal with problems as close to their place of occurrence as possible.

Navarro, Vicente. "The City and the Region: A Critical Relationship in the Distribution of Health Resources." AMERICAN BEHAVIORAL SCIENTIST 14 (1971): 865-92.

> Confronts the difficult and complex problems of (1) overconcentration of resources in urban centers as compared with surrounding rural and semiurban areas; and (2) competition and lack of a clear division of labor and graded hierarchy of services between urban services, particularly hospitals. Clearly links the solutions to political economic changes.

_____. "Regionalization and Planning of Personal Health Services: An Annotated Bibliography." Baltimore: Department of Medical Care and Hospitals, Johns Hopkins Univ., 1967. Available from the author, School of Hygiene and Public Health, 615 N. Wolfe St., Baltimore, Md. 21205.

> An extensive bibliography on regionalization of health services including items on methodologies used for regional allocations of health resources.

New York Academy of Medicine. "Hospitals: Isolated or Interpedendent?" In THE HOSPITAL AS A COMMUNITY FACILITY. Special issue of BUL. N.Y. ACAD. MED. 48 (December 1972): 1349-1514.

> Includes papers by Guillermo Arbona on the regionalized system in Puerto Rico; by Irial Gogan, "Cooperation of Hospitals in Canada: Regionalization, Mergers, and Shared Services"; and other papers on regionalization of hospitals by Kenneth H. Hannan, Sidney S. Lee, Stephen M. Morris, and Cecil G. Sheps.

Odell, Peter R. "A European View on Regional Development and Planning in Latin America." INT'L. REVIEW OF COMMUNITY DEVELOPMENT 17 (Spring 1971): 3-22.

> A useful overview of experience in a number of countries, recognizing the frequent problem of imbalanced economic "development" in a particular area (e.g., single-crop farming or mining) without attention to other economic possibilities and human needs. A useful table (p. 13) ranks centers of economic activity within countries and within Latin America as a whole.

Palec, Rudolf. "The Regional System and Post-graduate Medical Training in Czechoslovakia." MILBANK MEM. FUND Q. 44 (October 1966): 414-25.

Pellegrino, Edmund D. "Regionalization: An Integrated Effort of Medical School, Community, and Practicing Physician." In NEW DIRECTIONS IN PUBLIC POLICY FOR HEALTH CARE. Special issue of BUL. N.Y. ACAD. MED. 42 (December 1966): 1193-1200.

> An early statement presenting the rationale for the impending Regional Medical Programs legislation designed to work through the medical schools in the United States.

_____. "Role of the Community Hospitals in Continuing Education; The Hunterdon Experiment." JAMA 165 (May 25, 1957): 361-65.

> Of historical interest as it describes the conception and early experience of the famous Hunterdon County experiment in New Jersey, linking local community practitioners with a university medical center faculty through the staff of an upgraded local hospital.

Puerto Rico Commonwealth. Department of Health. OPERATION REGIONALIZATION IN PUERTO RICO: A PLAN FOR IMPROVING MEDICAL, HEALTH CARE, AND WELFARE SERVICES THROUGH REGIONAL COORDINATION. San Juan, 1957.

> An early prospectus of the plan for a regional health system. This statement identifies four major benefits to be expected from regionalization: (1) improved quality of service by diffusion of standards, knowledge, and expertise from professional schools to isolated areas; (2) the holding of costs to a minimum through avoidance of duplication and coordination of effort (though it was recognized that coordination itself costs); (3) comprehensive, preventive, and curative health services to be made available to all residents, whether urban or rural; and (4) encouraging local citizens to improve health conditions and health through their own efforts. The country's experience with this plan is discussed in the works by Seipp and Arbona, cited in this chapter.

Roemer, Milton I. "Planning Health Services: Substance versus Form." CA-NADIAN J. OF PUB. H. 59 (November 1968): 431-37.

> Good brief discussion of the health planning goals and the social process of overcoming vested interests to provide a full range of coordinated services. The author states, "The effective and efficient provision of these several types of service in communities, in my view, constitutes the substance of planning. The articulation of different communities and the transfer of services or patients across community borders constitutes regionalization." In offering this conception, the author cites an article by Paul Lembcke (ANNALS OF THE AMERICAN ACADEMY OF POLITICAL AND SOCIAL SCIENCE, January 1951, pp. 53-61).

Ruderman, A. Peter "Discussion of Papers on the Regionalization of Health Services." In HEALTH CARE RESEARCH: A SYMPOSIUM, edited by Donald E. Larsen and Edgar J. Love, pp. 115-18. Calgary, Alberta: Univ. of Calgary, 1974.

> Provocative, occasionally acerbic discussion of other papers in this volume.

Rummel, R.J. THE DIMENSIONS OF NATIONS. Beverly Hills, Calif.: Sage Publications, 1972.

> Valuable for assessing the potential of multivariate analysis for CNSHS, including factor analysis (given availability of data). Although 230 variables are included for many nations, this large volume has little current interest as to content since 1955 data were employed.

Saward, Ernest W., ed. THE REGIONALIZATION OF PERSONAL HEALTH SERVICES. Rev. ed. New York: Prodist (for the Milbank Memorial Fund), 1977. Appendixes.

> One of the most complete overviews of thought and experience on this topic with conference discussion by some of the leading US students of health services regionalization. A lengthy first chapter by David Pearson records history of US regionalization--the work of Joseph Mountain; the Hill-Burton Hospital Construction Act; Comprehensive Health Planning legislation and Regional Medical Program legislation; and the most recent act, intended to draw the skein together, The National Health Planning and Resources Development Act of 1975, Public Law 93-641. The appendixes include an invaluable summary of P.L. 93-641, and make available for the first time to the American reader the classic Dawson Report, one of the cornerstones of planning in the health services of the UK.

Schicke, R.K. "Die regionalisierte Gesundheitsversorgung Schwedens" [The regionalized provision for health of Sweden]. KRANKENHAUSARZT [Hospital doctor] 7 (1972): 402-10. In German.

Very useful, detailed description of the Swedish system, particularly focused on the graded hierarchy of services among hospitals.

Schultz, G.P. "Logic of Health Care Facility Planning." SOCIO-ECONOMIC PLANNING SCIENCES (Elmsford, N.Y.) 4 (September 1970): 383-93. 12 refs.

This study presents a logical model for the planning of health care facilities, aiming at a plan that maximizes net social benefit for the population of a metropolitan region. The health services utilize several orders of services and a facility hierarchy. The model states a method for determining the optimal scale and service area for each order. Net social benefit is computed from a set of basic functions that describe the demand for services, the unit cost of services, travel cost, and benefits derived.

Seipp, Conrad. "Puerto Rico, A Social Laboratory." LANCET 1 (June 22, 1963): 1364-68.

One of the most important pieces in the literature on regionaliza-tion. Draws on the Dawson Report, the writings of John Grant, and experience in Puerto Rico in which an attempt was made to merge medical and social services at the periphery and focus the center around the university health schools (medicine and public health) with these having real operating responsibility for delivery of services through the regionalized system throughout the island. Did not adequately anticipate the influences of the elitist, class-based private system of care which eventually undercut this promis-ing conception. See also next item.

_____. "The Regionalization of Health Care in Puerto Rico." Chapter 6 in a forthcoming book on coordination of health services, Univ. of North Carolina, Chapel Hill. Unpublished manuscript. Available from the author, Health Ser-vices Research Center, Univ. of North Carolina, Chapel Hill, N.C.

This eighty-page chapter provides perhaps the most perceptive and one of the most thoroughly documented studies of the Puerto Rican experience. Includes a table showing changes in socioeconomic and health conditions from 1940 to 1970. The regionalization ex-periment was unique in this setting because of the strong US co-lonialist forces and special tax arrangements with the United States. Thus it is not directly applicable to other UDCs, though many of the principles and some influences apply. Under the guidance of John Grant and others of "a small elite," including the author and Guillermo Arbona, a noble experiment in health services re-gionalization was undertaken in conjunction with "operation boot-strap," an industrialization-development effort designed to make the most of the population and climate--the major resources of the island. Although some aspects of the regionalization effort remain in the system, it must be counted as a failure. This in-depth case study details the conflicting ideologies and interests accompanying a market-oriented, capitalist "development" effort, as well as divergences in orientation internal to the medical, public health, and social welfare institutions and occupational groups. One of the richest, most valuable pieces in the literature on regionalization. The fundamental shortcoming was probably the failure to encourage a mass-based political-economic revolution to give direction, rather than a "small elite," however public in orientation.

Shannon, G.W., and Dever, G.E.A. HEALTH CARE DELIVERY: SPATIAL PERSPECTIVES. New York: McGraw-Hill, 1974.

As part of the historical background of this work the authors note that L.L. Finke, a German doctor, wrote in 1792 that differences between states and countries which influence disease patterns could be called "medical geography." In the view of these authors, medical geography has two parts: (1) ecology of disease, and (2) spatial arrangements in the planning and provision of care. "The spatial element, synonymous with the geography of health care, is an important aspect of the economic, the sociological, the epidemiological, the behavioral (psychological), and other factors that constitute the system of health care" (p. 6). Central place theory is considered an ideal way of viewing the arrangement of elements of a regional system. The less than ideal, but nevertheless quite fully regionalized systems of the USSR and Sweden are considered. The gross disparities between regions in the United States are considered, for example, in terms of primary care physicians and their characteristics. Only 2 percent of US doctors are blacks. Women are also much underrepresented. Discrimination is seen as an important factor in "health space."

THE SWEDISH REGIONALIZED HOSPITAL SYSTEM, PAPERS IN HONOR OF ARTHUR ENGEL. Stockholm: National Board of Health, 1967.

Arthur Engel, director of the National Board of Health for many years, achieved worldwide recognition as the main architect and enactor of the regionalized hospital system in Sweden. These papers honor him, following his retirement. The papers examine the concept, reflect on experience, and examine problems leading to the "7 crowns reform" in the early 1970s.

Taliaferro, J. Dale, and Remmers, W.W. "Identifying Integrated Regions for Health Care Delivery." H. SERVICES REPORTS 88 (April 1973): 337-43.

Considers the three main bases for defining regions: Imposed from without (administrative bases); derived from existing behavior patterns, such as health care utilization data (ecological bases); and prescribed on the basis of relevant administrative and ecological data and a theoretical system for improving the delivery of care. "The system we present is an attempt to modify some existing analytical techniques so as to produce a more desirable kind of regionalization procedure." The paper employs hospital use data by patient residence as taken from hospital billing records in Kansas to illustrate the suggested approach.

Trussel, Ray E., and Elinson, Jack. CHRONIC ILLNESS IN A RURAL AREA: THE HUNTERDON STUDY. Cambridge, Mass.: Harvard Univ. Press, 1959.

The complete report of the important Hunterdon County, New Jersey, experiment, linking a local hospital to a university medical center for purpose of in-service education for practitioners, assessment of quality of care, and upgrading of care generally.

United Kingdom. Department of Health and Social Security. "Regional Resource Allocation Formula, First Interim Report of the Resource Allocation Working Party." London, 1975.

Examines for the UK as a whole the disparities in medical resources by regions (a nearly universal problem--see Alan Maynard, cited in chapter 5). The better endowed areas are around London and the Thames. The report recommends emphasis on improvements in the northern regions. This recommendation may be political, however, because the Labour Government was in power, and the report favors the Labour-dominated northern regions, while the areas around the Thames tend to be conservative.

United Nations Research Institute for Social Development (UNRISD). "Sociology of Regional Development." A collection of working papers for discussion. Geneva, June 1968. Mimeographed. Available from UNRISD, 1211 Geneva, 27 Switzerland.

A short collection of papers by Antoni Kulinski, Riccardo Petrella, Z.J. Pioro, and others.

United Nations (UN). Department of Economic and Social Affairs. DECENTRALIZATION FOR NATIONAL AND LOCAL DEVELOPMENT. See chapter 2.

Warren, Sharon, and Williams, J.I. "What Role is There for Municipal Government in Health Regionalization?" CANADIAN J. PUB. H. 67 (March-April 1976): 105-8.

Considers that local governments in Canada could play a role in improving and democratizing care. However, given the negative attitudes of British physicians toward local government, the authors anticipate resistance from the medical profession in Canada to a more active role for local governments in organizing and delivering medical care.

Wheeler, K.E. "The Regional Health Authority: A Possible Approach to Rural Health Problems." INQUIRY 7 (1970): 15-31.

World Health Organization (WHO). ORGANIZATION OF LOCAL AND IN-
TERMEDIATE HEALTH ADMINISTRATIONS, REPORT OF A WHO EXPERT COM-
MITTEE. Technical Report Series, no. 499. Geneva, 1972.

> An important document in this field. Opens by citing earlier WHO
> Technical Reports of historical and background interest, especially
> number 83 (1954), "Local, Regional and Other Intermediate Or-
> ganizational Patterns"; and number 122 (1957), "Regionalization
> of Hospital Services." The report recognizes an increasing tendency
> towards the decentralization or regionalization of health services."
> The report offers several useful definitions, including the following
> two: (1) Region--A subdivision of a country for the purposes of
> planning for socioeconomic development; (2) Regionalization of
> health services--The rationalization of services so as to provide
> comprehensive health care to a community or group of communities.
> About a third of the report is devoted to administrative and man-
> agement concerns. The rest is devoted to the concept and struc-
> tural and functional aspects of regionalized health and medical care
> systems. Although good in recognizing cultural, resource, geo-
> graphic, and epidemiologic variations, the report is singularly in-
> adequate in its lack of recognition and discussion of variation in
> political economic forms and their impacts on such key aspects of
> regionalization as citizen participation and integrated authority for
> health.

_____. "Regionalization, A Selected Bibliography." Geneva: Community
Health Services/WP/71.3, 1971. Reproduced.

> A very useful (though not annotated) multilanguage bibliography on
> this subject.

Worth, R.M. "Institution Building in the People's Republic of China: The Rural
Health Center." EAST-WEST CENTER REV. (Honolulu) 1 (February 1965): 19-34.

> In China prior to 1949, the physical environment was heavily pol-
> luted, parasitic diseases were universal, infectious diseases were
> highly prevalent, and infant and child mortality rates were ex-
> tremely high. The first Chinese National Health Congress of 1950
> stated four specific health policies: (1) improve the health of pea-
> sants, workers, soldiers, (2) emphasize preventive medicine, (3)
> participate in mass health campaigns, and (4) join forces with tra-
> ditional practitioners. By 1955 most serious health problems had
> been alleviated and the most logical step forward was to develop
> local health centers. Meanwhile the membership of the Chinese
> Medical Association included traditional practitioners and Western-
> style doctors who were studying traditional medicine part-time. In
> 1958 came the communes, the Great Leap Forward, and the con-
> comitant health measures of (1) intensifying campaigns against para-
> sitic diseases, (2) building health centers in every commune and
> health stations in each village, (3) rotation of urban health workers
> to rural areas, and (4) an effort to gather private home remedies

to turn over to research institutions. At health centers, patients were free to choose between a Western doctor and a traditional practitioner, but the two doctors would consult with each other and treat each other as equals. There appears to be a pragmatic amalgamation of these two medical systems at the local level. Communication in this development scheme has involved radios, newspapers, meetings, plays, and other media, all of which provide reinforcement of party policies at the local level. It will be of interest to see whether China's mass communication system can reduce the birth rate to match the dramatic fall in the death rate.

_____. "Strategy of Change in the People's Republic of China: The Rural Health Center." In COMMUNICATION AND CHANGE IN THE DEVELOPING COUNTRIES, edited by W. Schramm and D. Lerner, pp. 216-30. Honolulu: East-West Center Press, 1967.

Preliberation China suffered from intense overcrowding in cities and villages, universal pollution by human and animal wastes, a mortality rate of 30 percent in the one-to-five-year group, and a high prevalence of insect-borne, parasitic, and infectious diseases. One of Mao's first steps toward a national health policy was to call for the unity of all medical workers of traditional and Western schools alike, and to emphasize disease prevention and mass health education. The next step was to develop local health centers for the 85 percent or so of the people in rural districts, and to restore traditional medicine to a place of prominence in the national scheme, thus allowing the Chinese people to retain pride in their heritage, and bridge the gap in identity between "old China" and "new China". Research institutes and schools of Chinese medicine were established and Western-style doctors given courses in traditional medicine. The rural health center became an established institution in every commune, with smaller health stations in the villages. Here, as well as in city hospitals, a patient was free to choose which type of physician, traditional or modern, he wished to be treated by. There appears to be a real communication between and a pragmatic fusion of these two medical systems at the local level; the situation illustrates a successful effort in development, achieved through the overwhelming force of the Communist mass communication system.

Zayed, Marlene. "Contrasting Case Studies of National Health Systems in Arab Countries." See chapter 4.

Zukin, Paul. "Planning a Health Component for an Economic Development Program." AJPH 61 (September 1971): 1751-59.

Although this article only mentions regional planning within the context of national planning, it is particularly useful in identifying the need to interweave health planning within regions and nations with socioeconomic planning generally. Provides a useful figure depicting stages in health planning and cites some illustrative experiences from Turkey, Malaysia, and Crete.

Chapter 7
METHODS

Methods derive from or are or should be closely determined by theory. Yet, the framework for CNSHS is in need of much further work. And presupposing such work, can we envision the implications for methods of a conflict perspective versus the implications of a consensual framework (see the introduction to chapter 5)? Perhaps the most general methodological implications of these differing perspectives are drawn out in the work of Mills included in chapter 5. The conflict approach clearly admits a value orientation and seeks to develop links between theory and practice. A researcher taking the consensual perspective is more likely to pretend to assume a value-free observational, nonaction stance. Also, the conflict view is likely to entail a greater commitment to wholistic understanding while the consensual approach may be biased toward discrete quantification. These are only some of the most general methodological implications of different theoretical approaches. These implications remain to be drawn out more completely in future scholarly work.

For now, it seems most helpful to draw upon Boulding's THE IMAGE, cited in Chapter 5, to recall that any social entity such as a research team or a ministry of health, has an image--a way of orienting itself and being known to surrounding social world of competing similar entities, possible supporters, antagonists, and so forth. The gathering, processing, and use of data are very important aspects of creating this image. While some of the work in this chapter (e.g., McGranahan) considers CNSHS data primarily in terms of technical shortcomings and opportunities, it is important to consider the sociopolitical and cultural context surrounding the generation and use of cross-national health systems data. Thus, failure of governments to report cholera or smallpox outbreaks, even attempts to hide a national disaster such as a massive famine (e.g., Ethiopia in 1972-74) become understandable, if unacceptable. Health statistics may be matters of national pride, as Haeroe points out in his chapter in the important book edited by Pflanz and Schach. Researchers attempting to use available data must take such considerations into account. Even in gathering original data, political considerations can become intertwined at every stage of the CNSHS research process (see items by Elling and Glaser, especially). While most methods texts are relevant to CNSHS (but are not included here as being too general for this introduction to this special field) they generally give almost no attention to the sociopolitical context of data generation and use, except perhaps in abstract discussions of "bias," and often this is treated simply as a statistical concept. Perhaps, the special methodological contribution of CNSHS is to heighten our awareness of sociopolitical as well as cultural factors in the research process. Because of the sociopolitical context of data generation and use and the difficulty in getting cross-national comparability (see Acheson, Chance, and Jacobson, among others), an approach contrasting in-depth case studies is preferable. In this approach one depends on fitting information together within a context to achieve what Weber termed "Verstehen" (understanding). See Elling and Kerr, cited in this chapter.

Acheson, Roy M., ed. COMPARABILITY IN INTERNATIONAL EPIDEMIOLOGY. New York: Milbank Mem. Fund, 1965. Also issued as part 2 of MILBANK MEM. FUND Q. 43 (April 1965). Index.

> Selected papers from the International Conference on Comparability in Epidemiological Studies, Fourth Scientific Conference of the International Epidemiological Association. Includes a very valuable introduction (pp. 11-18) by the editor giving an overview of the issues and approaches covered in the volume, for example, on the virtues and limitations of "portable" or "raw" data to develop reliable "language- and culture-free" coding systems (though such culture-freedom is never totally attainable nor even a sensible goal). A very rich and valuable collection with thirty-nine contributions. Perhaps section 6 in the first part, "Medical Care" is most relevant to CNSHS, but there are other papers with valuable general methodological points throughout.

Aday, Lu Ann, and Andersen, Ronald. DEVELOPMENT OF INDICES OF ACCESS TO MEDICAL CARE. Ann Arbor, Mich.: Health Administration Press, 1974.

Agency for International Development (AID). "Project Evaluation Guidelines." See chapter 5.

Aiken, Michael. "Comparative Cross-National Research on Subnational Units in Western Europe. Problems, Data Sources and a Proposal." See chapter 8.

> Considers the effects of within country variations on national data.

Alker, Hayward R., and Russett, Bruce M. "Indices for Comparing Inequality." In COMPARING NATIONS: THE USE OF QUANTITATIVE DATA IN CROSS-NATIONAL RESEARCH, edited by R.L. Merritt and Stein Rokkan, pp. 349-82. New Haven, Conn.: Yale Univ. Press, 1966.

> Important for considering the difficult but key question of how wealth and income are concentrated among an elite or how they are dispersed throughout a citizenry.

Allardt, E. "Implications of Within-nation Variations and Regional Imbalances for Cross-National Research." In COMPARING NATIONS: THE USE OF QUANTITATIVE DATA IN CROSS-NATIONAL RESEARCH, edited by R.L. Merritt and Stein Rokkan, pp. 337-48. New Haven: Yale Univ. Press, 1966.

> Valuable consideration of nearly all aspects of this general problem in the use of aggregated available data for comparing national units, be it in the health field or otherwise.

Altman, Isadore, et al. METHODOLOGY IN EVALUATING THE QUALITY OF MEDICAL CARE; AN ANNOTATED SELECTED BIBLIOGRAPHY, 1955-1968. See chapter 9.

Andrews, Frank M., and Withey, Stephen B. "Assessing the Quality of Life as People Experience It." Paper presented at the annual meetings of the ASA, Montreal, August 1974. Appendix. Available from the author through the ASA, Washington, D.C.

> Describes several sophisticated survey approaches for measuring perceived quality of life. Using survey data, this paper gives selected early results among national samples of the US population aged sixteen and over. The respondents' personal health and adequacy of doctors and hospitals in the area are only 2 of 123 items making up the specific concerns which are conceptually and statistically grouped into "criteria" which guide the person to evaluating "domains of concern." There is also the assumption that the quality of life as a whole can be summed up through the measures of the several domains put together. The paper includes some "maps" of the domains of concern. Major ones are self; other people; family; job; local area; and larger society. Economic aspects cross-cut several of these. "Smaller" domains of concern fit within certain of the larger ones (house in local area and religion). Provocative for conceiving of and measuring "health" in relation to other aspects of well-being. The appendix lists the items used according to which surveys included them.

Austin, Charles J. "Selected Social Indicators in the Health Field." AJPH 61 (August 1971): 1507-13.

Badgley, Robin F. "International Health Research Methods: Footnotes on Canadian Health Services." In CROSS-NATIONAL SOCIOMEDICAL RESEARCH: CONCEPTS, METHODS, PRACTICE, edited by Manfred Pflanz and Elisabeth Schach. Stuttgart, Germany: Thieme, 1976.

> A chapter illustrating the pitfalls of applying abstract cross-country statistical findings to a particular country, in this case Canada, and giving contextual qualifications necessary for a better understanding.

Methods

Baster, Nancy, ed. MEASURING DEVELOPMENT: THE ROLE OF ADEQUACY OF DEVELOPMENT INDICATORS. Portland, Oreg.: Frank Cass and Co., 1972.

Berg, Robert L. "Methodologic Problems in Construction of Health Status Indexes." Paper presented at the 8th int'l. scientific meetings of the IEA, Puerto Rico, September 17-23, 1977.

> Author's abstract: "With increasing research in the field of health status indexes, a number of important methodologic problems have emerged which require satisfactory resolution before such indexes can be applied to the allocation of scarce resources.
>
> Issues of reliability and validity have progressed along guidelines set down by psychologists particularly. This includes criterion validation, that is to say the established ways of measuring health status against which other measures can be compared. While physician evaluations of patients have often been used, it is clearly inadequate in certain fields such as social function.
>
> Content validation tests whether the measure tests what is supposed to be measured and includes such issues as whether the health status should be phrased in a positive or negative way, and the comprehensiveness of the functions measured (including descriptions of the quality of life). Construct validation refers to the comparative evaluation of different aspects of a construct when no single criterion is available.
>
> The assignment of weights to different conditions of life is the area of perhaps greatest discussion, whether they should be decided by direct or indirect means (such as equivalence, standard gambles, money or time tradeoffs); whether consumption expenditures should be included, and whether a correction factor should be added for uneveness of the distribution of morbidity and death in the population. Approaches will be recommended for meaningful international comparisons."

_____, ed. HEALTH STATUS INDEXES. Chicago: Hospital Research and Education Trust, 1973.

> Proceedings of a conference--papers and discussions of concepts, methods and utilization of health status indexes. Identifies models, and needs for standardized terminology and uniform data collection and analysis techniques. Recognizes need for improved general health status indicators as distinct from disease-specific indicators.

Bergner, Marilyn, et al. "The Sickness Impact Profile: Conceptual Formulation and Methodology for the Development of a Health Status Measure." INT'L. J. H. SERV. 6 (1976): 393-415. 33 refs.

> The development of a health status measure, the Sickness Impact Profile (SIP), is described in terms of both its conceptualization and its methodology. Discusses the need for a health status measure

that is sensitive, appropriate, based on sickness-related behavior, and culturally unbiased. An important contribution toward solving the problem of general versus disease-specific measures of health and illness. Since this approach was developed in relation to US experience, its applicability in CNSHS remains uncertain.

Bice, Thomas W., and Kalimo, Esko. "Comparisons of Health-related Attitudes: A Cross-National, Factor Analytic Study." SOC. SCI. MED. 3 (August 1971): 283-318.

The application of factor analysis to selected data from the International Collaborative Study of Medical Care Utilization.

Boelen, C. "Systematic Bedside Statistics Used as a Substitute for Vital Statistics at Present in Ethiopia." AFRICAN J. OF MED. SCI. 4 (January 1973): 59-66.

The absence of census and other basic demographic information sources can sometimes be partially made up for by special efforts. This article describes one such but does not take adequate account of out-of-hospital events.

Bogatyrev, I.D. "Establishing Standards for Outpatient and Inpatient Care." INT'L. J. H. SERV. 2 (1972): 45-50.

Development of norms of outpatient and inpatient care in the USSR is based on studies of the morbidity of different population groups. Analysis is made of general morbidity data on recorded visits to medical facilities and data on medical examinations. An average of 1,247 such visits and 195 cases of hospitalization (including confinements and abortions) were recorded per 1,000 urban population in five cities with a total population of 1.5 million. The total number of visits adequately reflected acute and chronic morbidity with marked clinical manifestations, but did not accurately reflect the extent of mild and early forms of chronic disease. Experienced physicians from research institutions in twelve major specialties examined 54,000 people from different communities. Additional investigations such as x-ray and laboratory tests were performed as necessary. Over 800 unknown incidences of disease or abnormal conditions for each 1,000 population were revealed during these examinations. These findings were used for the introduction of corrective factors in the determination of actual need in medical care.

Brenner, M. Harvey. "Fetal, Infant and Maternal Mortality During Periods of Economic Instability." INT'L. J. H. SERV. 3 (1973): 145-59. 67 refs.

From the author's summary: "One of the most sensitive indicators of the general socioeconomic level of a nation is the infant mortality rate. For industrialized societies, however, the problem of adapting to economic growth concerns less the level of economic growth than whether that growth is relatively smooth or chaotic. . . . The evidence indicates that economic recessions and upswings have played a significant role in fetal, infant, and maternal mortality in the last 45 years. In fact, economic instability has probably been responsible for the apparent lack of continuity in the decline in infant mortality rates since 1950." Three different methods of time series analysis were compared: long-term trends, three- to eleven-year trends, and cyclical trends.

Brooks, Charles H. "Path Analysis of Socioeconomic Correlates of County Infant Mortality Rates." INT'L. J. H. SERV. 5 (1975): 499-514. 49 refs.

Examines relationships between selected socioeconomic characteristics of counties and infant mortality rates. Data corresponding to 2,237 US counties are analyzed by path analysis. The percentage of blacks and low education are two variables which have appreciable direct effects on infant mortality. These two factors are also responsible in large measure for gross associations between low family income, sound housing, and rates of infant loss. Aside from the techniques of analysis, themselves of interest, this article is valuable to inform and qualify studies between countries based on such general health indicators as infant mortality.

Carr, Willine, and Wolfe, Samuel. "Unmet Needs as Sociomedical Indicators." INT'L. J. H. SERV. 6 (1976): 417-30.

The authors discuss the Meharry Medical College Study of Unmet Needs. The central hypothesis of the study is that comprehensive health programs will be more effective than traditional care in reducing unmet needs. Household interviews and clinical examinations provided the data base for determining unmet needs in the medical, dental, nursing, and social services areas. Three forms of services were compared in this study: (1) a neighborhood-based comprehensive care program with considerable outreach to homes and neighborhood activities; (2) a hospital-based comprehensive care program; and (3) the usual array of disparate sources (private office practices, hospital emergency room, etc.). A subsequent report by Janet S. Birch indicates that the neighborhood-based program generated the least unmet need and greatest satisfaction. But there was some hint that since truly comprehensive care also involves political organization and action among the low-income minority groups to correct pathogenic life conditions, federal funding under a conservative regime was cut. See Birch's chapter in the book edited by Gallagher (cited in chapter 5).

Cartwright, Dorwin P. "Analysis of Qualitative Material." In RESEARCH METHODS IN THE BEHAVIORAL SCIENCES, edited by Leon Festinger and Daniel Katz, pp. 421-70. New York: Dryden Press, 1953.

Thoughtful, especially relevant to the qualitative aspects of case studies. Appears in a generally valuable text-like collection.

Chance, Norman A. "Conceptual and Methodological Problems in Cross-Cultural Health Research." AJPH 52 (March 1962): 410-17.

Addresses conceptual, terminological, and data collection problems. Notes and gives examples of importance of appropriate translation of conceptual or cultural underpinnings of disease and treatment terms.

Chase, Helen C. "The Position of the United States in International Comparisons of Health Status." AJPH 62 (April 1972): 581-89.

A thorough consideration of the methodological problems and conceptual limits involved in using such general health indicators as infant mortality to compare the health statuses of nations' populations. The US National Center for Health Statistics criteria for including a country for comparison are identified and some forty-six countries are thereby compared. Between 1950 and 1969 Sweden remained in first place while the US slipped from sixth to fifteenth place.

_____. "Ranking Countries by Infant Mortality Rates." PUB. H. REPORTS 84 (January 1969): 19-27.

Chen, Martin K. "A Population Health Status Index Applicable to Disadvantaged States or Nations." Paper presented at the 8th int'l. scientific meetings of the IEA, Puerto Rico, September 17-23, 1977.

Author's abstract: "This paper describes a population health status index applicable to disadvantaged nations. The H-index uses data on average life expectancy at birth and percent of population with disability, however defined. It is useful in assessing the health status of developing countries relative to that of the more advanced nations selected to serve as the norm. The H values computed annually for the developing countries show the progress, or lack of it, toward the norm.

The statistical procedure used in deriving the H-index is contour analysis, by means of which the Euclidean distances of the disadvantaged nations in two-dimensional space to the centroid of the normative nations are reflected in the H values computed. The farther away from the centroid, the less resemblance the disadvantaged nation has to the norm and the lower its health status. A computational sample is given using five of the more healthy states in the U.S. as the norm, and even less healthy states as the disadvantaged states. The results demonstrate the feasibility of applying the H-index to the international community."

Methods

Coale, Ansley J. "The Determination of Vital Rates in the Absence of Registration Data." In RESEARCH METHODS IN HEALTH CARE, edited by John B. McKinlay, pp. 47-60. New York: Prodist, 1973.

Especially useful in population and mortality studies in UDCs.

Cochrane, A.L. "Rhondda Fach, South Wales." In COMPARABILITY IN INTERNATIONAL EPIDEMIOLOGY, edited by Roy M. Acheson, pp. 326-32. New York: Milbank Mem. Fund, 1965. 19 refs.

Crisply worded insight-rich description of an epidemiological survey in a geographically defined coal mining population. Reports the methods and measurement cautions and ways of getting around problems which this study taught the investigators. Especially interesting is a diagram showing the distribution of an epidemiological problem. The diagram shows for what portion of patients in a controlled trial it is ethical to randomize treatment, and for what portions it is unethical to treat and unethical not to treat.

Cochrane, C. EFFECTIVENESS AND EFFICIENCY: RANDOM REFLECTIONS ON HEALTH SERVICES. London: Nuffield Provincial Hospitals Trust, 1972.

Although randomized controlled clinical trials have become common in evaluating new drugs, in most other medical care situations this approach remains impracticable, or is unethical because a given procedure is assumed to be life saving or has been defined as "the treatment of choice." This work reviews the logic and successes of random controlled trials and discusses limits on their use. An important methodological contribution.

Cohen, Lois K., and Jago, John D. "Toward the Formulation of Sociodental Indicators." INT'L. J. H. SERV. 6 (1976): 681-98. 68 refs.

Author's summary: "The bases for the construction of sociodental indicators is discussed in the paper, considering several available indexes of oral health status (dental caries, periodontal disease, malocclusion, oral hygiene and other oral conditions) as well as measures of quality of services. Very little research exists relating any of the above measures to social indicators such as personal life style or cultural and ecological factors. Such expansion would enable dental indicators to be useful for purposes of policy decisions. Combining any dental indicators or set of indicators with a potential global social health index is discussed in terms of potential problems obscuring dentistry's cost to society. Dentistry, in addition, is offered as a system in microcosm - one which can be useful for purposes of polishing methodology for the social health indicator movement."

Committee on Maternal and Child Care. American Medical Association. "How is a Nation's Health Level Measured? Implications of Infant Mortality Rates." JAMA 189 (July 27, 1964): 321-25.

Davies, A. Michael, ed. USES OF EPIDEMIOLOGY IN PLANNING HEALTH SERVICES. PROCEEDINGS OF THE SIXTH INTERNATIONAL SCIENTIFIC MEET-ING OF THE INTERNATIONAL EPIDEMIOLOGICAL ASSOCIATION, AUGUST 29-SEPTEMBER 3, 1971, Primosten, Yugoslavia. 2 vols. Belgrade: Savremena Administracija, 1973.

> An eclectic collection, not all contributions fitting well under this title. Nevertheless, includes a number of valuable pieces on an often ignored link--epidemiology and planning of health services.

Department of International Health. Johns Hopkins University School of Hygiene and Public Health. THE FUNCTIONAL ANALYSIS OF HEALTH NEEDS AND SERVICES. London/New York: Asia Publishing House, 1976.

> Describes an operations research approach to studying health systems, primarily based on experience in India and other UDCs.

Duijker, H.C.J., and Rokkan, Stein. "Organizational Aspects of Cross-National Social Research." J. OF SOCIAL ISSUES 10 (1954): 8-24. Notes, refs.

> Begins by defining cross-national as distinct from "cross-cultural" and "international" research. Then examines in a most helpful way the logistical, team, and other organizational problems in-volved in (1) documentary studies (already aggregated statistics and reports); (2) current statistics studies (aggregation and reaggregation of comparable cases or records of events available through similar statistical systems); and (3) field and laboratory studies (the gather-ing of fresh comparable data). Type 3 studies are rarer and involve many more organizational problems. The discussion of type 3 is broken into four categories: (1) repetitive successive; (2) joint development-successive; (3) repetitive concurrent; and (4) joint development-concurrent. There is also some discussion of the Or-ganization for Comparative Social Research and its relations to UNESCO. A particular research is used as a case study to discuss organizational problems in more detail under these headings; com-munication problems; common versus nation-specific features; or-ganizational structure; problems of data utilization. A frank, in-sightful piece. Very valuable.

Elder, Joseph W. "Comparative Cross-National Methodology." In ANNUAL REVIEW OF SOCIOLOGY, vol. 2, edited by Alex Inkeles et al. Palo Alto, Calif.: Annual Reviews, 1976.

Elinson, Jack. "Insensitive Health Statistics and the Dilemma of the HSAs." AJPH 67 (May 1977): 417-18. 16 refs.

> A short editorial statement recognizing the difficulty for health systems agencies in the United States, the new regional health planning bodies created under the National Health Planning and Resources Development Act (Public Law 93-641), to achieve their

goal of improving health levels when these cannot now even be measured. Some of the key literature on measuring human functioning is cited and recent work by multidisciplinary teams of social and medical scientists is mentioned. Work by a McMaster University group in Canada is cited as reconfirming the value of household interviews when properly designed and administered in identifying self-reported illness which can be clinically confirmed. What such measures do not provide is identification of disease which can be clinically confirmed--hypertension, atherosclerosis, diabetes, and neoplasms--about which the afflicted person may not be aware.

_____. "Towards Sociomedical Health Indicators." Paper presented at the International Conference of Medical Sociology. Jablonna, Poland, August 20-25, 1973. Published in HEALTH, MEDICINE, SOCIETY, edited by Magdalena Sokolowska et al., pp. 267-80. Dordrecht, Netherlands and Boston: D. Reidel; Warsaw: PWN--Polish Scientific Publishers, 1976. 46 refs.

Thoughtful examination of the need for and problems involved in developing more general health indicators (as distinguishable from disease, death, disability, discomfort, dissatisfaction--the "5 Ds"). A sophisticated piece.

Elling, Ray H. "Political Influences on Research Methods." In CROSS-NATIONAL SOCIOMEDICAL RESEARCH: CONCEPTS, METHODS, PRACTICE, edited by Manfred Pflanz and Elisabeth Schach, pp. 144-55. Stuttgart, Germany: Thieme, 1976. Refs., pp. 170-72.

Notes the predominance of work on research methods at the broad levels of philosophic conceptions, social policy, and government financing, and the relative dearth of work on political influences on the detailed aspects. To partially fill this gap the author identifies interest groups at different levels, including ministries of health and WHO, and gives examples of how these interests may influence problem definition; formation of the research team; selection of study sites and sample; development of research instruments; and gathering, aggregation, analysis, presentation, and use of data.

Elling, Ray H., and Kerr, Henry. "Selection of Contrasting National Health Systems for In-depth Study." In COMPARATIVE HEALTH SYSTEMS, edited by Elling. Supplemental issue to INQUIRY 12 (June 1975): 25-40.

Recommends examining different countries at equal levels of economic wealth and education. Preliminary analysis of the correlation between infant mortality and physician-population ratios within resource levels suggests health planning strategies should differ according to level of development. Suggests a framework for contrasting countries with similar levels of overall resources but marked differences in general health indicators. Includes methodological cautions in using available secondary data.

Elling, Ray H., and Sokołowska, Magdalena, eds. MEDICAL SOCIOLOGISTS AT WORK. New Brunswick, N.J.: Transaction Books, 1978.

The development of a special field of scholarly and scientific work is examined through the work autobiographies of twelve international medical sociologists. Both support and resistance to innovative approaches in this new specialty of sociology is evidenced. The work highlights the relationship of the field to the parent discipline of sociology and the practical world of health institutions and personnel. The recent trend toward resocializing and rehumanizing medicine is viewed as a function of the development of well-founded work in this new field. Contributors: Jack Elinson, Ray Elling, Mark Field, Eliot Freidson, Margot Jeffreys, Yngvar Lochen, Hans Mauksch, Yvo Nuyens, Jorge Segovia, Judith Shuval, Magdalena Sokolowska, Robert Straus.

Fabrega, Horacio, Jr. "The Biological Significance of Taxonomies of Disease." J. OF THEORETICAL BIOLOGY 63 (1976): 191-216.

Goes beyond the relativistic point usually made in anthropological studies of illness beliefs to conceive of disease taxonomies as ways of a people adapting. In terms of CNSHS methods, the implication is that more than simple translation problems of single medical or disease terms are involved, especially if studies of those pursuing traditional medical approaches are included.

Fanshel, S., and Bush, J.W. "A Health-Status Index and Its Application to Health-Services Outcomes." OPERATIONS RESEARCH 18 (1970): 1021-66.

Discusses the development of a health-status index based on classes of functional states and value judgments of the probability of change in condition. The purpose of the index is to quantitatively define the output of a health system with respect to program planning and decision-making processes. Confronts head-on the important problem of general versus disease-specific measures of health.

Field, Mark. "A Sociological Perspective on Applied Multidisciplinary Research in the Third World." DEVELOPMENT ET CIVILISATION (Centre National de la Recherche Scientifique, Paris) Special issue no. 45/46 (September-December 1971): 100-110.

Considers the complexities of research involving people trained in different disciplinary and national cultures.

Flook, E. Evelyn, and Sanazaro, Paul J., eds. HEALTH SERVICES RESEARCH AND R & D IN PERSPECTIVE. Ann Arbor, Mich.: Health Administration Press, 1973.

An important collection by two veteran medical care researchers including methodological as well as substantive and historical works.

Forbes, Hugh Donald, and Tufte, Edward R. "A Note of Caution in Causal Modelling." AMERICAN POLITICAL SCIENCE REV. 62 (1968): 1258-63.

Forsyth, Gordon, and Logan, R.F.L. "Studies in Medical Care: An Assessment of Some Methods." In TOWARDS A MEASURE OF MEDICAL CARE, OPERATIONAL RESEARCH IN THE HEALTH SERVICE, A SYMPOSIUM, pp. 66-86. New York: Oxford Univ. Press, 1962.

Experience with some early medical care researches in the NHS in the UK.

Fox, Renee C. "An American Sociologist in the Land of Belgian Medical Research." In SOCIOLOGISTS AT WORK, edited by Phillip E. Hammond, pp. 345-91. New York: Basic Books, 1964.

An insightful autobiographical statement of resistances encountered when unpopular findings began to be reported.

Fraser, R.D. "Health and General Systems of Financing Health Care." MEDICAL CARE 10 (1972): 345-56. 30 notes and refs.

Author's summary: "The linear relationship between infant mortality, used as a proxy for the overall level of health, and the number of physicians per 10,000 persons, the number of hospital beds per 1,000 persons, and real Gross Domestic Product per capita is estimated with data for 18 well-developed countries in the post-war period. This relationship is then used to estimate the level of infant mortality that one would expect to find in a particular country given the value of the explanatory variables in that country. The size and sign of the residual, the difference between this expected level and the level of infant mortality actually found, is then used to assess roughly the effect on health of different general systems of financing health services. Recently published data on the percentage of health services financed or directly controlled by government, on the relative size of the health sector and on the proportion of health care resources allocated to the provision of nonpersonal, public health care, are then examined in relation to variations in infant mortality left unexplained by the initial explanatory variables. Of the latter three, only the last, the proportion of health care resources devoted to the provision of nonpersonal, public health appears to be a significant determinant of levels of health."

An important contribution. But see Badgley's critique (cited above, this chapter) of this method and the pitfalls of attempting to explain complex phenomena like infant mortality rates using a single-factor explanation such as expenditures for nonpersonal health. Badgley points out the necessary qualifications of a contextual sort specific to a given country if such relationships are to be applied with understanding. See also Fraser's later article analyzing data from twenty-five countries (cited in chapter 3.4).

Gilson, Betty S., et al. "The Sickness Impact Profile, Development of an Outcome Measure of Health Care." AJPH 65 (December 1975): 1304-10. 15 refs.

The sickness impact profile is a behaviorally based measure of sickness-related dysfunction which is being developed to provide an appropriate and sensitive measure of health status for use in assessing the effects of health care.

Glaser, William A. "The Process of Cross-National Survey Research." Presented at the Round Table Conference on Cross-National Survey Research of the International Social Science Council, Budapest, 1972. Published in CROSS-NATIONAL COMPARATIVE SURVEY RESEARCH THEORY AND PRACTICE, edited by Alexander Szalai et al., pp. 403-35. 30 notes and refs.

An excellent examination of organizational problems involved in mounting cross-national survey research. Notes the predominance of work under US auspices. Contents: organizational tasks, structure of cross-national surveys, from safaris to collaboration, purposes of the research and effects on organizational structure (information gathering, hypothesis testing, theory development, developing relations among researchers and their institutions), sponsorship, selection of countries, selection of research centers, leadership and coordination (centralized projects, conferences and committees, individual coordinators, teamwork during the analysis); conclusion.

Grundy, F., and Reinke, W.A. HEALTH PRACTICE RESEARCH AND FORMALIZED MANAGERIAL METHODS. Public Health Papers, no. 51. Geneva: WHO, 1973.

A text-like statement (193 p.) from the perspective of within-system operations research and systems analysis rather than cross-system sociopolitical analysis. Perhaps the best general work available from this perspective.

Hall, T.L. "Chile Health Manpower Study: Methods and Problems." INT'L. J. H. SERV. 1 (1971): 166-84.

Describes the principal methods used to assess future health manpower requirements in Chile and the ability of the country to meet them. The first phase of the study, completed in late 1970, represents the preparation of a dynamic model of the entire health sector. Techniques are described for assessing the potential economic burden of alternative manpower targets while at the same time minimizing the hazards of long-range projections of economic growth and costs. The paper concludes with a discussion of some of the problems faced in the Chile study.

Subsequent cataclysmic political economic changes in Chile throw this kind of quantitative modeling into serious question.

Methods

Holt, Robert T., and Turner, John E., eds. THE METHODOLOGY OF COMPARATIVE POLITICAL RESEARCH. New York: Free Press, 1972.

> While focused mostly on methods for the study of elections, has useful contributions for the assessment of the positions of parties and analysis of power and its distribution. Not specifically oriented toward health systems.

Horowitz, Irving Louis, ed. THE USE AND ABUSE OF SOCIAL SCIENCE: BEHAVIORAL SCIENCE AND NATIONAL POLICY MAKING. New York: E.P. Dutton, Transaction Books, 1974.

> The seventeen original essays in this volume are a provocative examination of the increasing involvement of social scientists in the formulation and execution of policymaking. A major contribution to the understanding of the political uses of social research.

Inkeles, Alex. "Fieldwork Problems in Comparative Research on Modernization." In ESSAYS ON MODERNIZATION OF UNDERDEVELOPED SOCIETIES, edited by A.R. Desay, chapter 2, pp. 20–75. New York: Humanities Press, 1972. 17 refs.

> Reports in considerable valuable detail the vicissitudes of organizing and doing survey research with local social science researchers in a multination study of modernization of individual's attitudes, values, and beliefs. This direct approach was chosen over "contracting out" the data gathering to a professional organization so as to better contribute to development of social science and to be sure of the quality of the data. Loaded with concrete examples of things others would want to anticipate and plan to improve if beginning a cross-national research involving field work. Covers every phase: theoretical approach, general research strategy, selecting the countries, selecting and training staff, constructing and translating the interview schedule, conducting interviews, response bias, communication and "drift" between counterpart teams. Highly recommended.

Jacobson, Eugene. "Methods Used for Producing Comparable Data in the OCSR Seven-Nation Attitude Study." J. OF SOCIAL ISSUES 10 (1954): 40–51.

> Reports on a study conducted under the aegis of the Organization for Comparative Social Research. Discusses how nonidentical elements were often deliberately included as being more equivalent or comparable than identical elements would have been in different cultural contexts. Also considers translation, selection, and training of interviewers.

Kalimo, Esko, and Bice, Thomas W. "Causal Analysis and Ecological Fallacy in Cross-National Epidemiological Research." SCANDINAVIAN J. OF SOCIAL MED. 1 (1973): 17–24.

This paper has two interrelated purposes. The first is to examine the usefulness of a statistical technique derived from a causal model, that is, path analysis of cross-national epidemiological data. With this method, the data are analyzed according to the causal relations among the variables specified by the theory, thereby tying together the statistical analysis of the data and the testing of causal hypotheses. The second purpose of the study is to scrutinize the importance of the analytical unit in the interpretation of the results, based on individuals, with results calculated across the areas, using aggregate data. Because of the ecological fallacy, interpretations on individuals cannot usually be made on the basis of area level results. The results are demonstrated by using data from a cross-national study incorporating forty-eight subpopulations in seven countries.

Kalimo, Esko, et al. "Cross-Cultural Analyses of Selected Emotional Questions from the Cornell Medical Index." BRITISH JOURNAL OF PREVENTIVE AND SOCIAL MEDICINE 24 (November 1970): 229-40.

Kobben, A.J.F. "The Logic of Cross-Cultural Analysis: Why Exceptions?" In COMPARATIVE RESEARCH ACROSS CULTURES AND NATIONS, edited by Stein Rokkan, pp. 17-53. Paris and the Hague: Mouton, 1968.

A piece on deviant-case analysis which is a first step in the in-depth contrasting case study approach (see Elling and Kerr, cited above, this chapter). Appears in an important early collection of both substantive and methodological contributions to cross-national research.

Kohn, Robert. "Development of Cross-National Comparisons of Health Services Use." In CROSS-NATIONAL SOCIOMEDICAL RESEARCH: CONCEPTS, METHODS, PRACTICE, edited by Manfred Pflanz and Elisabeth Schach, pp. 12-24. Stuttgart, Germany: Thieme, 1976.

Covers the literature of this field recounting the growing complexity and sophistication of methods. Concludes, nevertheless, that there is need for a less piecemeal, fragmented approach, since use of one part of a system may mean something for other parts. He quotes Joshua Cohen of WHO who calls for a combination of gestalt and atomistic approaches.

Kohn, Robert, and White, Kerr L., eds. HEALTH CARE, AN INTERNATIONAL STUDY: REPORT OF THE WHO INTERNATIONAL COLLABORATIVE STUDY OF MEDICAL CARE UTILIZATION. London, New York, Toronto: Oxford Univ. Press, 1976.

See the methods of this landmark study, especially chapter 3 and appendix B.

Methods

Kpedekpo, G.M. "Planning and Design of Sampling Surveys with Particular Reference to the Epidemiological Survey of the Danfa Project in Ghana." GHANA MED. J. (Accra), 11 (December 1972): 377-82.

> Planning a sample survey begins with consideration of survey objectives, geographic coverage, methods of data collection, questionnaire design, sample design, selection and training of interviewers, and so forth. Consultation at the planning stage is essential. Possible sample designs include simple random, systematic, stratified, cluster, and multistage designs, or a combination of these. The author describes a sample design for an integrated multisubject health survey.

Krupinski, Jerzy. "Health and 'Quality of Life': An Epidemiological Study." Paper presented at the 8th int'l. scientific meetings of the IEA, Puerto Rico, September 17-23, 1977.

> A health and social survey was carried out in an industrial area of Melbourne (pop. 235,000). Using 1,036 households, the health of all members of the family was assessed by final-year medical students, supervised by physicians and psychiatrists. Subjects over the age of eighteen underwent automated multiphasic health screening. In the assessment of quality of life, distinction was made between the mode of life and its subjective perception. The mode of life was analyzed in terms of the social activities of the preceding week. The discrepancy between the desired kind of life and the actual situation was assessed using a specially designed questionnaire. The prevalence of psychological and psychosomatic disorders is related to this discrepancy.

Leeson, Joyce. "Social Science and Health Policy in Preindustrial Society." See chapter 3.3.

> Offers a thoughtful critique of the way the social sciences, particularly anthropology, have tended to serve colonialist and imperialist interests.

Lengyel, Peter, ed. SOCIAL SCIENCE, NATIONAL INTERESTS AND INTERNATIONAL ORGANIZATION. New York: E.P. Dutton, Transaction Books, 1974.

> This collection of essays from the INTERNATIONAL SOCIAL SCIENCE JOURNAL describes how social scientists communicate with the public and each other and the problems involved in such interaction. It examines the choice of research locations, the goals of research studies, the role of the social sciences in the third world, and looks at how an ethics of social science is becoming a formal reality.

Mabry, John, et al. "The Natural History of an International Collaborative Study of Medical Care Utilization." SOCIAL SCIENCE INFORMATION 5 (December 1960): 37-55.

Relates the early development of the effort eventuating in the monu-
mental volume finally published in 1976 as HEALTH CARE, AN IN-
TERNATIONAL STUDY (see Kohn and White, cited above, this
chapter).

McDonald, A.G., et al. "Balance of Care: Some Mathematical Models of the National Health Service." BRITISH MED. BUL. 20 (September 1974): 262-70.

McGranahan, Donald V. "Comparative Social Research in the United Nations."
In COMPARING NATIONS: THE USE OF QUANTITATIVE DATA IN CROSS-
NATIONAL RESEARCH, edited by R.L. Merritt and S. Rokkan, pp. 525-55.
New Haven, Conn.: Yale Univ. Press, 1966.

Classic statement of the problems of data collection and standardized comparative social statistics--especially the use of standards
of developed nations applied to preindustrial environments and the
use of UN system data. An important contribution by the director
of UNRISD.

Martini, Carlos J.M., et al. "Health Indexes Sensitive to Medical Care Variation." INT'L. J. H. SERV. 7 (1977): 293-309.

From the author's summary: "Data from the fifteen Hospital Regions
of England and Wales were used to determine the utility of health
outcome indexes, derived from existing health statistics, for monitoring the quality and effectiveness of health services. Outcome
measures reflect not only the impact of the system of care but also
the sociodemographic characteristics of the population. . . . Those
outcome measures related to provision of care in hospital appear to
be relatively more sensitive to variation in medical care than those
which are community based. This suggests that, at least for monitoring the effectiveness of medical care in the community, it may
be necessary to move away from the more traditional health indexes
toward measures that take into consideration the different patterns
of care and the social and behavioral aspects of health."

Matthews, V.L. "Assessing Health Resources." CANADIAN J. OF HEALTH
59 (1968): 375-79.

MEASURING SOCIAL WELL BEING, A PROGRESS REPORT ON THE DEVELOP-
MENT OF SOCIAL INDICATORS. Paris: OECD, 1976.

A valuable overview of problems of defining and measuring well-
being in a wide range of spheres such as work, education, housing,
leisure. The book includes a brief section on measures of health,
illness, and mortality which is all the more valuable for its inclusion in the context of other spheres of social well-being.

Merrit, R.L., and Rokkan, Stein, eds. COMPARING NATIONS: THE USE OF QUANTITATIVE DATA IN CROSS-NATIONAL RESEARCH. New Haven, Conn.: Yale Univ. Press, 1966.

> One of the most complete and valuable collections on methods questions involved in cross-national research, though no chapters focus specifically on health systems. The very good chapter by McGranahan (cited above, this chapter) considers some health or rather mortality data problems from the perspective of the limitations of official UN statistics.

Mitchell, R.E. "Survey Materials Collected in the Developing Countries--Obstacles to Comparisons." In COMPARATIVE RESEARCH ACROSS NATIONS AND CULTURES, edited by Stein Rokkan, pp. 210-38. Paris and the Hague: Mouton, 1968.

Moore, F.W., ed. READINGS IN CROSS-CULTURAL METHODOLOGY. New Haven, Conn.: Human Relations Area Files, 1961.

> A useful early collection of methods statements focused on cultural groups rather than nation states and concentrated on document analysis as available through the Human Relations Area Files.

Moriyama, Iwao M. "Problems in the Measurement of Health Status." In INDICATORS OF SOCIAL CHANGE: CONCEPTS AND MEASUREMENTS, edited by Eleanor Bernert Sheldon and Wilbert E. Moore, pp. 573-600. New York: Russell Sage Foundation, 1968.

> One of the best statements of the problem in a generally valuable collection. The presumptions involved in the overall work are those of "the end of ideology" school of thought in which socioeconomic development and improved life and living conditions for all is seen as a purely technical matter, rather than a matter of class struggle. This is a shortcoming, but the technical excellence of the contribution is high.

Munoz, Raul A., and Arbona, Guillermo. "The Puerto Rico Master Sample Survey of Health and Welfare." In THE COMMUNITY AS AN EPIDEMIOLOGIC LABORATORY: A CASEBOOK OF COMMUNITY STUDIES, edited by Irving I. Kessler et al., pp. 279-95. Baltimore: Johns Hopkins Univ. Press, 1970.

> In conjunction with the identification of health needs-demands as part of the important attempt to regionalize health and welfare services in Puerto Rico (see works by Seipp, Arbona, and Ferrer, cited in chapter 6) an extensive population-based survey was undertaken as described here. This chapter is particularly valuable for its frank detailing of the technical problems which seemed continually to plague the survey. It also lays out the fact that the health leadership was most often unwilling or unable to make effective use of information provided by the survey.

Murdock, George P. "The Cross-Cultural Survey." ASR 5 (1940): 361-70.

The founder of the Human Relations Area Files at Yale presents the logic and description of this powerful tool for cross-cultural (not necessarily cross-national) research. Of both historical and fundamental interest.

Mushkin, Selma J. "Evaluations: Use with Caution." EVALUATION 1 (1973): 30-35.

Among the cautions offered in this clear piece is the fact that global indicators like mortality are summary measures affected by numerous factors. Few of these factors, however important theoretically or actually (e.g., medical care), can reasonably be expected to have a major impact on the gross indicator.

_____. "Measuring Intercountry Expenditures for Medical Care." PUB. H. REPORTS 76 (August 1961): 655-58.

Myers, George C. "Mortality Statistics." In CROSS-NATIONAL SOCIO-MEDICAL RESEARCH: CONCEPTS, METHODS, PRACTICE, edited by Manfred Pflanz and Elisabeth Schach, pp. 82-93. Stuttgart, Germany: Thieme, 1976.

A thorough consideration of the pitfalls in the use of available mortality data, including infant and perinatal mortality. The article begins by noting some general similarities and differences in reporting of national total and infant and neonatal mortality (the article's focus, as opposed to specific causes of death) in different parts of the world. Then some uses of mortality data, such as surveillance and projection, are discussed. Then the procedures of recording and problematic aspects are covered, including purposes of registration, scope of registration, whether registration is centralized or not, and reports by residence or place of occurrence, the definition of the event, who is the informant, the reporting form, coding, and statistical handling of the information. There is a helpful time-scale scheme for classifying deaths in the prenatal and postnatal period. The effects of different definitions and practices are illustrated on data for Swedish infant deaths by comparing Swedish and WHO approaches.

Nishi, S. "The Development of Health Status Indicators in Japan for Health Planning." BUL. OF THE INSTITUTE FOR PUBLIC HEALTH (Tokyo) 20 (1971): 62-77.

One of the best statements of the health services planner's need for better general health indicators as opposed to disease-specific mortality or morbidity indicators. Gives some coverage of the literature internationally and the situation in Japan.

Nowak, Stefan. "The Strategy of Comparative Survey Research for the Development of Social Theory." Paper presented at the Round Table Conference on Cross-National Survey Research, sponsored by The International Social Science Council, European Coordination Centre for Research and Documentation in Social Sciences in Budapest, July 25-28, 1972. Published in CROSS-NATIONAL COMPARATIVE SURVEY RESEARCH: THEORY AND PRACTICE, edited by Alexander Szalai et al. Oxford, England, and New York: Pergamon, 1977.

> Important in linking theory and methods. Also considers use of different measures (e.g., ownership of cows versus cars or money) in different countries to represent wealth.

Olsen, Marvin E. "Multivariate Analysis of National Political Development." ASR 33 (October 1968): 699-712.

Pan American Health Organization (PAHO). SYSTEMS ANALYSIS APPLIED TO HEALTH SERVICES. Scientific Bul. no. 239. Washington, D.C., 1972.

> A within-country rather than cross-national perspective, but good for acquainting oneself with this approach.

Patrick, Donald L. "Constructing Social Metrics for Health Status Indexes." INT'L. J. H. SERV. 6 (1976): 443-53. 54 refs.

> Health status indexes must confront the question of who prefers which states of health under which circumstances. A useful scholarly consideration of a complex unsolved problem of developing adequate general health status indexes. The values implied in this statement reflect a neopositivist approach, flavored with individualism. Democratic socialist countries may be less concerned with personal variety in preferences and more concerned with adequate general standards. Thus the explicit strategy of seeking a context-independent measure may be quite unrealistic.

Patrick, Donald L. "Social Indicators in the Development of National Health Policy." Paper presented at the 105th annual meeting of the APHA, Washington, D.C., October 30-November 3, 1977.

> Author's abstract: "Social indicators are being developed to aid the formulation of national health policy through evaluation, priority setting, and resource allocation. Health status indicators, in addition to assessing physical, social, and psychological well-being, can be viewed as criteria for establishing and quantifying variation in the needs of different populations defined by social factors or geography. If the goal of health policy is to work toward equal opportunity for health-promoting circumstances, as well as for equal access to health care, then health status measures must be linked to indicators of housing, environment, work and other social conditions which influence the quality of life. This paper explores the implication that developing health measures emphasizing function,

performance, productivity, or dependence is in the public interest and discusses the assumption made by most researchers in the field of health indicators that the instruments being developed will be for the public good."

Peterson, Osler. "What is Value for Money in Medical Care? Experiences in England and Wales, Sweden and the U.S.A." See chapter 5.

Raises the question of how elements of different systems are to be defined and points, at least by implication, to in-depth case studies as the approach of choice.

Pflanz, Manfred. "Social Structure and Health: Methodological and Substantial Problems without Solutions." In HEALTH, MEDICINE, SOCIETY, edited by Magdalena Sokolowska et al., pp. 253-66. Dordrecht, Netherlands, and Boston: D. Reidel; Warsaw: PWN--Polish Scientific Publishers, 1971. 9 refs.

Clearly links epidemiologic research and information exchange from such research with government policy and other political interests. Points out that although measuring techniques for individuals are sophisticated, there is a lack of adequate theory and measurements of social structures bearing upon the studies of individual phenomena.

_____. "Problems and Methods in Cross-National Comparisons of Diagnoses and Diseases." In CROSS-NATIONAL SOCIOMEDICAL RESEARCH: CONCEPTS, METHODS, PRACTICE, edited by Manfred Pflanz and Elisabeth Schach, pp. 60-68. Stuttgart, Germany: Thieme, 1976.

A full and sensitive consideration of semantic and conceptual as well as organizational and social process issues in achieving "the three great Cs--completeness, correctness, comparability." These "are not marginal methodological issues but essential aspects of the research process."

Pflanz, Manfred, and Schach, Elisabeth, eds. CROSS-NATIONAL SOCIO-MEDICAL RESEARCH: CONCEPTS, METHODS, PRACTICE. Stuttgart, Germany: Thieme, 1976. Refs., index.

The contributions discuss comparisons of health systems and their components; comparability of statistics, records, and diseases; methodological aspects of research; planning, execution, and po-litical aspects of cross-national sociomedical research, considering both conceptual and practical problems. Based upon papers presented at the Hannover Seminar on this subject held March 5-8, 1974. Contributions by R. Andersen, R.F. Badgley, T.W. Bice, M. von Cranach, R.H. Elling, M.G. Field, D.G. Gill, A.S. Haeroe, E. Kabino, R. Kohn, G.C. Myers, M. Pflanz, N. Sartorius, E. Schach, J.T. Shuval, and K.L. White. Perhaps the most valuable methodological collection available in the field of CNSHS. The book is divided into four parts: (1) comparisons of

health services systems and their components; (2) comparability of
official statistics, records and diseases; (3) a diverse section treating surveys, measurement of attitudes, reliability, and research on
Canadian health services; and (4) planning, execution, and political aspects. The contributors are described. The conference
on which this book is based is summarized in "La Conférence de
Hanovre sur la méthodologie des recherches internationales en
socio-economie de la santé" by S. Sandier and E. Schach,
CAHIERS DE SOCIOLOGIE ET DE DEMOGRAPHIE MÉDICALES
14 (1974): 85–88.

Przeworski, Adam, and Teune, Henry. THE LOGIC OF COMPARATIVE SOCIAL
INQUIRY. New York: Wiley-Interscience, 1970.

Fundamental considerations in design and interpretation of comparative studies. Includes work by these same authors which first appeared as "Equivalence in Cross-National Research." PUBLIC
OPINION Q. 30 (1966): 551–68.

Public Health Service. Health Services and Mental Health Administration. National Center for Health Statistics. DISABILITY COMPONENTS FOR AN IN-
DEX OF HEALTH, DATA EVALUATION AND METHODS RESEARCH. Publication
no. 1000, series 2, no. 42. Washington, D.C.: GPO, July 1971.

"Recommendations of the Yale Data Conference." In COMPARING NATIONS:
THE USE OF QUANTITATIVE DATA IN CROSS-NATIONAL RESEARCH, edited
by Richard L. Merritt and Stein Rokkan, pp. 555–60. New Haven, Conn.:
Yale Univ. Press, 1966.

Important suggestions for improving secondary (available) data which
contributed to the World Handbook data and studies (see Charles F.
Taylor and Michael C. Hudson, cited in chapter 8).

Record, Jane Cassels. "Alternative Measures of Output for Medical Care Delivery Systems." Paper presented at the Seminar on Disease Costing, Univ. of
Ottawa, February 20, 1974. Available from the author, Kaiser Research Foundation, Portland, Oreg. Notes, refs.

Discusses approaches in the Kaiser Health Services Research Center
to answering two questions: (1) What portion of the physician's
work load can be shifted to new, less expensive types of health
manpower?, (2) How much cost saving would such a shift achieve
if fully carried out? Output is conceived as physician activities
or services which may or may not be shifted to other workers.
Medical procedures were coded and weighted according to the
California Relative Value Studies (CRVS). This paper presents a
"tree" for considering what sort of decisions might be made at different levels.

Reinke, William A. "Alternative Methods for Determining Resource Requirements: The Chile Example." INT'L. J. H. SERV. 6 (1976): 123-37.

> This technically oriented work based on data from 1970 or so fails entirely to take into account the intervening political economic upheavals and is not applicable to Chile today (1977). Probably the piece should not have been published but is included here with this comment to underline the shortcomings of supposedly "pure," "objective," highly quantifying "scientific" approaches to health systems when they make no serious effort to include a qualitative assessment of the political, economic, and cultural context from which the data are being abstracted.

Roemer, Milton I. EVALUATION OF COMMUNITY HEALTH CENTERS. Public Health Papers, no. 48. Geneva: WHO, 1972.

> Suggestive of both conceptual and methodological points in the study of local health services in different countries of the world.

Rommetveit, Ragnar, and Israel, Joachim. "Notes on the Standardization of Experimental Manipulations and Measurements in Cross-National Research." J. OF SOCIAL ISSUES 10 (1954): 61-68. Notes, refs.

> Discusses some general problems encountered in a social psycho-logical study of cohesiveness among groups of thirteen-year-old male aviation club members in seven European countries when a set of nonoperationally phrased hypotheses are to be experimentally tested in different cultural settings. From the author's summary: "We have attempted to show that conceptually identical experi-mental conditions, in some cases, can best be established by deli-berate and systematic deviations from traditional standardization procedures. . . . We suggest semantic studies of verbal behavior in different settings as a means for improving the cross-cultural comparability of control measures, especially important in the case where one has to substitute 'functionally equivalent' manipulations for identical stimulus situations."

Sackett, David L., et al. "The Development and Application of Indices of Health: General Methods and a Summary of Results." AJPH 67 (May 1977): 423-28.

> This research group from McMaster University, Hamilton, Ontario, suggests prerequisites for a health index: it should encompass "social and emotional health and function as well as physical func-tion," and also "good or even excellent function." An index should be applicable to free-living populations as well as those who are captive in medical care facilities; it should be sensitive enough "to detect important changes in health status or function"; it should be simple, acceptable, and of reasonable cost; it should have high reproducibility; and be amenable to quantitative manipulation. In the McMaster study these prerequisites were met by "responses to

a questionnaire, administered to an appropriate sample of citizens by lay-interviewers." The study shows that such responses can be sensitive, biologically sensible, and clinically credible.

The McMaster group has shown that reported illness in interview surveys is verifiable by medical judgment. In other words, there are few false positives in interview-reported illness. As Jack Elinson points out in a review of this and other work on health indicators (see above, this chapter) this household interview approach does not handle the problem of false negatives, that is, lack of information on diseases which are only clinically detectable, such as hypertension, atherosclerosis, and cancer.

Salkever, David S. "Economic Class and Differential Access to Care: Comparisons Among Health Care Systems." See chapter 4.

Provides detailed methodological cautions for a study of economic class and differential access to care in different health systems.

Sartorius, Norman. "The Cross-National Standardization of Psychiatric Diagnoses and Classification." In CROSS-NATIONAL SOCIOMEDICAL RESEARCH: CONCEPTS, METHODS, PRACTICE, edited by Manfred Pflanz and Elisabeth Schach, pp. 73-81. Stuttgart, Germany: Thieme, 1976.

Covers the program coordinated through the Mental Health Unit, WHO, Geneva, to (1) improve the International Classification of Diseases (ICD) as regards mental illnesses; (2) carry out training sessions for psychiatrists from different countries and different theoretical backgrounds by reliably and validly recording diagnoses and other aspects of mental health statistics; and (3) carry out the International Pilot Study of Schizophrenia. This important study was conducted in nine countries--Columbia, Czechoslovakia, Denmark, India, Nigeria, Taiwan, UK, United States, and USSR. It had three aims: (1) to develop standardized instruments and procedures for valid and reliable evaluation of functional disorders, especially schizophrenia; (2) to determine in what sense it can be said that such disorders exist in different parts of the world; and (3) to set up a network of collaborative research centers in different parts of the world. Among the interesting findings and many successes of this project was that there is greater agreement between psychiatrists of different nationalities and theoretical backgrounds on the Present State Examination (PSE) than on any other aspect of the data, such as history.

Scheuch, Erwin K. "The Cross-Cultural Use of Sample Surveys--Problems of Comparability." In COMPARATIVE RESEARCH ACROSS NATIONS AND CULTURES, edited by Stein Rokkan, pp. 176-209. Paris and the Hague: Mouton, 1968.

_____. "Cross-National Comparisons Using Aggregate Data: Some Substantive and Methodological Problems." In COMPARING NATIONS, THE USE OF QUANTITATIVE DATA IN CROSS-NATIONAL RESEARCH, edited by R.L. Merritt and Stein Rokkan, chapter 7, pp. 131-67. New Haven, Conn.: Yale Univ. Press, 1966.

Considers the pitfalls of available official data used to represent national entities within which there may be great variation. Considers accuracy of data, comparability of measurements, representativeness of the data for collective properties, and types of permissible inference. An important contribution.

Schwefel, Detlef. BEITRAEGE ZUR SOZIALPLANUNG IN ENTWICKLUNGS-LAENDERN [Contributions to social planning in developing countries]. Publications of the German Development Institute, vol. 8. Berlin: Bruno Hessling, 1972. 108 p. In German.

Social planning means planning for social justice. This statement remains vague as long as no concrete indicators of social justice are available. The article included here, "Indicators of Social Justice," presents a system of indicators which relate the three dimensions of social justice to one another: satisfaction of basic needs, social equality, and social security. An empirical comparison between Chile and Cuba is the frame of reference for the construction of a numerical index of social justice--referred to as 'S-J-score'. This S-J-score can be used in planning national and international development policies.

An essential aspect of social justice is the assurance of equal opportunity for everyone in regard to health and medical care. Need and performance in the health sector have to be analyzed. An international comparison indicates need and performance of the Turkish health sector, which serves here as an example and is analyzed with the aid of secondary material. The meaning of need and performance is defined by the national development plan. On the subsector level, the method of health sector analysis renders possible the making of more rational decisions concerning priorities in national or international development policies.

Siegmann, Athilia E. "A Classification of Sociomedical Health Indicators: Perspectives for Health Administrators and Health Planners." INT'L. J. H. SERV. 6 (1976): 521-38. 73 refs.

From the author's summary: "Mortality and morbidity rates, the traditional health indicators, by themselves no longer serve to assess health status in developed nations. Their deficiencies as indicators serve as background for a classification schema for sociomedical health status indicators that relates health definition frames of reference, measures of health status, and health problems. The role of a group of health indicators--sociomedical health indicators--in the current formulation of health status measures is assessed." A thorough, scholarly consideration of this difficult problem from a sociopolitical perspective.

Sivard, Ruth. WORLD MILITARY AND SOCIAL EXPENDITURES. New York: Institute for World Order, 1974, 1975, 1976, 1977.

Slater, Sherwood, et al. "The Definition and Measurement of Disability." SOC. SCI. MED. 8 (1974): 305-8.

Describes the measurement conceptions and plans in a very significant study in Yugoslavia of disability in males in the productive years. One of a few systematic attempts to develop a general measure of ill health. Sponsored by WHO, the study will include comparisons of assessments of disability by self, family, and physician, and will also have a more "biological" measure of incapacity based on a clinical medical assessment. This article appears in a special issue of SOC. SCI. AND MED. devoted to social science research in WHO.

Sokołowska, Magdalena. "Social Science and Health Policy in Eastern Europe: Poland as a Case Study." INT'L. J. H. SERV. 4 (1974): 441-51. 16 refs.

Characterizes some traits of Polish sociology, especially its pragmatic approach and its relationship with social practice. Discusses two methodologic models of practical applications of sociology as proposed in the Polish literature, the first based on the assumption that sociology should be integrated into all spheres of social life, and the second calling for a fundamental reorientation of sociology. Attempts to show how health is being incorporated in the applied social sciences and social engineering. Discusses the utilization of sociologic studies in various spheres of Polish practice, particularly in the area of health. One of the remarkable things made evident in this article is the involvement of Polish sociologists with the effective power apparatus of the society, while their Western counterparts, for the most part, only carry out critical analyses from the outside.

Starfield, Barbara. "Measurement of Outcome: A Proposed Scheme." MILBANK MEM. FUND Q. HEALTH AND SOCIETY 52 (Winter 1974): 39-50.

A contribution to the conception of the measurement of health status and other health outcomes.

Stolley, Paul D. "Assuring the Safety and Efficacy of Therapies." INT'L. J. H. SERV. 4 (1974): 131-45. 35 refs.

This article discusses problems in evaluating surgical procedures, increasing drug use, and adverse reactions to therapies, indicating limitations in current practices and pointing out where greater acceptance and application of the controlled clinical trial could improve the overall safety and efficacy of therapies. A minor epidemic of drug-induced cancer is described to illustrate the use of the epidemiologic method in detecting adverse effects and for providing evidence for the development of a more responsible public policy. New government regulations have been developed on the basis of epidemiologic detection coupled with the controlled clinical trial. Reviews current practices of drug advertising and recommends a greater attention to the ecologic consequences of drugs and food additives.

Studnicki, James. "The Minimization of Travel Effort as a Delineating Influence for Urban Hospital Service Area." INT'L. J. H. SERV. 5 (1975): 679-93. 25 refs.

> From the author's summary: "Using a study population of 16,080 live births occurring to residents of Baltimore City in 16 hospitals in 1969, this research measured the existing flow of these patients against the flow 'expected' in an optimal accessibility model (where each birth would occur at the hospital with the shortest travel time to the residence of the mother)."

Suchman, Edward A. EVALUATIVE RESEARCH: PRINCIPLES AND PRACTICE IN PUBLIC SERVICE AND SOCIAL ACTION PROGRAMS. New York: Russell Sage Foundation, 1968.

> Applies various categories--background, independent, intervening, dependent--to the complex problem of evaluating health services. Makes the important point that health administrators should not expect social scientists simply to evaluate goal achievement. Rather, social scientists should contribute to the formulation of goals as well as programs for their accomplishment if the evaluation is to be valid. A classic in the field of methodology for health services evaluation but focuses on programs and not whole systems or cross-national studies.

Szalai, Alexander, et al., eds. CROSS-NATIONAL COMPARATIVE SURVEY RESEARCH: THEORY AND PRACTICE. Oxford, England, and New York: Pergamon, 1977.

> A most valuable collection from the Round Table Conference on this subject, sponsored by the International Social Science Council, European Coordination Centre for Research and Documentation in Social Sciences held in Budapest, July 25-28, 1972. Although not specifically directed toward health systems, includes such valuable papers as those by Glaser and Nowak (cited above, this chapter) as well as others.

United Nations Research Institute for Social Development. CONTENTS AND MEASUREMENT OF SOCIO-ECONOMIC DEVELOPMENT, AN EMPIRICAL ENQUIRY. Report no. 70.10. Geneva, 1970.

> A very thoughtful statement on a difficult problem.

Vukmanović, Čedomir. "The System and Statistics in Yugoslavia Compared with Other Countries." In COMPARABILITY IN INTERNATIONAL EPIDEMIOLOGY, edited by Roy M. Acheson, pp. 291-301. New York: Milbank Mem. Fund, 1965.

Although directed primarily toward utilization data, and this in one country, one can see from this paper examples of the problems which had to be taken into account in the International Collaborative Study of Medical Care Utilization (see Kohn and White above, this chaper). For example, "while each visit was recorded, with information on age, sex, occupation, etc., tabulation of data was done only for the total number of visits and for those made by active insured persons" (p. 295). Thus one does not know of the breakdown of visits by characteristics of patients among the active insured, and one has no information on visits of the nonactive insured (though this may be just 5 percent of the Yugoslavia population). Nor is it clear from tabulations where the visits were made-- at home, at a health center, or hospital. The article suggests some possible solutions to such problems.

Wessen, Albert F. "On the Scope and Methodology of Research in Public Health Practice." Working paper for a consultation of experts on research in public health practice, WHO, Geneva, December 2-10, 1968, OMC/RES/68.17. 40 notes, refs. Available from the author, Department of Community Medicine, Brown University, Providence, R.I.

A valuable overview from the perspective of a medical sociologist, then chief, Behavioural Science Unit, WHO, Geneva. First the field is defined, including such characteristics as a population or defined community as the target of public health research. And some substantive concerns are discussed: assessment of health levels in a population, development and testing of new methods and programs of health services delivery, determinants of utilization, evaluation of programs and systems, sociological and economic analysis of the operation of health care systems, the provision of materials and other components of service systems (logistics, support, etc.), allocation of resources. In a second part (pp. 16-28) some conceptual issues are raised concerning (1) the nature of a system, (2) biological and social bases of public health, (3) the generalizability of findings across cultural, national, and historical lines, (4) need versus demand, (5) is there one right way of meeting public health problems? In a third section, some methods and approaches are considered: epidemiological techniques; record research, including record linkage; surveys; observation; economic research; mathematical modeling; operations research; and systems analysis. Many of these reflect the component units of the Division of Research in Epidemiology and Communications Science within which Behavioral Science was placed. A final section (pp. 37-40) faces some issues such as pressures for immediate payoffs from practically concerned ministries of health.

"Wie gute Statistiken ein schlechtes Gesundheitswesen produzieren koennen [How good statistics can produce a poor health system]." DEUTSCHES AERZTE-BLATT 72 (January 1975): 53-56. In German.

> Discusses the interesting problem of how a health service can come under greater political pressure if an improved reporting system, rather than poorer health conditions, leads to an apparent decline in health levels.

Wilberg, Hakan. "Images of the World in the Year 2000." In CROSS-NATIONAL COMPARATIVE SURVEY RESEARCH: THEORY AND PRACTICE, edited by Alexander Szalai et al., pp. 51-72. Oxford, England, and New York: Pergamon, 1977.

> Project Report 3, prepared for the International Social Science Council's Round Table Conference on Cross-National Survey Analysis, Budapest, July 25-28, 1972. Interesting application of the delphi method which has also been used to tap people's images of what the future of medical practice will look like.

Wishik, Samuel M., and Van der Vynckt, Susan. "The Use of Nutritional 'Positive Deviants' to Identify Approaches to Modification of Dietary Practices." AJPH 66 (January 1976): 38-42. 7 refs.

> Presents a method of identifying feasible local approaches to improved nutrition by locating and studying "positive deviants" in an otherwise malnourished population.

Woolley, P.O.; Hays, W.S.; and Larson, D.L. SYNCRISIS: THE DYNAMICS OF HEALTH, AN ANALYTIC SERIES ON THE INTERACTIONS OF HEALTH AND SOCIOECONOMIC DEVELOPMENT. Vol. 3: PERSPECTIVES AND METHODOLOGY. US HEW, Office of International Health, Div. of Planning and Evaluation, June 1972. Tables, refs.

> The overall methods and approach statement for a series with some twenty volumes covering different national health systems.

World Health Organization (WHO). MEASUREMENT OF LEVELS OF HEALTH, REPORT OF A STUDY GROUP. Technical Report Series, no. 137. Geneva, 1957.

> One of the most thorough considerations of the subject.

_____. STATISTICAL INDICATORS FOR THE PLANNING AND EVALUATION OF PUBLIC HEALTH PROGRAMMES. Technical Report Series, no. 472. Geneva, 1976.

Wotjun, Bronislaw S. "Application of the Balancing Equation to Test the Quality of Population Data for Political Subdivisions: Case of Upper Silesia." Paper presented at the session on population studies of the USSR and Eastern Europe,

MEDICAL CENTER LIBRARY

annual meeting of the Population Studies Society of America, Montreal, April 29–May 1, 1976. Available from the author through the Population Studies Society.

Discusses the approach of breaking a population down into its many components and seeking reliable estimates for each as a way of seeking an improved estimate of the total. This is applied to Upper Silesia.

Chapter 8

DATA SOURCES

The reader interested in using secondary information to compare or contrast national health systems and their socioeconomic, political, and epidemiologic contexts, has a large number of sources to search. No attempt is made here to treat approaches to gathering primary data; these are covered in chapter 7. Many of these sources will be national population and socioeconomic statistical reports available from each country's central office of statistics. See, for example, National Central Bureau of Statistics (Sweden), THE COST OF FINANCING SOCIAL SERVICES IN SWEDEN IN 1971.

Most ministries of health (or their counterparts, such as DHEW in the U.S.) issue annual reports on mortality, morbidity, on health personnel, and facilities. Only some examples of these sources are given here. See for example, Department of Health and Social Services, London, also annual statistical reports of census bureaus or their equivalent. For example, ANNUAL ABSTRACT OF STATISTICS, London: Central Statistics Office, Great George Street; or ANNUAIRE STATISTIQUE DE LA FRANCE, Paris: Institute Nationale de la Statistique et des Etudes Economiques; or JAPAN STATISTICAL YEARBOOK, Tokoyo: Bureau of Statistics, Office of the Prime Minister.

The majority of multinational statistical reports stem out of the UN system. The reader is advised to read through this section to see what the range of sources is. Searching for a certain source may not be rewarding as authorship, titles, and other information are not always as clear or standard as in other chapters. The reader is also advised to read a chapter such as that by D.V. McGranahan (see chapter 7) on the pitfalls and shortcomings of data gathered through the UN system. Many of these cautions will apply to other secondary data. Professional associations often provide useful data. For example, the AMA (Chicago) produces several publications useful as data sources for the United States: DISTRIBUTION OF PHYSICIANS IN THE U.S. (1977--annual); SELECTED CHARACTERISTICS OF THE PHYSICIAN POPULATION, 1963 AND 1967 (1968); and DISTRIBUTION OF PHYSICIANS, HOSPITALS, AND HOSPITAL BEDS IN THE US, VOL. 1: REGION, STATE, COUNTY (1966--). Professional associations in other countries generally issue similar statistical reports, or do so in cooperation with government agencies, for example, THE MEDICAL REGISTER (London) General Medical Council, (1972). Such items are pointed to here but are generally not separately listed in this chapter.

Data Sources

A general collection on the problems of data and methods in cross-national sociomedical research is given in the book edited by Pflanz and Schach (see chapter 7). The patterns vary a great deal, even when the data base is adequate. For example, most countries count a live birth when the child lives through the first hour or so. However, few countries count only those children surviving after twenty-four hours. Obviously this affects reporting of infant mortality rates.

Aiken, Michael. "Comparative Cross-National Research on Subnational Units in Western Europe. Problems, Data Sources and a Proposal." J. OF COMPARATIVE ADMINISTRATION 4 (February 1973): 437-71. Refs.

> Revision of a paper originally presented at the City University of New York. Colloquium on Comparative Urban Politics, New York, May 14, 1971. A number of publications are cited which list data sources, including Council for European Studies, A GUIDE TO SOURCES OF ECOLOGICAL AND SURVEY DATA FOR WESTERN EUROPE (1972). There is also a specific listing and discussion of data sources on cities and other subnational units for almost every West European country. Also reports on several scientific organizations and committees which have developed to pursue comparative studies. Proposes more joint research efforts and the setting up of a data pool.

Alford, Robert R. "Data Resources for Comparative Studies of Urban Administration." SOCIAL SCIENCE INFORMATION 9 (June 1970): 193-203.

Banks, Arthur S., ed. POLITICAL HANDBOOK OF THE WORLD: 1975. New York: McGraw-Hill, 1976.

> One of a series of volumes giving information on leaders, governmental form and organization, political parties, issues, news media, and foreign policy in 164 nations.

Boulding, Elise, et al. HANDBOOK OF INTERNATIONAL DATA ON WOMEN. New York: Sage Publications, 1976.

> Brings together the statistical analysis of women's position in the world gathered by international census teams of the UN during International Women's Year. The assembled data provide a cross-national basis for future research, proof of the under-enumeration of women in all areas of society, a new resource for policymakers seeking solutions to world problems, and the latest look at women as part of population, marriage, child bearing, and death.

BUSINESS ENVIRONMENTAL RISK INDEX. Triannual.

> As described in MOTHER JONES (Boulder, Colo.) 3 (January 1978): 8: "Each issue of BERI rates every major country on a 0-to-100 scale of how safe it is for your company to do business

in. . . . BERI's publisher is a business administration professor named F.T. Haner. . . . Haner says BERI's rating system is based on detailed assessments of various countries from a panel of more than 100 bankers, business men and government officials around the world. A complicated weighting system takes account of 15 factors including currency convertibility, a country's 'attitude' toward foreign investors and uppity local labor. Countries in the upper half of the scale tend to be our [US] NATO partners or Third World states that have firmly kept leftists in line, like Korea and Taiwan. The Philippines' rating has risen from 43 in 1973 to 56.1 in 1976 with the increasing repressiveness of the Marcos dictatorship. Denmark moved from 'moderate risk' into 'high' when it gave labor union representatives a voice in factory decisions. . . . A one-year subscription (three issues) [costs] $325. . . ."

No address is given for the publisher. This magazine might serve as a useful data source to rate countries as to how capitalist-oriented they are and how they relate in other ways to health services.

Canada National Department of Health and Welfare. Research and Statistics Directorate. COMPARISON OF SOCIAL SECURITY EXPENDITURES IN CANADA, AUSTRALIA, NEW ZEALAND, UNITED KINGDOM AND THE UNITED STATES, FISCAL YEARS 1961-62 TO 1966-67, INCLUSIVE. Ottawa, 1970.

Although dated, this is a valuable comparative data source for the indicated period.

Comecon Secretariat. STATISTICAL YEARBOOK. Moscow, 1975.

A source including health data such as life expectancy, infant mortality, and causes of death, as well as data on health personnel. Used among other sources by Michael Kaser in his data-rich book on health systems of Eastern European, Comecon countries (see chapter 3.2).

Foreign Area Studies Program. American University. AREA HANDBOOK FOR HAITI. Washington, D.C.: GPO, 1973.

One of a large series giving basic socioeconomic, political, governmental, cultural, armed forces, and some health information on many of the countries of the world. Primarily as background for US state department and other governmental foreign relations interests. An important data resource developed for a certain set of US governmental interests. Research for this volume was completed in February 1973.

Gold, Joseph. MEMBERSHIP AND NONMEMBERSHIP IN THE INTERNATIONAL MONETARY FUND A STUDY IN INTERNATIONAL LAW AND ORGANIZATION. Washington, D.C.: Int. Monetary Fund, 1974.

Data Sources

HANDBOOK OF INTERNATIONAL TRADE AND DEVELOPMENT STATISTICS, 1976. E/F.76.II.D.3. New York: UN, 1976.

> An important resource for national and international data on commercial, industrial, and economic activity and products.

"Health Information for International Travel." DHEW Pub. no. (CDC) 76-8280. Atlanta: Center for Disease Control, 1976. Booklet.

> Published as a supplement to MORBIDITY AND MORTALITY WEEKLY REPORT (a US-oriented data sheet) this internationally oriented publication lists shots required in going to and returning from nearly every country in the world. Also gives maps of endemic diseases such as yellow fever and malaria.

Hilton, Gordon. A REVIEW OF THE DIMENSIONALITY OF NATIONS PROJECT. Sage Professional Papers in Int'l. Studies, no. 02-105. Beverly Hills, Calif.: Sage, 1973. 80 p.

> A good source for data sources in that this booklet-sized study cites the sources used in attempts to categorize nations (mainly with foreign policy and international relations in view).

International Labour Organization (ILO). THE COST OF SOCIAL SECURITY. Geneva, 1949-- . Annual.

> A series with considerable valuable data on health care costs, coverage, use, and other health care information as well as other social welfare information.

International Social Security Association. SICKNESS INSURANCE: NATIONAL MONOGRAPHS. Geneva, 1956.

> A valuable historical resource series.

Jain, Shail. SIZE DISTRIBUTION OF INCOME, A COMPILATION OF DATA. Washington, D.C.: World Bank, 1975.

> A revised published version of the "World Bank Staff Working Paper . . ." (see below, this chapter). Some information was lost in the revision, for example, in the working paper the amount of income controlled by the upper 5 percent could be seen for many countries (e.g., Brazil, households, 1970: 36%) while in this published version only deciles are given ("upper" 10% of households in Brazil, 1970: 47%). Nevertheless, this is a valuable data source on a key problem on which it is otherwise difficult to obtain information. Gives some data for eighty-one countries. Provides extensive notes on sources and problems with information for each country.

Karlin, Barry. "Delivering Health Services in 54 Developing Countries: A Study of 180 Projects." Paper presented at the 105th annual meeting of the APHA, Washington, D.C., October 30–November 3, 1977. Available from the author through the APHA, Washington, D.C.

> During 1976 a large number of field projects were studied, including the services being offered, types of personnel who are permitted to deliver health services, and health care systems which have been organized. The study (1) describes the present status of a relatively large number of health projects; (2) determines the extent to which innovative practices are being pursued and their characteristics; (3) identifies possible trends in the delivery of health services; (4) searches for possible explanations for the variations uncovered; and (5) assesses unmet needs which obstruct efforts to improve health and health care. This article presents the major findings of the study, along with discussions of the methodologies employed.

Kohn, Robert, and White, Kerr L. eds. "Archive Tape Repositories." In HEALTH CARE, AN INTERNATIONAL STUDY: REPORT OF THE WHO INTERNATIONAL COLLABORATIVE STUDY OF MEDICAL CARE UTILIZATION. London, New York, and Toronto: Oxford Univ. Press, 1976.

Mickiewicz, Ellen, ed. HANDBOOK OF SOVIET SOCIAL SCIENCE DATA. New York: Macmillan, Free Press, 1973.

> Chapter 4, "Health," is authored by Mark Field.

National Center for Health Statistics. INTERNATIONAL COMPARISON OF PERINATAL AND INFANT MORTALITY: THE UNITED STATES AND SIX WESTERN EUROPEAN COUNTRIES. Series 3, no. 6. Washington, D.C.: USPHS, 1968.

National Central Bureau of Statistics (Sweden). THE COST OF FINANCING SOCIAL SERVICES IN SWEDEN IN 1971. Stockholm, 1973.

> An example of an important data source for this country allowing comparisons of expenditures between health and other service sectors also according to source of funds. It should be clear that not every country issues the same kind of report, nor do many countries have as fine a statistical system as does Sweden. However, most nations have census bureaus and ministries of health which issue periodic reports.

Nordic Council. YEARBOOK OF NORDIC STATISTICS, 1976. Stockholm: P.A. Norstedt, 1977.

> A valuable information resource published each year on Denmark, Finland, Iceland, Norway, and Sweden.

ON THE STATE OF PUBLIC HEALTH, ANNUAL REPORT OF THE CHIEF MEDICAL OFFICER OF THE MINISTRY OF HEALTH FOR THE YEAR 1920. London: HMSO, 1922.

> Listed here as an example of early official statistical reports issued by the ministry of health in a country (in this case the UK) which are valuable for historical studies of changes in different systems.

Pan American Health Organization (PAHO). HEALTH CONDITIONS IN THE AMERICAS, 1965-68. Scientific Publications NI. 207. Washington, D.C.: PAHO/WHO, 1970.

> One of a periodic series allowing comparison of health status and health services indicators between Latin and South American countries as well as North American countries.

POPINFORM. Available from Informatics Inc., 6000 Executive Boulevard, Rockville, Md., 20852.

> A collection of computerized population information and international data assembled by the Population Information Program of the George Washington University, Department of Medical and Public Affairs, Science Communication Division, under contract to AID. For on-line access by subscribers. A source of up-to-date published and unpublished studies on contraceptive technology, family planning programs, and population. Worldwide in scope. POPINFORM data bases are given below:
>
> 1. George Washington University, Population Information Program (PIP)
>   Includes citations with abstracts covering contraceptive technology, family planning programs, and population law and policy. Anticipated file size of 20,000 entries. PIP thesaurus is based on the National Library of Medicine's MeSH (Medical Subject Headings) and will provide greater in-depth indexing in the areas of contraception and contraceptive technology.
>
> 2. Columbia University, International Institute for the Study of Human Reproduction (CUIISHR)
>   Includes citations and in-depth indexing in the special field of family planning evaluation. Anticipated file size of 3,000 entries.
>
> 3. U.S. Dept. of Commerce, Bureau of the Census International Demographic Data Directory (IDDD)
>   Includes over 4,000 tables and bibliographic references to tables on demographic and vital statistics, statistics on family planning program activities, and selected economic and educational characteristics. (Worldwide data with primary emphasis on African, Asian, and Latin American countries). Estimated growth rate of 3,000

entries per year. Sources include census reports, UN
documents, sample surveys, journal articles, conference
reports on population and family planning, published
and unpublished papers.

4. Center for Disease Control, Family Planning Evaluation Division
(CDC-FPED)
Includes over 6,000 citations with abstracts and index
terms comprehensively covering US information on family
planning evaluation, pregnancy termination, complica-
tions associated with oral contraceptives, and IUDs.
Estimated growth rate is 1,200 entries per year. Sources
include journal articles, conference papers, published
and unpublished reports.

REPORT ON THE WORLD SOCIAL SITUATION, 1974. E.75.IV.6. New York:
UN, 1975.

An important world survey document of social and living conditions
country by country and by multinational regions. Many valuable
statistics and much useful qualitative information is provided. Previous issue for 1970, E.71.IV.13. The latest issue is for 1978,
issued in 1979.

Sivard, Ruth Leger. WORLD MILITARY AND SOCIAL EXPENDITURES. Leesburg,
Va.: WMSE Publications, 1974-- . Annual. Notes.

One of the most valuable annual general data sources for CNSHS,
published under the auspices of the Institute for World Order, New
York 10036. Includes data on physician-population ratios, public
health expenditures per capita, and infant mortality rates for nearly
every country. Also gives general economic data (GNP per capita,
etc.) and information on expenditures in such other sectors as military and education.

STATISTICAL ABSTRACT OF LATIN AMERICA. Los Angeles: Univ. of California, 1966.

One of an annual series giving primarily demographic and socioeconomic data but including selected health and health services
data by which countries can be compared.

STATISTICAL BULLETIN FOR LATIN AMERICA. New York: UN, vol. 3, 1969.

An example of a continuing series for one region of the world
giving primarily demographic and socioeconomic data but including
some health information.

SYNCRISIS: THE DYNAMICS OF HEALTH: AN ANALYTIC SERIES ON THE
INTERACTIONS OF HEALTH AND SOCIOECONOMIC DEVELOPMENT.

Washington, D.C.: U.S./HEW Office of International Health, Div. of Planning and Evaluation, June 1972-- . Ongoing.

> An important source of information with volumes on some twenty UDCs.

Taylor, Charles F., and Hudson, Michael C. WORLD HANDBOOK OF PO-LITICAL AND SOCIAL INDICATORS. New Haven, Conn.: Yale Univ. Press, 1972.

> An extremely important resource for socioeconomic, political, and some health and health system data on countries of the world, based mainly on UN sources. Complete as of 1965 with unfortunately only partial updating after 1970. Data is available through local universities participating in the Interuniversity Consortium for Po-litical Research based at the University of Michigan, Ann Arbor. Handbooks describe exactly the raw data, and the coding and careful definitions of items are provided as well as descriptions of limitations of the data. For an example of the use of this source for comparing health systems see Elling and Kerr, cited in chapter 7.

United Nations (UN). DEMOGRAPHIC YEARBOOK, 1976. New York, 1977.

> The most valuable general source for worldwide and country-by-country socioeconomic, population and health data. The data limi-tations, however, must be seriously considered. See D. McGranahan, cited in chapter 7.

U.S. Department of Commerce. Bureau of the Census. Foreign Demographic Analysis Division. INTERNATIONAL POPULATION STATISTICS REPORTS. Series P-90, P-91, and P-95, no. 64, Washington, D.C.: GPO.

> No. 64 in Series P-95 published in April, 1968 is only one of this valuable series going back some twenty years and giving information on a variety of sociodemographic aspects of populations in other countries. This particular one is entitled "Wages in the USSR, 1950-66: Health Services."

U.S. Department of Health, Education and Welfare. Social Security Administration. SOCIAL SECURITY PROGRAMS THROUGHOUT THE WORLD--1969. Social Security Administration, Research Report no. 31. Washington, D.C.: GPO, 1969.

> Describes programs for 51 countries.

Wittkopf, Eugene R. WESTERN BILATERAL AID ALLOCATIONS: A COMPARA-TIVE STUDY OF RECIPIENT STATE ATTRIBUTES AND AID RECEIVED. Sage Professional Papers in Int'l. Studies, no. 02-005. Beverly Hills, Calif.: Sage, 1972. 64 p.

WORLD BANK ATLAS. Washington, D.C.: World Bank, 1974. Booklet.
1 note.

> Sections and countries of the world are colored according to various
> socioeconomic information, and tabular material is provided along
> with maps. To be issued in updated form in subsequent years. The
> 1974 issue gave GNP, amount and average annual growth rate;
> and population and GNP per capita, and growth rate of these.

"World Bank Staff Working Paper on Size Distribution of Income." Washington,
D.C.: World Bank, 1975.

> An internal working document available with staff permission. Pro-
> vides distribution of income by households and certain other units
> for many countries. Data are from a variety of sources and there
> are many gaps. Although such information is extremely difficult
> to obtain, it is very important because disparities or equity within
> countries are a very important dimension related to health status.
> A version of this paper was published (see Shail Jain, above, this
> chapter).

WORLD FERTILITY PATTERNS. Washington, D.C.: AID, Office of Population,
1977.

> Provides fertility data by five-year age groupings from fifteen to
> fifty for countries of the world from the 1960s or later if available.
> Data are given in tabular form as well as graphically for each
> country. Sources for statistics are provided.

World Health Organization (WHO). FIFTH REPORT OF THE WORLD HEALTH
SITUATION. Geneva, 1973.

> Includes data and general information on WHO regions and on most
> countries within regions. A most important resource for beginning
> study of any particular system. Issued for five-year periods.

_____. PUBLIC HEALTH PAPERS. Geneva, WHO.

> This series of publications ranges from book-length to pamphlet size
> and covers a number of health system topics such as the rural hos-
> pital, and principles of health planning in the USSR. Some sixty
> items had been issued by 1977.

_____. TECHNICAL REPORT SERIES. Geneva, WHO.

> Now close to 600 issues on topics ranging from auxiliary health
> personnel to side effects of drugs.

_____. WORLD HEALTH STATISTICS ANNUAL. (Vols. 1-20, prior to 1961,
have the title, "Epidemiological and Vital Statistics Report.) Geneva.

Divided into different volumes each year--one covering mortality and morbidity and one covering health facilities and personnel--this is one of the major data resources on health conditions and services in countries of the world.

World Health Organization. Eastern Mediterranean Regional Office (WHO/EMRO). BASIC COUNTRY INFORMATION. Circular no. 10. Alexandria, Egypt, 1975.

Each of the six WHO regional offices (see WHO, chapter 11) publishes comparable compendia of basic information on countries of their regions.

WORLD POPULATION ESTIMATES. Washington, D.C.: Environmental Fund. Annual. Notes, data sources.

Published in the form of a single large table giving regions of the world and countries within regions. In 1974 information included population estimate; growth rate; crude birth rate; crude death rate; population under fifteen as a percent of the total; per capita energy consumption; population growth rate 1958-63; birth rate, 1965. Subsequent years have included such items as percent urban and rate of urban growth.

Zayed, Marlene. "Contrasting Case Studies of National Health Systems in Arab Countries." Farmington: Program in Cross-National Studies of Health Systems, Department of Community Medicine, Univ. of Connecticut, 1977. Reproduced.

A valuable student research paper comparing the regionalization of health services in Arab nations, particularly Syria and Saudi Arabia. Has information on most Arab countries' health systems. Available from the CNSHS program or through interlibrary loan from the University of Connecticut Health Center Library, Farmington 06032.

Chapter 9

BIBLIOGRAPHIES

Aday, Lu Ann, and Eichorn, Robert L. THE UTILIZATION OF HEALTH SERVICES: INDICES AND CORRELATES, A RESEARCH BIBLIOGRAPHY. DHEW Pub. no. (HSM) 73-3003. Washington, D.C.: GPO, 1972. No author index.

> Originally prepared by Aday for the Health Services Research and Training Program at Purdue University, Lafayette, Indiana, this well-indexed and classified bibliography has detailed annotations done in a thoughtful manner. Important resource with 203 items. Limited in focusing primarily on US studies.

Akhtar, Shahid, ed. HEALTH CARE IN THE PEOPLE'S REPUBLIC OF CHINA: A BIBLIOGRAPHY WITH ABSTRACTS. Introduction by J. Wendell MacLeod. Ottawa, Ontario: IDRC, 1975. Author and subject index.

> This 182-page bibliography taken from the IDRC data base on alternative primary health care delivery presents information on the approaches taken in the PRC. It is the most complete and valuable bibliography available on the PRC. The introduction summarizes the Chinese experience in health care. Annotations are given for 560 items. Includes the following appendixes:
>
> 1. Articles identified but not received for processing (173 items)
> 2. A selection of articles published in the CHINESE MEDICAL JOURNAL, Peking, 1960-74
> 3. Sources of information about Chinese documents
> 4. Names and addresses of select authors and institutions

_____. LOW-COST RURAL HEALTH CARE AND HEALTH MANPOWER TRAIN-ING: AN ANNOTATED BIBLIOGRAPHY WITH SPECIAL EMPHASIS ON DE-VELOPING COUNTRIES. Vol. 1. Ottawa, Ontario: IDRC, 1975. 3 indexes.

> The first volume in a series of annotated bibliographies on low-cost rural health care and health manpower training. These volumes will be published irregularly. (For volume 2 see Frances Delaney, this chapter.) With 700 carefully annotated references this is possibly the most valuable bibliography available for CNSHS even though it focuses on auxiliary and new types of health wo/manpower

in recognition of the problems of countries in which the bulk of
the population lacks access to physicians and hospitals. Contents:
(1) Reference Works; (2) Organization and Planning; (3) Primary
Health Care--Implementation; (4) Primary Health Manpower--Train-
ing and Utilization; (5) Formal Evaluative Studies.

Altman, Isadore, et al. METHODOLOGY IN EVALUATING THE QUALITY OF
MEDICAL CARE; AN ANNOTATED SELECTED BIBLIOGRAPHY, 1955-1968.
Pittsburgh: Univ. of Pittsburgh Press, 1969.

Bibliography on evaluation research methodologies--both general
works and specific evaluation studies pointing to problems and
resolutions through concrete methodological examples. Draws almost entirely on US experience.

Badgley, Robin F., et al. "Selected Bibliography on Social Science and Health
in Canada." MILBANK MEM. FUND Q. 49, pt. 1 (April 1971): 277-314.

Focused more on medical sociology in Canada than on organization
or comparative studies of the Canadian health services system, but
includes works of these sorts.

"Bibliography on Medical Education in the Developing Countries, 1956-1964."
J. MED. ED. 40 (October 1965): 931-47.

Biological Sciences Communication Project. DELIVERY OF HEALTH CARE SER-
VICES IN LESS DEVELOPED COUNTRIES, A LITERATURE SEARCH. Washington,
D.C.: George Washington Univ. Medical Center, Biological Sciences Com-
munication Project, June 1973.

A ninety-five item annotated bibliography produced for the APHA
project Development and Evaluation of Integrated Delivery Systems
(DEIDS). A broadly oriented work. The following item is more
specialized.

_____. DELIVERY OF HEALTH CARE SERVICES IN LESS DEVELOPED COUN-
TRIES WITH EMPHASIS ON INTEGRATION OF FAMILY PLANNING WITH MA-
TERNAL AND CHILD HEALTH, A LITERATURE SEARCH. Washington, D.C.:
George Washington Univ. Medical Center, Biological Sciences Communication
Project, February 1973. 3 indexes.

An extensive annotated bibliography (178 items) including a country-
by-country analysis concerning most UDCs and LDCs as well as
general topics related to the title. A most valuable resource.
Done for the APHA project Development and Evaluation of Integrated Delivery Systems (DEIDS).

Center for Health Administration Studies. Univ. of Chicago. LIST OF PUB-
LICATIONS. Chicago, 1977.

An extensive list of medical researches developed over the years. Many are directly relevant to CNSHS. Included are the Michael M. Davis lecture series with a number of talks by international experts.

Centre de Récherches et de Documentation sur la Consommation. BIBLIOGRA- PHIE DES ETUDES D'ÉCONOMIE MÉDICALE ET MÉDICO-SOCIALES. Paris: C.R.E.D.O.C. and the Group de Recherche Universitaires, 1965. In French.

Although dated, this bibliography helps with items on health ser- vices in France and items on other countries in French as well as in other languages.

Clarkson, J. Graham. COMPREHENSIVE BIBLIOGRAPHY: MEDICAL CARE; HOSPITALIZATION; AND PUBLIC HEALTH IN SASKATCHEWAN. Iowa City: Univ. of Iowa Program in Hospital Administration, 1966.

CURRENT BIBLIOGRAPHY OF EPIDEMIOLOGY: A GUIDE TO THE LITERATURE OF EPIDEMIOLOGY, PREVENTIVE MEDICINE AND PUBLIC HEALTH. Bethesda, Md.: National Library of Medicine. Ceased publication December 1977.

The purpose of this bibliography was to provide a comprehensive and continuing index to the current periodical medical literature for practitioners and investigators in community medicine and for others concerned with the etiology, prevention, and control of disease. The bibliography is divided into two parts, each arranged in alphabetical order. Section 1, "Selected Subject Headings," includes references related to some 200 topics, such as birth rate, child health services, communicable disease control, environmental health, hygiene, nutrition surveys, preventive dentistry, sanitation, and WHO. Section 2, "Diseases, Organisms, and Vaccines," in- cludes the current references related to the etiology, prevention, and control of specific diseases. Topics here include abortion, birth injuries, deficiency diseases, gynecologic diseases, kwashiorkor, and trypanosomiasis. Since each reference cited here appears at least once in INDEX MEDICUS, a separate author index is not required. Each volume consisted of twelve monthly issues accom- panied by an annual cumulation at the end of the year. Back volumes can be ordered from the Superintendent of Documents, US Government Printing Office, Washington, D.C. 20402, at $22.50 per volume.

Davis, Lenwood G. URBAN GROWTH, DEVELOPMENT AND PLANNING OF AFRICAN TOWNS AND CITIES. Columbus: Ohio State Univ., Department of Black Studies, 1977. 27 p.

Delaney, Frances. LOW-COST RURAL HEALTH CARE AND HEALTH MAN- POWER TRAINING: AN ANNOTATED BIBLIOGRAPHY WITH SPECIAL EM- PHASIS ON DEVELOPING COUNTRIES. Vol. 2. Ottawa, Ontario: IDRC, 1978.

This is a 170-page work. For the first volume of this series, see Shahid Akhtar, above, this chapter.

Elling, Ray H., ed. CROSS-NATIONAL STUDY OF HEALTH SYSTEMS BY COUNTRY AND WORLD REGIONS, INCLUDING SPECIAL PROBLEMS. Detroit: Gale Research, 1980. Index.

The companion volume to this. Following the introduction, provides annotations of numerous items. Chapter 2, Special Problems, has the following seventeen sections: Allied Health Personnel, Brain Drain, Citizen Participation, Dental Health, Education (Medicine, Nursing, Other), Geriatric and Organized Home Care, Health Planning, Hospitals and Other Health Organizations, Liberation Movements and Health Services, MCH, Mental Health, Nomads and Other Special Groups, Nutrition, Occupational Health, Population-Family Planning, Traditional and Modern Care, and Health Services Utilization; Chapter 3, Countries on Which Considerable Work Has Been Done, covers Canada, Cuba, PRC, Sweden, UK, United States. Other chapters are (4) Africa; (5) Americas; (6) Eastern Mediterranean; (7) Europe; (8) Southeast Asia; and (9) Western Pacific.

_____. HEALTH SYSTEMS AND HEALTH PLANNING IN INTERNATIONAL PERSPECTIVE, AN ANNOTATED BIBLIOGRAPHY. Council of Planning Librarians Exchange Bibliography no. 265. Monticello, Ill., March 1972.

Annotated in three sections: (1) one by the editor on approaches to health planning in different countries; (2) a short section by S. Leonard Syme on the relevance of cross-national social epidemiologic studies to health planning; and (3) a section by E. Richard Weinerman on medical care systems first published in the Asilomar conference volume of MEDICAL CARE (May-June 1971) (see Weinerman, chapter 5).

ENVIRONMENT. Geneva: WHO, 1977.

List of Publications of the WHO and the International Agency for Research on Cancer. Category headings: environment (general); air pollution; water and wastes; housing and urban planning; education and training; radiation; publications of the Int'l. Agency for Research on Cancer. Some 120 items are listed.

Foltz, Ann-Marie. "Sociology of Medical Care in Norway, A Critical Bibliography and Questions for Research." New Haven, Conn.: Yale Univ. School of Pub. H., May 31, 1971. Mimeographed. Available from the author, Department of Epidemiology and Public Health, Yale School of Medicine, New Haven, Conn.

A valuable annotated selection of sixty-nine items concluding with questions deserving further study.

Garfin, Susan Bettelheim. "Comparative Studies: A Selected, Annotated Bibliography." In COMPARATIVE METHODS IN SOCIOLOGY, ESSAYS ON TRENDS AND APPLICATIONS, edited by Ivan Vallier, pp. 423-67. Berkeley and Los Angeles: Univ. of California Press, 1973.

Gish, Oscar, ed. HEALTH MANPOWER AND THE MEDICAL AUXILIARY: SOME NOTES AND AN ANNOTATED BIBLIOGRAPHY. See chapter 3.3.

Gray, G.I. HEALTH SERVICES RESEARCH AND DEVELOPMENT ABROAD: A SELECTED BIBLIOGRAPHY. Bethesda, Md.: Capital Systems Group, July 1971. 161 p. Indexes.

> This bibliography was developed from a project entitled "Systematic Inventory of Active Non-U.S. Information Sources and Preparation of Bibliography of Foreign Literature in Health Services Research and Development in 1965-1970." Describes a sample of literature selected from the larger mass of documentation identified and examined during the course of this study. The sources were approximately one hundred different indexing/abstracting journals and bibliographies; literature provided or suggested by health specialists in the United States and abroad; special computer searches using the MEDLARS system of the National Library of Medicine and the Excerpta Medica automated Biomedical Data Bank; and direct searching of the contents of specific journals considered to be most important in the field of health services research. Non-English documents are annotated in English. There are 521 annotated references listed under the following headings: (1) economics and planning, (2) health care services, (3) manpower and training, (4) methodology and technology, and (5) bibliographies and services.

Heald, K.A., and Cooper, J.K. ANNOTATED BIBLIOGRAPHY ON RURAL MEDICAL CARE. Document no. R-966-HEW. Santa Monica, Calif.: RAND Corp., April 1972. 35 p.

> This bibliography on rural health care has been compiled for persons interested in health problems of rural America. A total of 180 annotated references are categorized according to the following subject areas: manpower supply and distribution; demand for health services; factors affecting physician placement; physician shortage; and related topics.

Huard, P., and Wong, Ming. "Bio-bibliographie de la Médecine chinoise" [Biobibliography of Chinese medicine]. BUL. SOCIÉTE DES ÉTUDES INDO-CHINOISES (Saigon) 11 (1956): 181-246. In French.

> Bibliography of Chinese medicine includes an index to principal authors (from the past twenty-five centuries), and an annotated title index, both compiled alphabetically. Separate indexes list authors by historical period and by subject. Brief bibliography of twentieth-century work on China is included.

Bibliographies

Inkeles, Alex, and Holsinger, Donald B., eds. EDUCATION AND INDIVIDUAL MODERNITY IN DEVELOPING COUNTRIES. Leiden, Netherlands: E.J. Brill, 1975.

Jumba-Masagazi, A.H.K. THE SOCIOLOGY OF FAMILY HEALTH, A BIBLIOGRAPHY AND A SHORT COMMENTARY. Information Circular no. 5. Nairobi, Kenya: East African Academy, May 1971.

> The academy serves as a research information center for Kenya, Tanzania, and Uganda. Following eight pages of introductory notes and commentary and almost one hundred pages of citations (not annotated). Perhaps the most extensive listing of works on health in Africa to date of publication. Includes a nine-page list of periodicals. The work concludes with several pages of names and addresses of health and scientific research and related agencies in many parts of the world which conduct research related to African health.

Koch-Weser, Dieter. "Informal Draft Bibliography, Internations Programs." Boston: Department of Preventive and Social Med., Harvard Med. School, July 1975. 11 p.

> Headings and number of items for each are foreign medical graduates, 11; health planning, 11; international health, 24; international medical education, 6; Latin American development, 8; population, 3. There follow a number of individual countries or world areas with generally four or five items for each. Not annotated.

Kohn, R., and Radius, S. "International Comparison of Health Services Systems, An Annotated Bibliography." INT'L. J. H. SERV. 3 (1973): 295-309.

> Lists publications facilitating cross-national comparisons of health services systems. Research for the work included a Medical Literature Analysis and Retrieval System (MEDLARS) search of the National Library of Medicine. Includes only English-language sources. It consists of an annotated bibliography of selected books, including both national and cross-national studies. Subject areas as well as individual entries are selective. The bibliography will be kept up to date, and in the future will incorporate new publications, non-English sources, and suggestions from readers. A valuable contribution with thirty-one items under the cross-national, and thirty-seven items under the national categories.

Litman, Theodore. THE SOCIOLOGY OF MEDICINE AND HEALTH CARE: A RESEARCH BIBLIOGRAPHY. San Francisco: Boyd and Fraser, 1976.

> While focused mainly on the United States, this work includes a number of references (not annotated) on other countries, especially the UK, Western Europe, Canada, Australia and New Zealand, Latin America, China, Scandinavian countries, and USSR, Cuba,

and India and other developing countries. There are also sections
on frameworks and methods for comparative study of health systems.

Little, Virginia. SOCIAL SERVICES FOR THE ELDERLY, INTERNATIONAL.
Philadelphia: Temple Univ. Press, expected 1980.

A valuable annotated resource.

Logan, Michael H. "Selected References on the Hot-Cold Theory of Disease."
MEDICAL ANTHROPOLOGY NEWSLETTER. (Washington, D.C., American
Anthropology Association) 6 (February 1975): 8-11.

Categorical but not annotated bibliography. Categories: Latin
America, Mexico, Guatemala, Costa Rica, Nicaragua, Haiti,
Puerto Rico, Peru, Bolivia, United States.

Moodie, P.M., and Pedersen, E.B. THE HEALTH OF AUSTRALIAN ABORI-
GINES: AN ANNOTATED BIBLIOGRAPHY. Service Publication no. 8. Univ.
of Sydney, School of Pub. H. and Tropical Med., 1971.

National Center for Health Services Research. NCHSR RESEARCH BIBLIOGRAPHY.

A newly published research bibliography provides ready access to
all National Center for Health Services Research interim and final
reports submitted to the National Technical Information Service between July 1, 1976, and June 30, 1977, for public announcement
and sale. NCHSR series publications and staff papers also are included. Indexes are based upon key search terms such as author,
institution, title, and subject. Citations include document title,
performing institution and address, authors, subject field, report
date, page number, contract or grant number, abstract, purchase
order number, and price. Available on request from NCHSR, Rm.
7-44, 3700 East-West Highway, Hyattsville, Md. 20782.

_____. RESEARCH SUMMARY SERIES, RECENT STUDIES IN HEALTH SERVICES
RESEARCH. DHEW Pub. no. (HRA) 77-3162. Washington, D.C., 1977.

Summarized researches on medical care organization, primarily US
work. Also lists data files available for secondary analyses, including the WHO/International Collaborative Study of Utilization
(see Kohn and White, cited in chapter 7).

Navarro, Vicente. "Regionalization and Planning of Personal Health Services:
An Annotated Bibliography." See chapter 6.

Pirro, Ellen B. "Cross National Research: A Selected Bibliography." In COM-
PARING NATIONS, THE USE OF QUANTITATIVE DATA IN CROSS-NATIONAL
RESEARCH, edited by R.L. Merritt and S. Rokkan, pp. 561-69. New Haven, Conn.:
Yale Univ. Press, 1966.

Bibliographies

An important social science research bibliography oriented toward methods. Contains 200 unannotated items. Not specifically health related. Categories: general and theoretical works; techniques of data analysis; content analysis; survey research; elite analysis; some comparative applications of research techniques.

The Population Council. "Family Planning Developments in China, 1960-1966: Abstracts from Medical Journals." STUDIES IN FAMILY PLANNING 4 (August 1973): 197-215.

Abstracts are presented for virtually all articles dealing with abortion, sterilization, contraceptive devices, and related subjects that appeared in medical journals in the PRC between 1960 and 1966 and that are available in the United States. Leo A. Orleans, who compiled the abstracts and wrote the introduction, is China research specialist in the Reference Department of the Library of Congress, Washington, D.C. He is the author of EVERY FIFTH CHILD: THE POPULATION OF CHINA.

Quaethoven, P. "Health Organization in the European Economic Community, An Annotated Bibliography." INT'L. J. H. SERV. 2 (1972): 513-23.

Includes over forty publications, divided into five groups: (1) general, (2) costs, (3) social security, (4) professional staff, and (5) national health care. The first group includes comparative analyses dealing with either the EEC as a whole or some EEC countries. The section on costs covers only two articles, indicating the lack of publications in this field at the time. Special attention has been given to social security as one of the major issues of health organization in Europe. Because the free movement of persons, services, and capital is one of the most difficult problems in the EEC, professional staff has been listed as a specific topic. A few studies dealing with problems of national health care are included. Includes both books and articles after 1969. Each deals with at least one EEC country. HOSPITAL ABSTRACTS (London), INFORMATIONSDIENST KRANKENHAUSWESEN (Duesseldorf and Berlin), and HEALTH ECONOMICS (Amsterdam) have been used as sources.

RECURRING BIBLIOGRAPHY: EDUCATION IN THE ALLIED HEALTH PROFESSIONS. Columbus: Ohio State Univ., College of Med., Ohio MEDLARS Center, 1969-- . Annual.

This annual bibliography includes those articles listed in INDEX MEDICUS from April through March of the following year. References cited focus primarily on education in the health professions and the reader is referred to the following related recurring bibliographies developed by the National Library of Medicine, Washington, D.C.: BIBLIOGRAPHY ON MEDICAL EDUCATION, INDEX TO DENTAL LITERATURE, INTERNATIONAL NURSING INDEX, and CURRENT BIBLIOGRAPHY OF EPIDEMIOLOGY. In this

recurring bibliography, citations are listed in subject categories
such as allied health personnel, community health aides, dental
assistants, dietetics, health manpower, hospital administration,
nutrition, physicians' assistants, psychiatric aides, and public health
administration. An author index is provided. Copies are obtain-
able from the Ohio MEDLARS Center, College of Medicine, Ohio
State University, Columbus.

Roemer, Milton I. "Bibliography." In his HEALTH CARE SYSTEMS IN WORLD
PERSPECTIVE, pp. 285-93. Ann Arbor, Mich.: Health Administration Press,
1976.

A valuable, categorized but not annotated listing of some 200 items
by one of the outstanding scholars of comparative health systems.
The first, most valuable category from the point of view of CNSHS
is "Multinational and Comparative Studies of Health Services" with
some 60 items. Subsequent items are grouped mostly by individual
country.

Roemer, Milton I., and Roemer, Ruth. HEALTH MANPOWER POLICIES UNDER
FIVE NATIONAL HEALTH CARE SYSTEMS: INSIGHTS FOR THE UNITED STATES
FROM THE EXPERIENCE OF AUSTRALIA, BELGIUM, CANADA, NORWAY, AND
POLAND. DHEW Pub. no. (HRA) 78-43. Hyattsville, Md.: USPHS, Health
Resources Administration, Div. of Medicine, 1978. 60 p.

Roemer, Ruth, and Roemer, Milton I. HEALTH MANPOWER IN FOUR COUN-
TRIES, AN ANNOTATED BIBLIOGRAPHY. Foreword by Betty A. Lockett.
DHEW Pub. no. (HRA) 75-46. Bethesda, Md.: Health Resources Administration,
Division of Medicine, 1974. 189 p.

Includes works on Australia, Belgium, Canada, and Norway. One
of the most important contributions to bibliographic work in CNSHS.
Annotations are very detailed. For each country works are categorized into (1) general system; (2) education; (3) functions and
supply [of health manpower]; and (4) regulation. An opening section entitled "Global Aspects" has forty-five items. The authors
provide a preface. The foreword indicates that this work was pre-
paratory to the authors' field studies in each country.

SOVIET MEDICINE: A BIBLIOGRAPHY OF BIBLIOGRAPHIES. DHEW Pub. no.
(NIH) 74-575. Bethesda, Md.: John E. Fogarty Int'l. Center, NIH, 1973.

Gives 525 references to bibliographies dealing with various aspects
of medicine and public health in the USSR. Includes only titles
available at the National Library of Medicine or the Library of
Congress.

Starkweather, D.B., and Taylor, Shirley J. "Health Facility Mergers and Combinations: An Annotated Bibliography." Chicago: American College of Hospital Administrators, 1970. Reproduced.

Bibliographies

Strauss, Marvin D. BIBLIOGRAPHY ON CONSUMER PARTICIPATION. Cincinnati: Department of Community Health Organization, Univ. of Cincinnati, 1972.

> Unannotated but still-valuable selection of some 140 items including a number related to health affairs and institutions--primarily in the United States.

United Nations (UN). PUBLICATIONS IN PRINT, CHECK LIST ENGLISH, 1977. New York, 1977. Annual.

> Lists all UN sales publications available up to September 30, 1976. Periodicals such as POPULATION AND VITAL STATISTICS REPORT, STATISTICAL INDICATORS OF SHORT TERM, and the J. OF DEVELOPMENT PLANNING are listed along with yearbooks, proceedings, books, reports, studies, and pamphlets. Many items have an indirect bearing on health and health systems; some have a rather direct bearing, such as the REPORT OF THE UN CONFERENCE ON THE HUMAN ENVIRONMENT, Stockholm, June 5-16, 1972; the REPORT OF THE WORLD FOOD CONFERENCE, Rome, November 5-16, 1974; or THE DEMAND FOR WATER. A number of studies relate to the development efforts and problems in particular regions and countries, for example, VARIOUS COUNTRIES IN THE MIDDLE EAST, 1973. Statistical and economic bulletins are listed for Asia, Latin America, and other parts of the world. Category 4, "Social Questions," is perhaps most closely related to CNSHS. Some issues of the INT'L. SOCIAL DEVELOPMENT REV. are important, such as issue number 3, "Unified Socio-Economic Development and Planning: Some New Horizons." The series entitled "Organization and Administration of Social Welfare Programmes" is also an important publication. Countries covered in the 1977 list are UK; Norway; Romania; United Arab Republic; USSR.

U.S. Department of Health, Education, and Welfare. INTERNATIONAL MIGRATION OF PHYSICIANS AND NURSES: AN ANNOTATED BIBLIOGRAPHY. Bethesda, Md.: Health Resources Administration, Bureau of Health Resources Development, Div. of Med., January, 1975.

Wilensky, Harold L. "Bibliography." In his THE WELFARE STATE AND EQUALITY: STRUCTURAL AND IDEOLOGICAL ROOTS OF PUBLIC EXPENDITURES, pp. 139-47. Berkeley and Los Angeles: Univ. of California Press, 1975.

> An extensive list of books, reports, and articles including some items related to the health aspects of social welfare. Not annotated.

World Health Organization (WHO). MEDICAL EDUCATION, AN ANNOTATED BIBLIOGRAPHY, 1946-1955. Geneva, 1958.

World Health Organization. Strengthening Health Services Division WHO/SHS. REGISTER OF HEALTH SERVICES DEVELOPMENT PROJECTS. Geneva.

Issue number 5 (January 1977) is introduced by a note from the editor, Mme. E. Israel: "Starting with this issue of the leaflet, the preamble has been discontinued. The recapitulation of projects appearing in previous lists also does not appear, nor does the glossary of terms related to the set of forms for the collection of data at the end of the leaflet. These chapters were found to be repetitive and may be referred to in previous issues by those interested."

Those wishing to describe a project to others can write to WHO/HSDP Register, SHS; 1211 Geneva 27, Switzerland, for forms. Those wishing to receive the leaflets can request them from the same address. Projects described in the January 1977 issue are the Eastern Clinic, MOBAI (via Baiima) Sierra Leone; Basic Health Services, Cap Bon, Tunisia; Basic Health Services, Nepal; Rural Health Care, Costa Rica; National Institute of Health Administration and Education, India; Dana Sehat, A Developmental Approach to Raise Health Standards, Solo, Indonesia; Integrated Health Services, Miraj, India; Strengthening National Health Services, Indonesia.

Zhuk, A.P. PUBLIC HEALTH PLANNING IN THE USSR. DHEW Pub. no. 76-999. Bethesda, Md.: John E. Fogarty Int'l. Center, 1976.

Includes an extensive bibliography, not annotated. Translated from Russian.

Chapter 10

JOURNALS

There are no journals devoted primarily to CNSHS. The journal closest to this field is the INT'L. J. H. SERV. edited by Vicente Navarro at the Johns Hopkins School of Hygiene and Public Health. Included here, then, are a number of international disciplinary journals in the social sciences, journals concerned with socioeconomic development, and medical care research journals which include cross-national or international articles from time to time. The reader will find other journals listed in other chapters of this book. No attempt has been made to include all of them here.

ADMINISTRATION AND SOCIETY. Beverly Hills, Calif.: Sage Publications, 1969-- . Quarterly. Edited by William B. Eddy and Gary S. Wamsley.

Covers administration, bureaucracy, public organization, and public policy and the impact these have on politics and society.

AFYA: A JOURNAL FOR MEDICAL AND HEALTH WORKERS. Nairobi, Kenya: African Medical Land Research Foundation. Monthly. Edited by H. DeGlanville.

Medical journal for paramedical personnel. The issues of AFYA feature articles on diagnostic methods and treatment procedures for lower- and middle-level health workers. Articles on topics such as nutrition, hygiene, integrated health projects, and health centers are written in very simple instructional terms with appropriate illus-trations. Although comments and articles deal with epidemiological conditions peculiar to East Africa, the journal is of interest to medical and health workers in other developing regions. AFYA is available at a cost of Sh. 10/- (for 12 issues) from the editor, P.O. Box 30125, Nairobi, Kenya.

AGEING INTERNATIONAL. Washington, D.C.: Int'l. Federation on Aging, 1974-- . Quarterly. Edited by Charlotte E. Nusberg.

A newsletter including abstracts of scientific articles and other works.

Journals

ALTERNATIVES, A JOURNAL OF WORLD POLICY. New York: Institute for World Order, 1975-- . Approx. 4/yr. Edited by Sherle Schweninger.

An off-shoot of the Institute for World Order (New York) Models Project (WOMP). ALTERNATIVES has become the leading forum for the discussion of world order concerns and alternative features. Being avowedly normative and policy-oriented, this journal encourages contributions that deal with critical global issues within the framework of the search for a just world order and the transformations necessary for its realization. Contributions should be sent to Professor Rajni Kothari, general editor, ALTERNATIVES, Institute for World Order, 1140 Avenue of the Americas, New York, N.Y. 10036.

AMERICAN JOURNAL OF PUBLIC HEALTH, Washington, D.C.: American Pub. H. Assn., 1911-- . Monthly. Edited by Alfred Yankauer.

Formerly AMERICAN J. OF PUBLIC HEALTH AND THE NATIONS HEALTH. Covers the public health field from environmental considerations to psychology. Written for the "educated layman" with parts dealing with socioeconomic issues and public health methods. Frequently includes articles on medical care, population, nutrition, and other spheres of concern relevant to CNSHS.

AMERICAN JOURNAL OF SOCIOLOGY. Chicago: Univ. of Chicago Press, 1895-- . Bimonthly. Edited by Charles E. Bidwell.

Professional and scholarly coverage of advanced thinking and empirical research in the various areas of sociology and social psychology. Presents articles on field work and research on specific social problems. Includes signed book reviews, bibliographic listings of current books, and a yearly listing of Ph.D. information in sociology.

AMERICAN SOCIOLOGY REVIEW. Washington, D.C.: American Sociological Assn., 1936-- . Bimonthly.

Official journal of the American Sociological Association including articles on theory, methodology, case studies, and field work. It tends to be highly technical in presentation.

BRITISH JOURNAL OF PREVENTIVE AND SOCIAL MEDICINE. London: British Medical Assn., 1947-- . Quarterly.

BRITISH MEDICAL BULLETIN. London: British Council Med. Dept., 1943. Triannual.

CAHIERS DE SOCIOLOGIE ET DÉMOGRAPHIE MÉDICALES. Paris: Centre de Démographie et Sociologie Médicales, 1961-- . Quarterly.

CANADIAN JOURNAL OF PUBLIC HEALTH. Ottawa, Ontario: Canadian Pub.
H. Assn., 1909-- . Bimonthly.

> Provides for disciplines in the public health field "scientific and
> other reports and articles of professional interest." Topics discussed
> (a small part in French) vary from health needs of Eskimos to the
> effects of urbanization.

CANADIAN NURSE. Ottawa, Ont.: Canadian Nurse's Association, 1905-- .
Monthly.

> Available in both English and French editions, articles range from
> technical to popular. Editorials deal with current topics and aim
> at stimulating interest in the profession's problems.

COMPARATIVE MEDICINE--EAST AND WEST. Garden City, N.Y.: Neale
Watson Academic Publications, 1977. Quarterly.

> A new journal intended to bring together scholarly opinion as well
> as research contributions on health systems. A continuation in new
> form of CHINESE MEDICINE.

COMPARATIVE POLITICAL STUDIES. Beverly Hills, Calif.: Sage Publications,
1968-- . Quarterly. Edited by James A. Caporaso.

> Contains theoretical and empirical research articles by scholars en-
> gaged in cross-national study, and includes research notes and an-
> notated bibliography.

COMPARATIVE POLITICS. New Brunswick, N.J.: Transaction Periodicals
Consortium, Rutgers Univ., 1968-- . Quarterly. Edited by Arnold A. Rugow.

> An international journal containing articles devoted to comparative
> analysis of political institutions and behavior. Articles range from
> the patterns of emerging nations to contrasts in the structures of
> established societies.

CONTACT. Geneva: Christian Med. Commission of the World Council of
Churches, 1970-- . Irregular.

> Periodic bulletin of the Christian Medical Commission of the World
> Council of Churches, 150 Rte. de Ferney, 1211, Geneva 20. Issue
> number 38 was issued in March 1977 and focused on the health
> problems of periurban slum dwellers in the burgeoning shack towns
> of the world. Earlier issues dealt with "Under Fives Clinics in the
> Tropics," "The Chimaltenango Clinic" in Guatemala, and so forth.
> A very creative and informative publication. A rich source for
> CNSHS.

CULTURE, MEDICINE AND PSYCHIATRY. AN INTERNATIONAL J. OF COM-
PARATIVE CROSS-CULTURAL RESEARCH. Dortrecht, Netherlands, and Boston:
D. Reidel, 1977-- . Quarterly. Edited by Arthur M. Kleinman.

> Serves an international and interdisciplinary forum for three inter-
> related fields: medical and psychiatric anthropology; cross-cultural
> psychiatry; and related cross-societal clinical and epidemiological
> studies. It publishes original research, theoretical papers, and
> review articles on subjects in each of these fields. Interdisciplinary
> work which attempts to bridge anthropological and medical perspec-
> tives and methods, which contributes toward a comparative cross-
> cultural science of illness and health care, and which is clinically
> relevant is especially encouraged. Research on the cultural con-
> text of normative and deviant behavior, including the anthropology,
> epidemiology, and clinical aspects of that subject, is also welcomed.

CURRENT SOCIOLOGY. The Hague, Netherlands: Published for the Int'l.
Sociological Assn. and UNESCO by Mouton and Co., 1959-- . Triannual.

> The purpose of this journal is to present international overviews of
> developments taking place in the past decade in the field of so-
> ciology.

DEVELOPMENT AND CHANGE. London: Published for the Int'l. Center for
Training and Research in Development Studies Institute of Social Studies, by
Sage Publications, St. George's House, 1969-- . Quarterly.

> Focuses on critical analysis and dialogue on current issues of de-
> velopment theory, with particular emphasis on third-world problems.

DEVELOPMENT DIALOGUE. Uppsala, Sweden: Dag Hammarskjold Foundation,
Oevre Slottsgatan, 1972-- . Semiannual. Edited by S. Hamrell and O. Nordberg.

> Has occasional health services articles, but is more important for
> the general problems of development, including health, and the
> policies and actions of wealthy countries and international bodies
> as well as policies and actions of third world countries.

ETHICS IN SCIENCE AND MEDICINE. New York: Pergamon Press, 1973-- .
Quarterly.

> Formerly SCIENCE MEDICINE AND MAN.

ETHNOMEDICINE: J. FOR INTERDISCIPLINARY RESEARCH. Hamburg, West
Germany: Helmut Buske Verlag, 1971-- . Irregular.

> Intends to lead to close relationships between the biological sciences
> and social sciences with articles in the fields of primitive medicine,
> natural history, health, and environment. Includes articles, short
> notes, reports, and reviews primarily in German and English.

HEALTH SERVICES RESEARCH. Chicago: Hospital Research and Educational Trust, 1961-- . Quarterly.

> Publishes research on hospital and health services organizations from a variety of disciplinary sources. US oriented.

HUMAN RELATIONS. New York: Published for Tavistock Institute of Human Relations by Plenum Press, 1947-- . Monthly.

> Journal of Studies towards the integration of the social sciences. Concerned with "identification of conditions which will render decision making more opposite and social action more effective." Articles include reports on research or monographs on theory and procedural design. Primarily devoted to psychological and sociological aspects of group process, systems, and interpersonal relations and interactions.

INQUIRY. Chicago: Blue Cross Assn., 1963-- . Quarterly.

> "A journal of medical care organization, provision, and financing." A professional journal for those engaged in planning and administration of health care services, including research articles on these problems. Published a supplemental volume entitled COMPARATIVE HEALTH SYSTEMS 12 (June 1975).

INTERNATIONAL DENTAL JOURNAL. Bristol, England: John Wright and Sons, 1950-- . Quarterly. Edited by F.E. Lawton.

> An example of a number of journals devoted to individual health professions, offering a publication outlet mainly to practitioners in the particular profession in different nations. These journals occasionally include articles examining the organization of services or provisions for education for the particular profession in one or more countries.

INTERNATIONAL DIGEST OF HEALTH LEGISLATION. Geneva: WHO, 1949-- . Quarterly.

> Articles on "health laws, regulations and studies in comparative health legislation."

INTERNATIONAL JOURNAL OF COMPARATIVE SOCIOLOGY. Leiden, Netherlands: Published for the Department of Sociology, York Univ., by E.J. Brill, 1960-- . Quarterly.

> "Coverage of world-wide developments in sociology. Includes scholarly studies evaluation and descriptive reviews, and samplings of materials from non-Western areas. Occasionally an entire issue devoted to a single topic which draws information from differing cultures."

Journals

INTERNATIONAL JOURNAL OF COMPARATIVE SOCIOLOGY. Dhanwar, Kannataka, India: Kannataka Univ., Dept. of Social Anthropology, 1960-- . Semiannual.

INTERNATIONAL JOURNAL OF HEALTH EDUCATION. Geneva: Int'l. Union for H. Education, 1958-- . Quarterly. Edited by Annette Le Meiour-Kaplun.

> The official journal of the International Union for Health Education. Published in a four-language edition--English, French, Spanish, and German. Although directed toward personal health and education and social psychology more than toward health systems, there are occasional articles with special importance for CNSHS.

INTERNATIONAL JOURNAL OF HEALTH SERVICES. Farmingdale, N.Y.: Baywood Publishing Co., 1971-- . Quarterly. Edited by Vicente Navarro.

> The most important journal for CNSHS. Offers an international forum for new thinking on the concepts, problems, and techniques in the planning, administration, and evaluation of health services systems. Provides a means for the exchange of information among professionals working in a variety of political, social, and economic areas.

INTERNATIONAL JOURNAL OF SOCIAL PSYCHIATRY. London: Avenue Publishing Co., 1955-- . Quarterly.

> An interdisciplinary journal covering aspects of various social and behavioral sciences of interest to workers in the fields of mental health, social service, and sociological theory.

INTERNATIONAL JOURNAL OF URBAN AND REGIONAL RESEARCH. London: Edward Arnold, 1975-- . Monthly. Edited by Michael Horbe.

> A scholarly research journal. Includes book reviews as well as original articles.

INTERNATIONAL SOCIAL DEVELOPMENT REVIEW. New York: Published for the UN Dept. of Economic and Social Affairs by UN Publications, 1969-- . Irregular.

> Formerly INTERNATIONAL SOCIAL SERVICE REVIEW and HOUSING, BUILDING AND PLANNING and POPULATION BUL.

INTERNATIONAL SOCIAL SCIENCE JOURNAL. Paris: UNESCO, 1949-- . Quarterly.

> Presentation of an authoritative international conspectus of articles on selected topics by distinguished personages in their field. Broad topics selected include legal learning, social research, administration, controlling the human environment, and medical sociology.

INTERNATIONAL STUDIES QUARTERLY. Beverly Hills, Calif.: Published for the Int'l. Studies Assn. by Sage Publications, 1957-- . Edited by Jonathan Wilkenfeld.

> "A multi-discipline medium devoted to research of a problem-oriented nature (including both theoretical and policy concerns) on transnational phenomena."

JOURNAL OF ASIAN AND AFRICAN STUDIES. Leiden, Netherlands: E.J. Brill, 1966-- . Quarterly.

> Issues center on specific subjects in developing countries of Asia and Africa with emphasis on sociology but including contributions from political science, history, anthropology, and related social science areas.

JOURNAL OF BIO-SOCIAL SCIENCE. Oxford, Engl.: Published for the Galton Foundation by Blackwell Scientific Publications, 1969-- . Quarterly.

> Material deals with social aspects of human biology including reproduction and its control, gerontology, ecology, genetics, and applied psychology.

JOURNAL OF CHRONIC DISEASES. Elmsford, N.Y.: Pergamon Press, 1955-- . Monthly.

> Devoted to the problems and management of chronic illness in all age groups. Often includes articles on health services organization and social aspects.

JOURNAL OF COMMUNITY HEALTH. New York: Published for the Assn. of Teachers of Preventive Med. and Community H. by Human Sciences Press (subsidiary of Behavioral Publications), 1975-- . Quarterly.

> Original articles on the practice, teaching, and research of community health. Includes articles on health care delivery, preventive medicine, new forms of health manpower, analysis of environmental factors, and health insurance programs.

JOURNAL OF COMPARATIVE SOCIOLOGY. Ottawa, Ontario: Canada Sociological Research Center, 1973-- . Annual. Edited by S.S. Anant and A.S. Sethi.

> The goal of this journal is to present contributions from a variety of professional fields in a cross-cultural perspective. Each issue of the journal is devoted to a specific problem and contributors look at the problem from a purely international point of view. The inaugural issue presents a comparative analysis of health care systems. The 1974 issue deals with ethnic groups and ethnic relations.

JOURNAL OF CROSS-CULTURAL PSYCHOLOGY. Beverly Hills, Calif.: Published for the Int'l. Assn. of Cross-Cultural Psychology by Sage Publications, 1970-- . Quarterly. Edited by Walter J. Lonner.

"Encourages an interdisciplinary approach to problems in cross-cultural behavioral and social research."

JOURNAL OF HEALTH AND SOCIAL BEHAVIOR. Washington, D.C.: American Sociological Assn., 1960-- . Quarterly. Edited by Mary Goss.

Formerly J. OF H. AND HUMAN BEHAVIOR. Explores the relationship between health and sociology in such topics as community mental health, smoking, drug use, medical care organization, deviant behavior, attitudes and behavior of physicians, and the relationship between socialization and medical care utilization.

JOURNAL OF HEALTH POLITICS, POLICY AND LAW. New York: Duke Univ. Press, 1976-- . Quarterly. Edited by Ralph A. Stroetz.

Has an outstanding medical care and social science board of editors and offers great promise for CNSHS.

JOURNAL OF THE HISTORY OF MEDICINE AND ALLIED SCIENCES. New Haven, Conn.: Dept. of History of Medicine and Allied Sciences, Yale Univ., 1946-- . Quarterly.

Specializing in scholarly articles by recognized authorities. Has an emphasis on articles for both medicine and biology.

JOURNAL OF INTERAMERICAN STUDIES AND WORLD AFFAIRS. Beverly Hills, Calif.: Published for the Univ. of Miami Center for Advanced Int'l. Studies by Sage Publications, 1959-- . Quarterly. Edited by John P. Harrison.

"Deals with Latin-American (including Caribbean) social, economic, political and cultural aspects as well as inter-relationships between the Americas and the rest of the world community."

JOURNAL OF MEDICAL EDUCATION. Washington, D.C.: Assn. of American Med. Colleges, 1926-- . Monthly.

Includes articles on preparation in medical study, the medical school experience, intern and resident education, and graduate and postgraduate medical education. Reports activities of faculty, students, administrators, and practicing professionals in medicine. Has occasional articles on medical education internationally.

JOURNAL OF TROPICAL PEDIATRICS AND ENVIRONMENTAL CHILD HEALTH. London: JMP Services, 1955-- . Bimonthly. Edited by D.B. Jelliffe.

Covers a wide spectrum of current research together with informal opinion and comment in the field of child health and nutrition, with worldwide contributions. Does not receive support from advertising from commercial firms. The editor is professor of Pediatrics and Public Health, Univ. of California, Los Angeles.

LANCET. London: Lancet Ltd., 1866-- . Weekly.

One of the medical journals most quoted by the world press. Articles remain technical on medical methods, results, but include discussions which reflect the relationship between medicine and current human problems.

MEDICAL CARE. Philadelphia: Published for the APHA, Med. Care Section by J.B. Lippincott Co., 1967-- . Monthly.

One of the most important resources for CNSHS. A multidisciplinary research journal primarily oriented to US medical care financing and organization problems but with articles on other systems. The official journal of the Medical Care Section, APHA.

MEDICAL CARE REVIEW. Ann Arbor: Univ. of Michigan School of Pub. H., Bureau of Pub. H. Economics, 1944-- . Monthly.

Formerly PUBLIC HEALTH ECONOMICS AND MEDICAL CARE ABSTRACTS. An abstracting and indexing service.

MILBANK MEMORIAL FUND QUARTERLY: HEALTH AND SOCIETY. New York: Milbank Memorial Fund, 1923-- .

Articles devoted to multidisciplinary, cross-institutional aspects of contemporary health care. Includes such topics (by authorities in their fields) as cross-national comparisons on social policy in disability, teaching community health, national health insurance, planning for health facilities in the United States and in UDCs and other countries.

MODERN CHINA: AN INTERNATIONAL QUARTERLY. Beverly Hills, Calif.: Sage Publications, 1975-- . Edited by Philip C.E. Huang.

"Encourages a new interdisciplinary scholarship and dialogue on China's on-going revolutionary experience."

NCHSR ANNOUNCEMENT. Hyattsville, Md.: NCHSR, 1977-- . Annual.

Intended for use by journal editors in medical care and public health as well as others in these fields, this news bulletin provides brief items on publications and research in progress. Several items in the January-December 1977 issue relate to the international conferences, for example, one on payment for drugs in different NHIs, and publications on health systems in different countries.

NEW ENGLAND JOURNAL OF MEDICINE. Boston: Mass. Med. Society, 1812-- . Weekly.

> One of the most authoritative general medical journals. Frequently used as reference by the popular press, it concerns itself with basic health problems such as cancer, heart disease, as well as information on the nation's progress in health and health services. Brief editorials on medical topics and technical correspondence are included. Has occasional articles comparing aspects of other health systems with the situation in the United States.

NURSING RESEARCH. New York: Published for the American Nurse's Assn. and the National League for Nursing by American J. of Nursing Co., 1952-- . Bimonthly.

> Stresses original research activities. Articles report on studies of nursing education, professional attitudes, experimental studies on nursing procedures, and clinical studies on nursing practices.

NUTRITION ABSTRACTS AND REVIEWS. Farnham Royal, Slough, Engl.: Commonwealth Agricultural Bureau, 1931-- . Monthly.

PAN AMERICAN HEALTH. Washington, D.C.: PAHO, Pan American Sanitary Bureau, 1969-- . Quarterly.

> This popularly worded, usually attractively illustrated magazine is informative of health conditions and their history in the Americas. Volume 9, number 2 (1977), for example, has an article on immunizing children in La Paz; an article on the history of public health in the Americas, especially of PAHO and early leading figures; an article on improving control of diarrhea as a way of attracting more tourist dollars; and a fascinating recall article by a former head of PAHO, Dr. Fred L. Soper, on eradicating the aegypti mosquito in Brazil.

POLICY AND POLITICS. London: Sage Publications, 1972-- . Quarterly. Edited by Bleddyn Davies and Ken Young.

> "A multidisciplinary journal publishing empirical and discursive papers in the fields of local and urban governments service delivery systems, urban policy analysis and political behavior."

SCANDINAVIAN JOURNAL OF SOCIAL MEDICINE. Stockholm: Published for Nordisk Socialmedicinsk Foerening [Scandinavian Assn. for Social Medicine] by Almquist and Wiksell Int'l., 1973-- . Triannual.

> Formerly ACTA SOCIO-MEDICA SCANDINAVICA.

SOCIAL POLICY. New York: Social Policy Corp., 1970-- . Bimonthly.

Includes articles on education, sociology, economic welfare, community development, and health (quantitative, qualitative, personal). Often gives a radical approach to social action and community control. Articles cover current topics of interest such as national health insurance, advocacy planning, student activism, black studies, and welfare rights.

SOCIAL PROBLEMS. Buffalo, N.Y.: Society for the Study of Social Problems, State Univ. of New York at Buffalo, 1953-- . 5 issues/yr.

Research articles present current data on such topics as deviant behavior, comparisons of role behavior, and the differences in activities and occupational pursuits between the sexes. A "Revue Essay," providing an overview of information on a selected subject, is a regular feature.

SOCIAL PSYCHIATRY. New York: Springer Verlag, 1966-- . Quarterly.

Intends to provide a medium for prompt publication of scientific contributions concerned with effects of social conditions upon behavior and the relationship between psychiatric disorder and the social environment.

SOCIAL SCIENCE AND MEDICINE: AN INTERNATIONAL JOURNAL. Elmsford, N.Y.: Pergamon Press, Journals Dept., 1967-- . 18 issues/yr. Edited by Peter McEwan.

One of the most important resources for CNSHS. Publishes articles in English, French, German, and Spanish, depending on the language of the author. Extensive book reviews, proceedings, and monograph supplements. Now done in special issues under editors for each area: anthropology, sociology, psychology, and so forth.

SOCIOLOGICAL METHODS AND RESEARCH. Beverly Hills, Calif.: Sage Publications, 1972-- . Quarterly. Edited by Edgar F. Borgatta and George W. Bohrnstedt.

"Focuses on the assessment of the scientific status of sociology with articles on systematic research, reviews and contributions to methodology."

SOCIOLOGY. London: Published for the British Sociological Assn. by Oxford Univ. Press, 1967-- . Triannual.

A highly specialized journal with valuable book reviews and articles. Documented contributions vary, including subjects from a study of toys to an article on compositions.

SOCIOLOGY OF WORK AND OCCUPATIONS: AN INTERNATIONAL JOURNAL. Beverly Hills, Calif.: Sage Publications; London: St. George's House, 1974-- . Quarterly. Edited by Marie Haug.

"An international forum for sociological research and theory in the substantive areas of work and occupations."

WASHINGTON PAPERS. Beverly Hills, Calif.: Published for Georgetown Univ., Center for Strategic and Int'l. Studies by Sage Publications, 1972-- . 10 issues/yr., mailed in groups. Edited by Walter Laquent.

"Evaluation of major events affecting (and affected by) current developments in U.S. foreign policy and world affairs. . . . Offers analyses by authorities on policy implications of recent events."

WORLD DEVELOPMENT. Elmsford, N.Y.: Pergamon Press, n.d.-- . Monthly.

Publishes articles with a broad perspective on problems of socio-economic developments.

WORLD FEDERATION OF PUBLIC HEALTH ASSOCIATIONS. Washington, D.C. Irregular.

This nongovernmental voluntary association which cooperates with WHO, publishes bulletins of this title on various health-related topics. For example, it issued a series of bulletins prior to the International Conference on Primary Health Care held in Alma Ata, USSR, September 6-12, 1978, cosponsored by WHO and UNICEF. Bulletin number 2 defined the role of UNICEF in the conference and reported on plans for similar conferences in each of WHO's six regions. The issue noted that PAHO chose to contribute through a report of ministers of health, without nongovernmental agencies present. Perhaps in response, this association cosponsored with the Canadian Public Health Association an international congress: Primary Health Care: A Global Perspective, Halifax, Nova Scotia, Canada, May 23-26, 1978.

WORLD HEALTH. Geneva: WHO, 1948-- . Monthly.

A popular-type magazine on a wide range of health topics, but including descriptions of health services organization projects or general strategies in different countries.

WORLD HEALTH ORGANIZATION BULLETIN. Geneva: WHO, 1947-- . Quarterly.

The scientific periodical of WHO. Contains technical articles reporting results of laboratory, clinical, or field investigations of international significance on subjects within the scope of the WHO.

WORLD HEALTH STATISTICS ANNUAL. Geneva: WHO, 1957-- . Annual.

A major data source on mortality and health personnel and facilities.

WORLD HOSPITALS. London: Int'l. Hospital Federation, 1964-- . Quarterly.

Chapter 11
ORGANIZATIONS

This chapter is divided into two sections, 11.1, "Publications about Organizations" and 11.2, "List of Organizations."

Items in the first section tend to describe the character of the major agencies such as WHO; foundations; nongovernmental voluntary associations; professional public health, medical, nursing, social science, and other associations; governmental aid and assistance agencies; and research institutes (see works by Goodman and Wasserman). But some items (e.g., those by Quimby and the Roses) on politics and policy in WHO analyze the organizations. There are too few of these works.

The second section makes no attempt to list every organization, institute, agency or association relevant to CNSHS. For example, by no means have all relevant governmental aid agencies (e.g., Canada's and Sweden's) or research settings been listed. Some of those listed have conducted research on CNSHS such as the Center for Health Administration Studies, University of Chicago, headed by Odin Anderson. The Institute for European Health Studies Research at the Catholic University, Leuven, Belgium, headed by Jan Blanpain, is important for West European studies. Generally, the field is dominated by individual researchers and scholars in a wide variety of settings, and people are known by their written work rather than their institutional location. NEP-CNSHS is described as a relatively new development.

An organization which is adequately covered by a descriptive work listed under 11.1 may not be specifically listed in 11.2. For example, WHO is covered by several publications under 11.1 including its own 25th anniversary statement, THE WORK OF WHO. There is no listing for WHO in 11.2. Thus the reader interested in an overview of organizations in the field is urged to peruse both sections.

11.1 PUBLICATIONS ABOUT ORGANIZATIONS

Association of American Medical Colleges. INFORMATION FOR LIAISON OFFICERS FOR INTERNATIONAL ACTIVITIES. Washington, D.C.: Assn. of American Med. Colleges, Division of Int'l. Med. Education (DIME), October 1973.

A somewhat dated but still suggestive pamphlet describing WHO and its regional offices; US official international health officers; foundations and associations with concerns for and activities in international health and other information. In 1976, DIME was merged with the Educational Resources Division of AAMC.

_____. ORGANIZATIONS UTILIZING AMERICAN PHYSICIANS ABROAD. Washington, D.C.: American Assn. of Med. Colleges, 1971. Pamphlet.

Bell, D.E. "World Health and the Role of the U.S., A Message from A.I.D." J. MED. ED. 41 Supplement (September 1966): 20-23.

Burns, Allan C. "United States Private Agencies' Contributions to Population Programs." INT'L. J.H. SERV. 3 (1973): 661-65.

A review of the participation of private organizations in population programs, indicating that the private foundations were supporting such work well before the academic community or the federal government. The contribution of the private sector in absolute amounts is slowly increasing with time, but, due to the entry into this field of governmental agencies such as the US AID, UN Fund for Population activities, and WHO, the percentage of support for population work which is contributed by the private foundations has declined annually.

Calder, Nigel. "The Controversy about World Health Research." NEW SCIENTIST 25 (January 28, 1965): 207-8.

Reflects on the policy questions and politics of moves to establish a major research arm of WHO. For a history and analysis of these moves, see H. and S. Rose (this chapter).

Elling, Ray H. "Political Influences on Research Methods." See chapter 7 on the politics of research in WHO.

Ferguson, Donald C. "The International Development Research Centre and the Health Sciences." CANADIAN J. PUB. H. 64, monograph supplement (October 1973): 5-10.

Describes the purposes and organization of this important center and particularly of its Population and Health Sciences Division which had sponsored important projects and issued useful materials (see esp. Akhtar, cited in chapter 9, "Bibliographies").

Goodman, Neville M. INTERNATIONAL HEALTH ORGANIZATIONS AND THEIR WORK. Philadelphia: Blakiston, 1952.

The most informative and valuable survey to date of publication. Primarily of historical interest. Brought up to 1970 in a revised edition; see the following item.

_____. INTERNATIONAL HEALTH ORGANIZATIONS AND THEIR WORK. Foreword by Marcolino G. Candau. Edinburgh and London: Churchill Living-stone, 1971. Index.

> Contents: "Why International Health?"; "Early Efforts: The Story of Quarantine"; "The Story of Quarantine Since 1851"; "The International Office of Public Health"; "The Health Organization of the League of Nations, 1921-46"; "Health Work of the United Nations Relief and Rehabilitation Administration (UNRRA)"; "WHO Origins"; "WHO: Politics, Administration, and Finances"; "WHO: General Work"; "WHO: Communicable Diseases"; "WHO: Non Communicable Diseases and Other Work"; "Regional Health Organizations, Old and New"; "Other Inter-governmental Agencies Concerned With Health"; "Voluntary Agencies and International Health"; "Past, Present and Future."

INTERNATIONAL HEALTH AND MEDICAL NEWS SERVICES. 23 chemin des Palettes, 1212 Grand-Lancy, Geneva, Switzerland. Tel. (022) 94 94 00. Edited by David Alan Ehrlich.

> This proposed publication may include (1) condensations of recently published papers and books; (2) research in progress (to help others who are embarking on related projects); (3) new books; (4) meetings; (5) correspondence on issues and new ideas; (6) notes about institutions and the people, such as new courses, new chairs, promotions of personnel, and publications; and (7) any interesting item, including cuttings from the lay press that are considered useful.

Lengyel, P., ed. SOCIAL SCIENCE, NATIONAL INTERESTS, AND INTERNATIONAL ORGANIZATIONS. New Brunswick, N.J.: Transaction Books, 1974.

New England Program for Cross-National Studies of Health Systems (NEP-CNSHS). Univ. of Connecticut Health Center, Farmington, Ct. 06032. Ray Elling, Coordinator.

> This defacto interuniversity multidisciplinary consortium has as its purpose the encouraging of cross-national studies of health systems by faculty, students, and associated research colleagues. It has held periodic meetings (traveling seminars) in each of the participating universities with a speaker and business discussions as a part of each meeting. It has twice sponsored the month-long (May-June) Comparative Health Systems Institute at Boston University. It has encouraged joint research projects as well as publication in this field. Members of the Steering Group in addition to the coordinator are: Mark Field, Ph.D., Department of Sociology, Boston University; Charles Hayes, M.D., Department of Community Medicine, University of Massachusetts; Dieter Koch-Weser, M.D., Department of Preventive and Social Medicine, Harvard University; Basil J.F. Mott, Ph.D., School of Health Sciences, University of

New Hampshire; Victor Sidel, M.D., Department of Social Medicine; George Silver, M.D., School of Medicine and Public Health, Yale University; Albert Wessen, Ph.D. Departments of Community Medicine and Sociology, Brown University; Alonzo Yerby, M.D., School of Public Health, Harvard University; Michael Zubkoff, Ph.D., Community Medicine, Dartmouth University; Manfred Pflanz, M.D., Department of Epidemiology and Social Medicine, Hannover School of Medicine, FRG (serves as advising correspondent).

Quimby, F.H. THE POLITICS OF GLOBAL HEALTH. See chapter 3.4 on the political issues involved in and facing WHO.

Ravenholt, Reimert T., et al. "World Fertility Survey: Findings and Implications." Paper presented at the 105th annual meetings of the APHA, Washington, D.C., October 30-November 3, 1977.

Rochester, J. Martin. INTERNATIONAL INSTITUTIONS AND WORLD ORDER: THE INTERNATIONAL SYSTEM AS A PRISMATIC POLITY. Sage Professional Papers in Int'l. Studies, no. 02-025, Beverly Hills, Calif.: Sage Publications, 1974. 72 p.

Rose, H., and Rose, S. SCIENCE AND SOCIETY. Middlesex, Engl.: Pelican Books, 1970.

Tackles the dilemma of scientific knowledge as shaping and being shaped by society. Notes the sophistication of controls and management of science policy as well as the underlying fear of the destructive potential of scientific discovery. Includes a chapter on the politics of establishing the research division (RECS, now defunct) in WHO headquarters.

Salas, Rafael M. "The United Nations Fund for Population Activities." INT'L. J. H. SERV. 3 (1973): 679-87.

Taylor, Carl E. "Challenge to International Agencies." INT'L. J. H. SERV. 5 (1975): 489-97. 10 refs.

Author's summary: "International health agencies face major changes requiring basic adjustments in approaches and values. The ethical issues include moral criteria for allocating scarce resources, relation of health to population growth and development, iatrogenic social consequences of health measures, and inappropriate transfer of technology. A proposed new style of international health work is summarized in five principles and ten guidelines. The principles are: development from below; a role shift from adviser to collaborator; sequential research, demonstration, and implementation; concentration on problems of motivation; and partnership in approaches to mutually shared complex problems."

Wasserman, Paul. HEALTH ORGANIZATIONS OF THE UNITED STATES, CA-
NADA AND INTERNATIONALLY. 3d ed. Washington, D.C.: McGrath, 1974.

A valuable general directory by a professional librarian.

Wegman, Myron E. "A Salute to the Pan American Health Organization." AJPH
67 (December 1977): 1198-1204. 9 refs.

The author, one-time director of PAHO, recounts the history and
growth of the oldest international health agency on the occasion
of its seventy-fifth anniversary (December 2, 1977). Beginning
with a budget of $5,000, PAHO's budget for 1978 is $31 million
in a composite budget of $63 million including the regular budget
from WHO, UN development program funds, and other grants.
This is seen as a large growth but still a small amount considering
the problems faced. The author notes that it is hard to assess the
success or failure of the organization in terms of impact on health
levels in any quantitative terms. But he concludes with the personal view that "the great hope of the world is in understanding
among peoples. Mutual interest in striving for improved health is
certainly one of the most ready common denominators. The success,
progress, and vigor of PAHO are, I believe, positive signs and its
seventy-fifth anniversary is, therefore, an occasion for a general
rejoicing."

World Health Organization (WHO). THE WORK OF WHO. OFFICIAL RECORDS
OF THE ORGANIZATION. No. 205. Geneva, 1972. The address for WHO
headquarters is 1211 Geneva, 27 Switzerland.

General review of WHO activity in the field of research, information exchange, planning. Covers specific diseases and projects
undertaken in different regions of the world. Published in preparation for the twenty-fifth anniversary of WHO. The six regional offices of WHO and their locations are (1) AMRO (PAHO),
Washington, D.C.; (2) AFRO, Brazzaville; (3) EMRO, Alexandria;
(4) EURO, Copenhagen; (5) SEARO, New Delhi; (6) WPRO, Manila.
The following is a brief organization self-description of WHO and
the Int'l. Agency for Research on Cancer (a special agency of
WHO based in Lyons, France):

"The World Health Organization (WHO) is one of the specialized
agencies in relationship with the United Nations. Through this
organization which came into being in 1948, the public health
and medical professions of more than 150 countries exchange their
knowledge and experience and collaborate in an effort to achieve
the highest possible level of health throughout the world. WHO
is concerned primarily with problems that individual countries or
territories cannot solve with their own resources--for example, the
eradication or control of malaria, schistosomiasis, smallpox, and
other communicable diseases, as well as some cardiovascular diseases and cancer. Progress towards better health throughout the

world also demands international cooperation in many other activities; for example, setting up international standards for biological substances, for pesticides and for pesticide spraying equipment; compiling an international pharmacopoeia; drawing up and administering the International Health Regulations; revising the international lists of diseases and causes of death; assembling and disseminating epidemiological information; recommending nonproprietary names for drugs; and promoting the exchange of scientific knowledge. In many parts of the world there is need for improvement in maternal and child health, nutrition, nursing, mental health, dental health, social and occupational health, environmental health, public health administration, professional education and training; and health education of the public. Thus a large share of the Organization's resources is devoted to giving assistance and advice in these fields and to making available--often through publications--the latest information on these subjects. Since 1958 an extensive international programme of collaborative research and research coordination has added substantially to knowledge in many fields of medicine and public health. This programme is constantly developing and its many facets are reflected in WHO publications."

Yankauer, Alfred. "Seventy-Five Years of International Health." AJPH, 67 (December 1977): 1139-40.

This editorial commemorates the seventy-fifth anniversary of the oldest international health agency, the Pan American Sanitary Bureau, later named PAHO (or AMRO in its affiliation with WHO). Especially good in recounting the history of the political situation in the Americas with US imperialism deeply determining the work of PAHO. Refers to an article in this same issue by Myron Wegman saluting PAHO and recounting its history. Notes a healthy shift toward local citizen involvement and determination of health services as the present stated policy of PAHO to help in avoiding the imperialist irrelevancies of US-type high technology in situations where these do not attack the main problems and cannot be supported.

Zahra, Albert, and Strudwick, Richard. "The Role of the World Health Organization in Health Related Aspects of Family Planning." INT'L. J. H. SERV. 3 (1973): 701-07.

11.2 LIST OF ORGANIZATIONS

Center for Health Administration Studies. Graduate School of Business. Univ. of Chicago, 5720 Woodlawn Ave., Chicago, Ill. USA 60637.

This center, directed by Professor Odin Anderson has a long record of research on US medical care problems, particularly in the voluntary health insurance field. Since moving from New York to

Chicago (about 1965) it has broadened its studies to include cross-national work, particularly US-Swedish comparisons. It sponsors a yearly lecture series in honor of Michael M. Davis. These are published in booklet form. Most of these have been noted health services researchers or administrator-planners who have reflected on experiences in other countries. The center issues a brochure listing its numerous publications.

The Center for Research on Utilization of Scientific Knowledge (CRUSK). Established 1964. Institute for Social Research, Univ. of Mich. P.O. Box 1248, Ann Arbor, 48106.

Seeks to create new knowledge about how knowledge is used. The center is concerned with uses of scientific knowledge from both social and natural sciences, utilization of this knowledge, and research on these topics. CRUSK is currently conducting programs in the areas of public policy and knowledge, planning and technology assessment; organizational development; health and medical knowledge utilization; utilization process; and program evaluation and action research. Much of the center's output is in the form of short reports in articles and unpublished papers. One may order a personal selection of short reports from different packages. Topic 8.1 of the short reports is medical knowledge and 8.2 is social problems. Another type of output consists of full-length, unpublished project reports, and manuals in knowledge utilization. The work of this agency is not especially related to CNSHS, but the problem of knowledge use is central to the business of improving health systems.

Centre de Recherches et de Documentation sur La Consommation (C.R.E.D.O.C.) 45 Boulevard de La Gare, Paris 75634.

Part of the National Institute for Statistics and Economic Studies of France. The Medical Economics Division of C.R.E.D.O.C. conducts and fosters a number of studies of health and health care in France and some cross-national work as well. The center issues a periodical, CONSOMMATION--ANNALES DE C.R.E.D.O.C.

The Harvard Institute for International Development (HIID). (Description from flyer of this title).

HIID "is Harvard University's center for programs of service, research and training related to developing countries. HIID is multidisciplinary in its approach and staffing, with direct ties to the Faculties of Arts and Sciences, the Graduate School of Education, the Graduate School of Design, the Harvard School of Public Health and Harvard Medical School.

The Institute provides technical assistance to government agencies in five specialized fields - education, public health, urban and regional planning, rural development and public managment and policy. Projects emphasize collaborative counterpart relationships and training to reduce dependence on outside expertise and to promote institutional self sufficiency.

The Institute conducts a braod program of research, much of it in collaboration with institutions in the Third World. Its field projects offer useful research insights and the resulting research, in turn, helps to strengthen the Institute's technical assistance."

Institute for European Health Services Research. 18 Mgr. Ladenzeplein, 3000 Leuven, Belgium.

A consortium of several departments of the Catholic University of Leuven committed to health services research. A reproduced, un-dated (about March 1975) statement entitled "What is the Institute for European Health Services Research?" is available from the in-stitute describing its organization and publications available and expected. Most of the work is on EEC countries. Professor Jan Blanpain is director.

Institute of Child Health. 30 Gulford Street, London.

From an announcement sheet on the Child to Child Programme: "Many United Nations organizations like UNICEF, WHO, UNESCO, FAO, and ILO agree that 1979 will be the International Year of the Child. UNICEF will be the leading organization. The In-stitutes of Education and Child Health in London and the Ministry of Overseas Development of the U.K. are developing the programme which is described here. There will be many other programmes in 1979.

This programme is for the children most in need in the world. These are the children under five living in the rural areas and poor towns of developing countries. There are 350 million children in the world without essential services in health, nutrition and edu-cation. This programme will try to use the services of the school child to help the healthy development of the pre-school child."

The rest of the announcement sheet describes the ways various people can help and the projected timetable.

International Epidemiological Association.

A scientific body which held its 8th papers meeting in Puerto Rico, September, 1977. The President was Kerr L. White, School of Hygiene and Public Health, 115 Wolfe St. Baltimore, Md. (Secre-tariat changes periodically. Most recent address: Dr. A.I. Adams. Div. of Health Services Research. 9 Young St., Sidney, N.S.W. 2000, Australia.)

International Health Section, APHA, 1015 Eighteenth Street, N.W., Washington, D.C. 20036.

Newly formed in 1976, this section could possibly become an important scientific forum for the encouragement of CNSHS. Its first chairman was Carl E. Taylor, Johns Hopkins School of Hygiene and Public Health. Dieter Koch-Weser, associate dean for international programs, Harvard Medical School, headed a policy and goals committee which delivered a report to the 1977 meeting of the section as part of the APHA meetings in Washington, D.C. Inquiries can be made by phone at (202) 467-5000.

International Labour Organization (ILO) Geneva.

One of the UN special agencies. Published studies of health services as related to social security insurance (see works by Roemer in chapter 3.4 and Fulcher in chapter 3.1). Concerned with special population groups such as indigenous peoples and their health and living conditions. Publishes a number of reports and studies related to occupational health.

International Sociological Association (ISA) Secretariat: P.O. Box 719, Station "A", Montreal, Quebec, Canada H3C 2V2.

Holds international scientific meetings every four years. The last, the Ninth World Congress of Sociology, was held in Uppsala, Sweden, August 14-19, 1978. The ISA is an NGO (Non Governmental Organization) affiliate of WHO and is usually represented at World Health Assembly meetings each May in Geneva. The ISA has a number of research committees, one (no. 15) is the Medical Sociology Research Committee, chaired by Mark Field, which fosters CNSHS as well as other medical sociological research. A volume entitled COMPARATIVE HEALTH SYSTEMS, edited by Ray H. Elling, derived from a papers session of this title at the 1974 meetings, published as a special issue of INQUIRY 12 (June 1975). Sessions and chairpersons of the Medical Sociology Research Committee which were scheduled for the Uppsala meetings are "Health and Social Development," Yvo Nuyens; "Traditional and Modern Health Care Systems and Their Interrelationships," Ray Elling; "Medical Sociology in Sweden and in Scandinavia." Sonja Calais; "The Political Context of Health Services," Peter New and Elliott Krause; "Cross Cultural Definitions and Measurements of Disability and Comparison of Models for Delivery of Rehabilitation Services," Gary Albrecht; "Primary Care in the Developing World," Margot Jeffreys; "Health Occupations: Socialization and Delivery of Health Care," Judith Shuval and Lois Cohen; "The Relevance of Social Science Research to the WHO," Albert Gebert. Papers from the "Traditional and Modern. . ." session are to appear in 1979 as a special issue of the journal, COMPARATIVE MEDICINE--EAST AND WEST.

International Studies Association. Univ. Center for International Studies, Univ. of Pittsburgh, Pittsburgh, Pa. 15260.

A multidisciplinary professional organization whose members are actively involved with one or more aspects of international studies. Among members are spokespersons for governments, foundations, universities, business firms, and other entities that seek advisers for the development of coherent programs, the evaluation of existing programs, and the nurturing of new thrusts in international studies. ISA welcomes professionals eager to test new approaches and new organizational formats. In addition to its annual convention, ISA offers a number of publications including the INTERNATIONAL STUDIES QUARTERLY, the INTERNATIONAL STUDIES NOTES, and the INTERNATIONAL STUDIES NEWSLETTER that are distributed to all members. The association is organized into eight geographical regions and eleven subject area sections. These subunits hold workshops, luncheons, and symposia and circulate their own printed materials. The organization is not specifically directed toward CNSHS but papers on cross-national studies of health-related topics are presented at annual meetings.

International Voluntary Services, Inc. (IVS). 1717 Massachusetts Ave., N.W. Suite 605, Washington, D.C. 20036.

IVS is a private, independent, nonprofit agency which supplies technical assistance for development projects in developing countries; mainly in the form of skilled volunteer technicians recruited internationally.

Joint Center for Studies of Health Programs, Institute of Social Medicine, University of Copenhagen, Copenhagen, Denmark.

Conducts a cooperative and comparative study and training program with the School of Public Health, Univ. of California, Los Angeles. Erik Holst is director in Denmark, Lester Breslow at UCLA.

Sandoz Institute for Health and Socio-Economic Studies. Rte de Florissant 5, Geneva, Switzerland.

Sponsors a number of health services conferences and studies. Recently jointly sponsored a self-help symposium with the Joint Center for Studies of Health Programs. This was published as: Leven, Lowell S., et al. SELF-CARE, LAY INITIATIVES IN HEALTH. New York: Prodist, 1976, and includes an annotated bibliography.

The Scandinavian Institute of African Studies. P.O. Box 2126, S-750 02 Uppsala, Sweden.

Issues the following kinds of publications with a significant number of works having appeared in each category: research reports; rural development series; annual seminar proceedings; studies of law in

social change and development; other books; and women in developing countries. Most items are in English; a few are only in Swedish.
Most items are valuable for general context, for example, Seminar
Proceedings No. 10 entitled "Multinational Firms in Africa." Few
items are directly on CNSHS.

Study Group on Health Systems Research, Univ. of Munich, ISB, Marchionistrasse
15, Munich, Germany.

The group is seeking the assistance of scientists and institutions
around the world in its attempt to produce a worldwide report on
the actual state of the art in health systems research. According
to Wolfgang Koepcke who is a group member, 5,000 publications
on health systems research have been collected and the group has
attempted to make contact with about 1,500 scientists and institutions all over the world. The results of the work will be published and the English version of the report is expected to be available in the near future.

United Nations International Children's Fund (UNICEF). Henry R. Labouisse,
Executive Director. U.N., New York, N.Y. 10017.

One of the UN special agencies. Concerned with much more than
education, this agency is deeply involved with maternal and child
health in all its aspects. At times it has been a driving force
stimulating other agencies to explore new approaches. Such was
the case in the important "UNICEF/WHO Joint Study of Alternative Approaches to Meeting Basic Health Needs in Developing
Countries" (see Djukanovic and Mach, cited in chapter 3.3).

U.S. Agency for International Development (USAID). Main State Bldg. Washington,
D.C. 20523.

A U.S. bilateral foreign aid agency which has sponsored the series of
studies by the Office of International Health, USPHS, of health systems in some twenty countries. (See SYNCRISIS, cited in chapter
3.3). AID's main health related interests have probably been in population-family planning (see Ravenholt, cited above, 11.1).

World Bank (International Bank for Reconstruction and Development). 1818 H.
Street N.W., Washington, D.C. 20433.

Has developed an interest in and considerable work on health and
its relations with economic development in recent years. Has published a HEALTH SECTOR POLICY PAPER and also has a number
of activities related to population-family planning.

World Federation of Public Health Associations. 1015 Eighteenth Street, Washington, D.C. 20036.

See chapter 10 (same title) for description of a series of bulletins
issued by this organization concerning the WHO/UNICEF series of
world regional conferences on primary health care which started in
1978.

AUTHOR INDEX

In addition to authors, this index includes all editors, compilers, translators, and other contributors to works cited in the text. Alphabetization is letter by letter.

Author Index

Beck, R.G. 97
Becker, Ernest 104
Beckford, George L. 7, 50
Beeley, Linda 77
Behm, Hugo 8
Bell, D.E. 238
Belmar, Roberto 97
Benjamin, B. 98
Berfenstam, Ragnar 153
Berg, Robert L. 176
Bergner, Marilyn 176
Beveridge, W. 32
Bice, Thomas W. 177, 186, 193
Bidwell, Charles E. 226
Biological Sciences Communication
    Project 214
Bjorkman, James 136
Black, Cyril E. 8
Blankenship, L.V. 106
Blanpain, Jan 82
Blasier, Cole 9
Bloor, Michael J. 104
Board, L.M. 50
Bodenheimer, Thomas S. 154
Boelen, C. 177
Bogatyrev, I.D. 177
Bohrnstedt, George W. 235
Bonnet, Phillip D. 98
Borgatta, Edgar F. 235
Boudreau, Thomas J. 154
Boukal, J. 154
Boulding, Elise 204
Boulding, Kenneth E. 99
Bourmer, Horst 61
Bowers, John Z. 62
Brand, Jeanne L. 32
Brenner, M. Harvey 99, 177
Breslow, Lester 99
Bridgman, Robert F. 117, 154
Brinkerhoff, Merlin B. 100, 107
Brockington, Fraser 32, 62
Brookfield, Harold C. 9
Brooks, Charles H. 178
Brown, E. Richard 9

Bryant, John H. 51, 62, 100
Brzeski, Andrzej 101
Btesh, Simon 63
Burdett, H.C. 32
Burns, Allan C. 238
Bush, J.W. 183
Bush, Patricia J. 72

C

Calder, Nigel 238
Caldwell, John C. 9
Campos, P.C. 69
Canada National Department of
    Health and Welfare. Research
    and Statistics Directorate 205
Candau, Marcolino G. 10, 51, 58,
    63
Caporaso, James A. 227
Carr, Willine 178
Carr-Saunders, A.M. 10
Cartwright, Anne 101
Cartwright, Dorwin P. 178
Cassel, John 102
Center for Health Administration
    Studies. Univ. of Chicago 214
Centre de Recherches et de Docu-
    mentation sur la Consommation
    215
Chadwick, Edwin 32
Chance, Norman A. 102, 179
Charron, K.C. 41
Chase, Helen C. 179
Chase-Dunn, Christopher 5, 10,
    19, 21
Chen, Martin K. 179
Christian Medical Commission 51
Christie, Ronald V. 78, 82
Cibotti, R. 10
Clark, Henry T., Jr. 154
Clarkson, J. Graham 215
Cleaver, Harry 102
Cline, William 10
Clyde, D.F. 32
Coale, Ansley J. 180
Cobb, S. 116
Cochrane, C. 180

Author Index

Fendall, N.R.E. 52
Ferguson, Donald C. 238
Ferrer, Rinaldo 159
Festinger, Leon 178
Feuerstein, Marie-Therese 53
Field, Mark G. 42, 83, 109-110, 183, 193, 245
First International Congress on Group Medicine 65
Flook, E. Evelyn 183
Follman, Joseph, Jr. 42
Foltz, Ann-Marie 216
Forbes, Hugh Donald 184
Foreign Area Studies Program. American University 205
Forsyth, Gordon 184
Foster, George M. 53, 110
Foulon, Alain 84
Fox, Renee C. 104, 131, 184
Frank, Andre Gundar 5, 6, 12
Frankenberg, Ronald 110
Frankenhoff, Charles A. 53
Fraser, R.D. 42, 66, 84, 111, 184
Freidson, Eliot 104, 111, 140, 183
Friedman, John 159
Fry, John 42, 66, 81, 84-85
Fucaraccio, A. 13
Fulcher, Derick 43
Furnia, Arthur H. 60

G

Gallagher, Eugene B. 112, 144
Gantt, W. Horsley 34
Garfin, Susan Bettelheim 217
Garlick, J.P. 53
Gass, Mary 113
George, Susan 13
Georgopoulos, Basil S. 112
Gill, D.G. 193
Gilles, H.M. 53
Gilson, Betty S. 185
Gish, Oscar 53-54, 112, 217
Gittelsohn, A. 146
Gitter, A. George 112
Glaser, Barney 104
Glaser, William A. 43, 66, 85, 112, 185

Glasgow, John 159
Godber, Sir George 45
Godlund, S. 159
Goffman, Erving 104
Gold, Joseph 205
Goldman, Franz 34
Gonzales, C.L. 54
Goodman, Neville M. 238-39
Goss, Mary 232
Gouldner, Alvin W. 13
Goulet, Denis 13
Gramsci, Antonio 118
Grant, John B. 34, 160
Gray, G.I. 217
Greenhill, Stanley 113
Griffith, D.H.S. 13
Grmek, M.D. 39
Gross, P.F. 160
Grossman, Gregory 101
Grundy, F. 185
Grzegorzewski, Edward 113

H

Haber, Lawrence D. 113
Haeroe, A.S. 193
Hage, Jerald 95
Haines, Anna J. 34
Halebsky, Sandor 106
Hall, T.L. 185
Hammond, Phillip E. 184
Hamrell, S. 228
Handler, Philip 4, 14
Hannan, Kenneth H. 164
Hansma, J. 40, 49
Haraldson, Sixten 160
Hardin, Garrett 14
Harrison, John P. 232
Hart, Julian Tudor 82, 104, 113
Harvey, David 14, 114
Haug, Marie 235
Hays, W.S. 201
Hayter, Teresa 15
Heald, K.A. 217
Hechter, Michael 161
Heilbronner, Robert L. 4, 5, 15
Heller, P.S. 161
Helt, Eric H. 114
Henild, Svend 15
Hess, J. 106

Author Index

Author Index

TITLE INDEX

This index includes the titles of all books cited in the text. In some cases, titles have been shortened. Alphabetization is letter by letter.

Title Index

Title Index

SUBJECT INDEX

This index contains subject areas of interest within the text. Main entries of emphasis are underlined. Alphabetization is letter by letter.

Subject Index

F

Subject Index

Subject Index

M

Makere Medical School (Uganda), community medical program of 69

Malaria
control of in India 59
effect on economic development 17
health benefits of control of 14
maps of 206
politics of control 102–3
population growth and control of 19

Malaya, medical care and health service systems in 83

Malaysia, regionalization of medical care in 171

Malnutrition 29
in Africa 23
in Burma 91
effect on economic development 17
foreign aid in increasing 26
in Nigeria 57
as a result of bottle feeding and commercial foods 17
See also Food supply; Hunger

Malthus, Thomas Robert 14–15
reassessment of 20

Manchuria, plague prevention in 36

Marx, Karl
on capitalism 18, 19
contradictions of 22
on population 14–15

Marxian perspectives
in a critique of the Russian health system 112
of epidemiology 138–39
health and health services viewed from 101, 128, 144, 145
in medical sociology 110–11
of the National Health Service 114
of women and health care 109–10

Maternal and child welfare 95–96
in Africa 115
in Australia 35
bibliography on 214
comparative studies of 84, 86
in India and Burma 91
organizations concerned with 247
priority needs of in UDCs 117

Mechanic, David 145

Medical anthropology 110, 131–32
journals concerned with 228

Medical care and health service systems
bibliographies on 213–23
comparative studies of 81–92, 96, 109, 124, 126, 132, 133–34, 143, 145–46, 146–47
bibliography of 218
control of 45
data sources for the study of 203–12
decision–making in 113, 142–43
demands vs. needs in 115
economics and finance of 31, 33, 40, 41, 42, 43, 44, 45, 47, 49, 59–60, 61, 63, 65, 66, 68, 70, 72, 73, 79, 84, 86, 89, 90, 97, 98, 99, 104, 106, 111, 114, 117, 121, 127, 130–31, 132, 135, 146, 149, 152, 158, 163, 184, 191, 196, 207
journals concerned with 229
economic security and 44, 65
expanding functions of 131
following World War II 34
forecasts of 201
framework statements on 93–148
general works on 31–80
in developed countries 40–49
historical and early studies of 31–40
in underdeveloped countries 10, 13–14, 29, 50–60, 64, 66, 74, 87, 94, 116–17
government regulation of 47, 73
group services in 65–66, 74, 124
information systems in 114–15
influence of political economy, population, and resources on 5–29
introduction to 1–4

Subject Index

Medical sociology. See Sociology
Medical statistics. See Medical research
Medical technology centers 114-15
Medicare 97
Medicine, social. See Socialized medicine
Medicines, rates of usage of 72-73. See also Drugs
Mediterranean Sea area, medical care and health service systems in 148
    bibliography on 216
Meharry Medical College Study of Unmet Needs 178
Menstruation 105
Mental health 78
    bibliography on 216
Mental illness 104
    care and treatment in 105
        comparative studies of 84
    economics of 99
    standardization of diagnosis and classification of 196
Mentally handicapped, planning services for 137
Michigan, regionalization of rural medical services in 163
Michigan, University of. Institute for Social Research. The Center for Research on Utilization of Scientific Knowledge 243
Middle East
    health policy making in 142-43
    hospital organization in 112
    See also names of Middle Eastern countries (e.g. India)
Midwifery 135
Migration, geographic 27
    disease and 16
    of health workers 63
    of physicians 29
Military 6
    world expenditures for 26, 198, 209
Minority groups, medical care and health service systems of 178
Mobility, socioeconomic, as a factor in improving living conditions 23

Modernization
    comparative research on 186
    in Japan and Russia 8
    See also Industrialization
Morbidity
    establishment of standards for measuring 177
    failure to serve as a health indicator 197
    medical and sociological concepts of 133
    See also Disease
Mortality 27, 70
    the business cycle and 107
    during periods of economic instability 177-78
    fostered by bottle feeding and commercial foods 17
    infant and child 23, 42, 66, 84, 178
        comparative studies of 207
        correlation with physician-population ratios 182
        data sources on 209
        ranking of countries by 179
        in Sweden 142, 191
        use and complications of statistics on 179, 180, 184
    in West Africa 9
    measurement of 189
    problems of and failures with data on 190, 191, 196
    social and economic factors affecting 98, 178
    studies of in UDCs 180
    of white males 142
Mountain, Joseph 166
Multinational corporations 14
    African economic development and 7
    commercial food programs of in UDCs 17
    impact on UDCs 7
        in agricultural production 7-8
        decapitalization factors 6
        protection and defense factors of 21
    responsibilities of 21
    role of in Latin America 18, 26

Subject Index

Occupational health. See Industrial health

Old age, as a social problem 105. See also Aged

Organization for Comparative Social Research 181, 186

P

Pacific Ocean area, bibliography on health systems of 216

Pakistan
argument against aid to 14
medical care and health service systems in 60
See also Bengal

Pan American Health Organization 241, 242

Paraguay, medical care and health service systems in 72

Paramedical personnel. See Health personnel

Parasitic diseases
economic development and 28
in the tropics 53
See also Schistosomiasis

Parsons, Talcott 145

Peace Corps, health personnel in 75

Pediatrics
the community and 78
journals concerned with 232-33
in Nigeria 57
in UDCs 59

Peru, resistance to hospital use in 110

Petroleum
embargo (1974) 7
the world food crisis and 7, 13

Pharmaceutical industry. See Drug industry

Philippine Islands, medical care and health service systems in 88
community medicine 69

Philippines, University of, community medical program of 69

Physician-patient relationship 86, 104, 112, 126, 145
models and modeling 106
in socialized medicine 45

in the United Kingdom 42, 101-2

U.S., Russian comparisons 42

Physicians 40, 121
access to under public insurance 97
as agents of social control 145
blacks as 168
in Chile 133
in China 98-99
in community medicine 126, 129
comparative studies of the roles of 46
continuing education for 62, 134
distribution of 62, 92, 123-24
the general practitioner 42, 63, 64
recruitment of 114
income of 48
in India and Burma 91
licensing of 84
methods of payment of 34, 43-44, 46, 66-67, 68, 85, 86, 87, 90, 122, 127, 129-30
migration of 29, 75
bibliography on 222
to Canada 47
number of related to infant mortality 66, 182, 184
organization and orientation of 45
organizations utilizing in foreign countries 238
peer review of 90
politics and 67, 98-99, 122
practice privileges of in EEC countries 46
ratios of to the general population 48, 209
role of 32, 89
in rural health 60, 217
in the Scandinavian countries 41
studies on shifting the work load of 194
substitutes for 134-35
in UDCs 52
women as 62, 128-29, 168
See also Medical education

Physician's assistants 134
bibliography on 221

Subject Index

Subject Index

ZW 84.1 E46c 1980
Cross-national   ref

3 0081 004 269 373